Human **Biology** *and Health Studies*

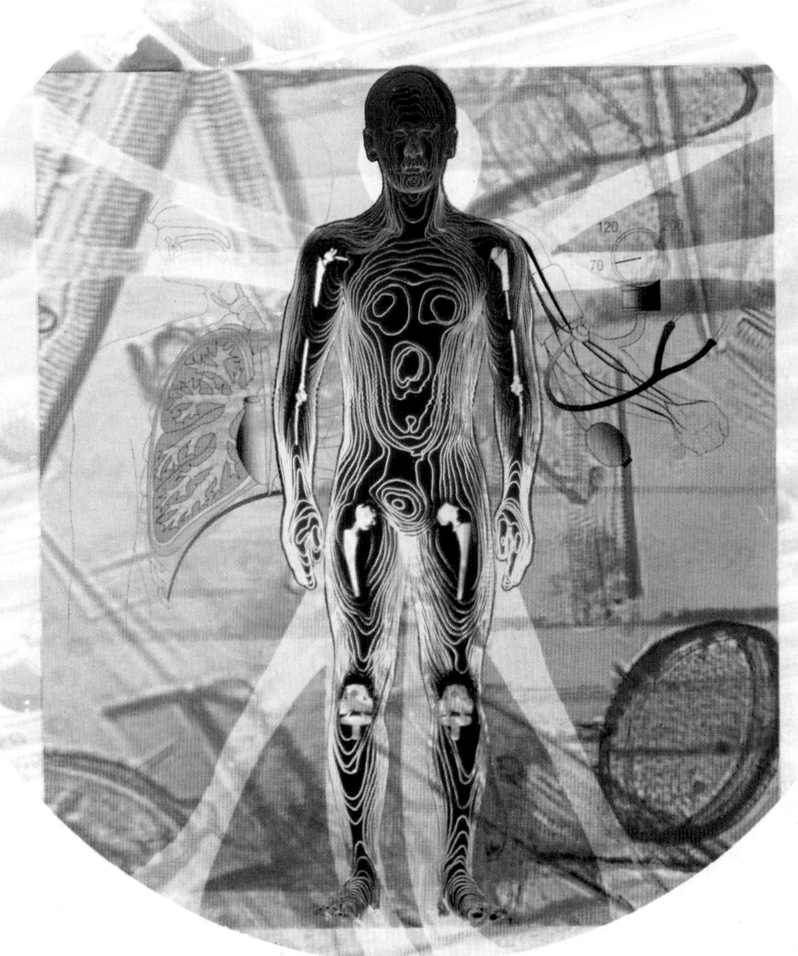

Peter Givens *and* ***Michael Reiss***
Editor ***Martin Rowland***

Nelson

Thomas Nelson and Sons Ltd
Nelson House Mayfield Road
Walton-on-Thames Surrey
KT12 5PL UK

First published by Thomas Nelson and Sons Ltd 1996

I Ⓣ P Thomas Nelson is an International Thomson Publishing Company

I Ⓣ P is used under licence

ISBN 0-17-490004-X

NPN 9 8 7 6 5 4

Acknowledgements
Acquisitions: Sonia Clark
Administration: Jenny Goode
Staff editor: Simon Bell
Editorial: Liz Jones
Marketing: Jane Lewis
Production: Hamish Adamson
Staff design: Maria Pritchard
Design and illustrations: TJ Graphics

Printed in Croatia

The GCSE Human Biology and Health Studies Team

Authors
Peter Givens is Head of Science at Alton College and teaches GCSE and A-level Biology courses.
Michael Reiss is Senior Lecturer in Biology at Homerton College, Cambridge. Previously he was Head of Social Biology at Hills Road Sixth Form College. He is also a Chief Examiner and a regular consultant to SCAA. He is the author of many well-known Nelson textbooks including *Practical Biology* and *Biology: Principles and Processes.*

Editor
Martin Rowland is Head of Advanced Education and Creative Arts at Ealing Tertiary College. He is a Principal Examiner and his publications include *Bath Science 16-19: Biology.*

Advisers
Chris Hodges teaches Human Physiology and Health GCSE at Worthing Sixth Form College and is a Reviser for SEG Human Physiology and Health. She also teaches at Davison High School for Girls.

Vic Pruden is Chief Moderator for SEG Human Physiology and Health and is also their Chief Examiner for Single and Double non-modular Science. He is also SEG KS4 Curriculum Consultant.

Professor N. G. McHale is based at the Department of Physiology, the Queen's University of Belfast. He advised on behalf of The Physiological Society.

Safety adviser
Phil Bunyan is a science inspector.

List of practicals

Contents

Introduction

This book contains the facts and concepts that you will need to pass a course in Human Physiology and Health, Health Studies or Science (Health Studies) at GCSE or equivalent level. You will find these facts and concepts listed in the syllabus you are following. Together they are called the **subject content** of the syllabus.
However, simply reading this book will not enable you to achieve your highest potential on your course. To do this, you must be able to show that you possess a number of skills. These skills are also listed in the syllabus you are following where they are called **Assessment Objectives** (in GCSE syllabuses) or **Performance Criteria** (in GNVQ courses). These skills include:

- **recall** – your ability to remember names, facts, terms, concepts and principles;
- **understanding** – your ability to use names, facts, terms, concepts and principles in their correct context;
- **application** – your ability to relate what you know to new situations;
- **interpretation** – your ability to obtain, and comment on, information from a variety of forms, e.g. tables, graphs, diagrams, photographs, comprehension passages;
- **translation** – your ability to convert information from one form to another, e.g. plot tables of numbers as graphs, describe graphs by written passages;
- **communication** – your ability to select relevant information and present it clearly (including good use of English);
- **practical skills** – which you will demonstrate in a laboratory or in completing a mini research project;
- **examination skills** – your ability to gain maximum marks in a timed GCSE examination or GNVQ external test.

If you think of other skills you possess, you will realise that you developed your skills by practising them. You will only achieve your highest potential on your course if:

- you are aware of the skills by which you will be assessed;
- you are aware of the way in which the assessment works;
- you practise the assessment skills until you become proficient at them.

Become aware of the skills by which you will be assessed

To do this you will need a copy of the syllabus you are following. Your teacher may give you a copy of one, but do not rely on this. Obtain your own copy of the syllabus by writing to the examination board that is validating your course to buy one. The addresses are given on page viii.

Use your own copy of the syllabus constantly to remind yourself of the skills you must develop. These are usually listed before the subject content of the syllabus. Also, use the syllabus as a checklist to record that you are covering the subject content in your studies.

DO: refer to the skills (assessment objectives or performance criteria) throughout your course; tick off each part of the subject content as you cover it. Ask your tutor if you seem to be missing bits of the syllabus in your studies.

Become aware of the way in which the assessment works

You will need to do three things.

- Read your copy of the syllabus to learn how each assessment component works and the skills it tests. For example, you might find that some components assess mainly recall whereas others assess your ability to handle data or to express your ideas clearly. Many syllabuses give you this information in a grid so that it is easy to understand.
- Study past examination papers so that you see which skills they are assessing. Do not at this stage worry about whether or not you can answer them, just make a note of which skills they are assessing. Bear in mind that syllabuses do change so that past papers are not always relevant to new syllabuses. For new syllabuses, examination boards publish Specimen Papers: you will need these if your syllabus is new.
- If you are taking a GCSE course, study the mark schemes that are published by your

examination board. These show you exactly how the examination papers were marked by the examiners – you may be surprised to find out how easy it is to obtain some marks!

DO: make sure that you understand which skills are assessed in each component of your examination; study published mark schemes so that you can see how marks are awarded in examinations.

Copies of past question papers and of the mark schemes can be obtained from the addresses given on page viii. You may find it is cheaper to buy these than to photocopy them from your college or school library.

Practise the assessment skills until you become proficient at them

Above all, this is the most important thing you can do to improve your grade. Unfortunately, no one else can do this for you.

The key to successful practise is to do a little often. Thirty minutes each day is better than three hours on Saturday or Sunday morning. Unfortunately, you might not enjoy practising your skills at first, particularly if it is a skill in which you lack confidence.

DO: become aware of the strengths and weakness of your skills; practise your weak skills and not just your strong ones; make sure you are doing something other than just reading, e.g. writing, drawing, plotting a graph; set time aside each week to organise your new notes and practise recall of new information; work somewhere that is without distractions and interruptions.

How this book can help you

Key words
The key words are emboldened where they are defined. You should make sure that you practise recall of these emboldened terms and that you understand their meaning.

Summaries
Each chapter has a summary. You can use these summaries to make sure that you have grasped the main points of each chapter. By re-reading them, you can help your recall of the content of the chapter.

In-text questions
Each chapter contains a number of in-text questions. These are designed to test your understanding or recall of material in the chapter and to help you to develop other skills. You might be tempted to skip these questions or to give up too quickly and turn to the answers at the end of the book. Try to avoid doing this. By attempting these questions you will help to develop your understanding.

Self-check questions
A selection of questions, mostly from past examination papers, is given at the end of the book. Outline mark schemes are also given. These questions have been chosen from a variety of examination boards to show you the style of question used. They have also been chosen so that they give you an opportunity to develop a range of skills. Use these question when you are practising your skills.

Note: Answers to self-check and in-text questions are given in the form that Examination Boards use for their mark scheme, i.e. a semi-colon (;) separates answers which gain an individual mark and a solidus (/) separates alternative answers for the same mark. Use of this notation will help you to understand mark schemes which GCSE Examination Boards publish. (Publication of mark schemes began for the June 1991 examinations)

Diagrams, photographs, graphs and tables
Information has been presented in a variety of ways. This has been done to help you to develop the skills of interpretation and of translation of information. The illustrations are referred to in the written text, but you can also use them to practise your skills after you have read the text.

Examination Boards from whom you can obtain copies of the syllabus, past examination papers (or specimen papers, for new syllabuses) and mark schemes are given over page.

Examination boards

Midland Examining Group (MEG), UCLES, Publications Department, 1 Hills Road, Cambridge CB1 2EU

Northern Examining and Assessment Board (NEAB), Publications Department, Manchester M15 6EU

Southern Examining Group (SEG), SEG, Publications Department, Stag Hill House, Guildford GU2 5XJ

University of London Examinations & Assessment Council (ULEAC) ULEAC, Publications Department, Stewart House, 32 Russell Square, London WC1B 5DN

Safety

Note to teachers/lecturers on safety

When practical instructions have been given we have attempted to indicate hazardous substances and operations by using standard symbols and appropriate precautions. Nevertheless you are legally required to carry out your obligations as specified by the Health and Safety at Work Act, Control of Substances Hazardous to Health (COSHH) Regulations and the Management of Health and Safety at Work Regulations. To do this, you must follow the requirements of your employer's Health and Safety Policy at all times.

In developing investigations, students could be encouraged to carry out their own risk assessments, i.e. they could identify hazards and suitable ways of reducing the risks from them. However, they must be checked by the teacher/lecturer and do not remove the legal obligation of the teacher/lecturer to consult and act upon appropriate risk assessments.

The teachers/lecturers should be familiar and up to date with current advice from professional bodies.

Note to students on safety

It is essential to take great care in a laboratory at all times. In fact, you are required by law to do so (Health and Safety at Work Act) and to comply with all safety instructions issued at your place of study.

Here are some suggested rules that all students in a laboratory should follow.

1. You should only be in a laboratory if a qualified supervisor is present.
2. Never rush about or throw things in the laboratory. Keep the bench and nearby floor clear of obstructions, with bags and coats well out of the way.
3. Follow instructions precisely; check bottle labels carefully; only touch or use equipment and materials when told to do so by the teacher/lecturer; never remove anything from the laboratory without permission.
4. Wear eye protection when told to do so and keep it on until all practical work is finished and cleared away.
5. When using a Bunsen burner, make sure that ties, long hair, etc. are tucked away or tied back.
6. When working with dangerous liquids or heating things always stand so you can quickly move out of the way if you need to.
7. Never taste anything or put any substance or object in your mouth in the laboratory. If you get something in your mouth spit it out at once, wash your mouth out with lots of water and tell the teacher/lecturer.
8. Always wash your hands thoroughly after handling chemicals or animal and plant material.
9. If you get burnt or splashed by a chemical, wash the affected part at once with lots of water. Report the incident to the teacher/lecturer.
10. Never put waste solids in the sink. Put them in the waste bin unless the teacher/lecturer instructs you otherwise.
11. Wipe up all small spills and report bigger ones to the teacher/lecturer.
12. Report any accident or breakage to the teacher/lecturer.

Student notes on safety adapted from *ASE Safeguards in School Science*, 10th Edition.

CHAPTER 1

Cells, tissues and organs

In this chapter you will learn about the structure of animal and plant cells and about the role of some of their components. You will also learn how cells are organised into a hierarchy of tissues, organs and organ systems.

Cell structure

All living organisms are made of smaller units called **cells**. Animal and plant cells can be seen fairly easily using an optical microscope (also called a light microscope). Figures 1.1 and 1.2 show light micrographs (photographs taken using a light microscope) of typical plant and animal cells, together with representative diagrams illustrating the visible structures.

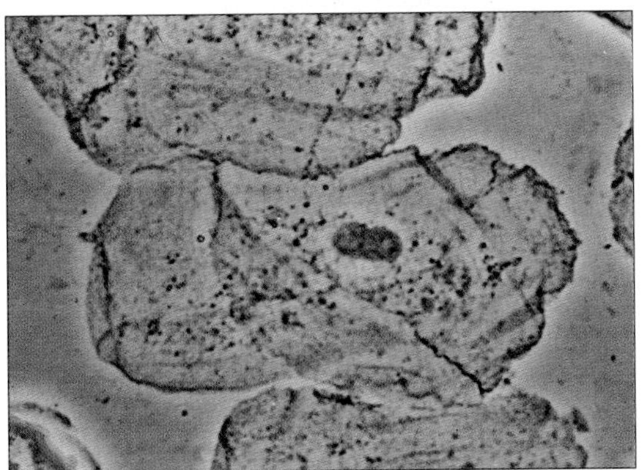

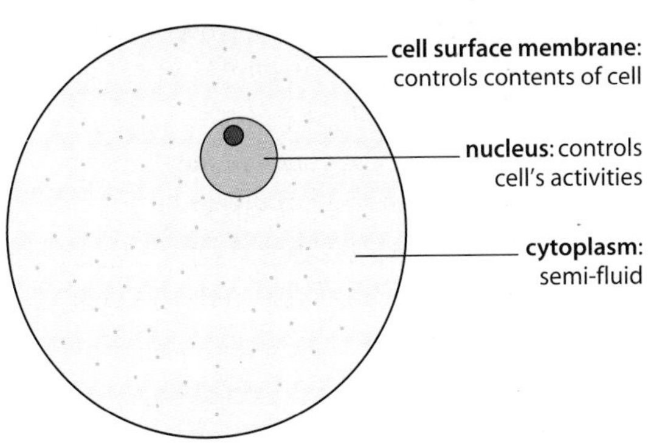

Figure 1.1 A typical animal cell. **Top:** cheek cells as viewed under a light microscope.

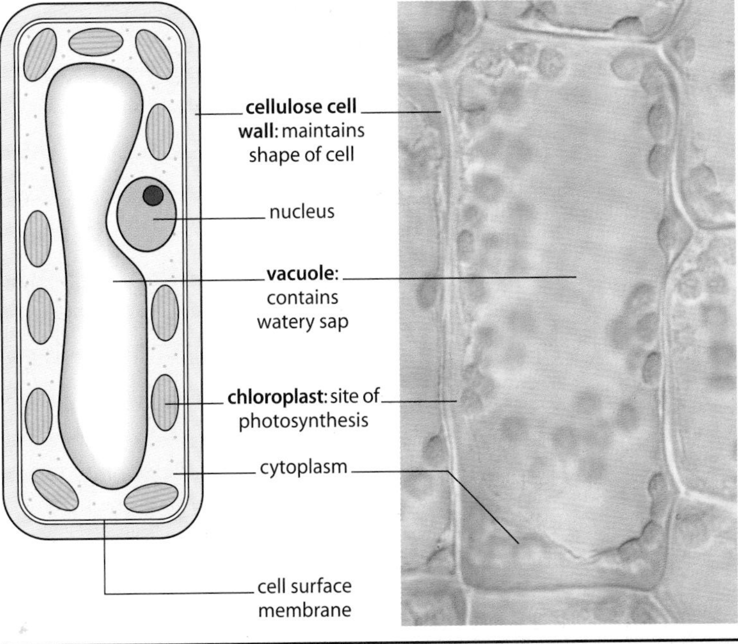

Figure 1.2 Left: a typical photosynthetic plant cell. **Right:** a leaf palisade cell as viewed under a light microscope.

Q1: Use Figures 1.1 and 1.2 to list three ways in which an animal and a plant cell are: (a) similar to each other; (b) different from one another.

Cell organelles

Electron microscopes are much more complicated instruments than optical microscopes and you are unlikely ever to see one. They are very useful because the electrons they use can distinguish between (resolve) much smaller objects than can light. As a result, electron microscopes show us much more detail of cell structure than optical microscopes. The extra detail shown by an electron microscope is called **cell ultrastructure**.

Figure 1.3 shows an electron micrograph (photograph taken using an electron microscope) of a typical animal cell, together with a representative diagram illustrating the cell ultrastructure. If you compare this with Figure 1.1, you will see the extra cell detail that an electron microscope is able to show compared with an optical microscope. Notice that the cytoplasm is now seen to be full of structures that are too tiny to be seen with an optical microscope. These structures are called **organelles** ('little organs') and their functions are described in the annotations to Figure 1.3.

Q2: Which of the cell organelles shown in Figure 1.3 contain membranes?

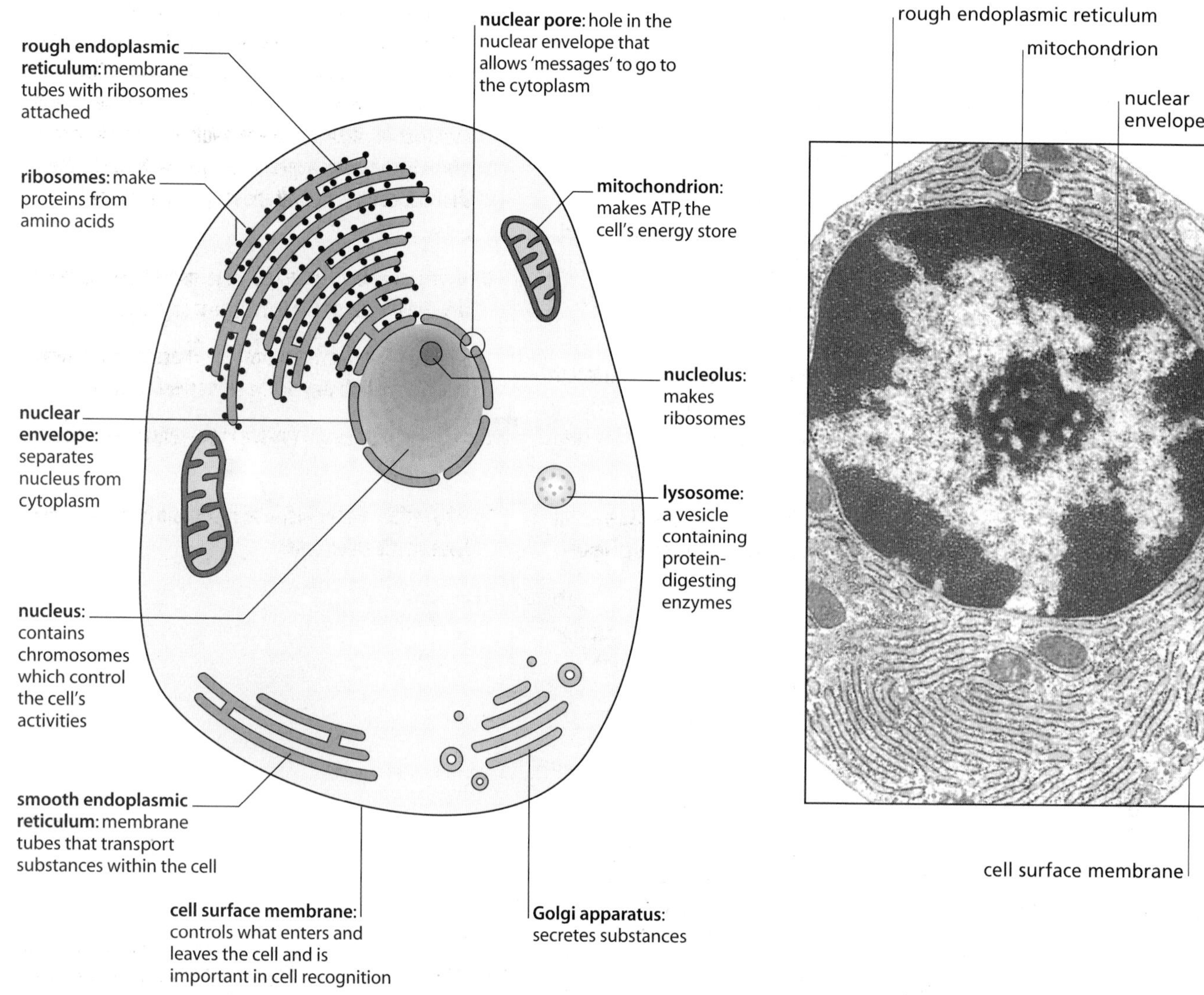

rough endoplasmic reticulum: membrane tubes with ribosomes attached
ribosomes: make proteins from amino acids
nuclear pore: hole in the nuclear envelope that allows 'messages' to go to the cytoplasm
mitochondrion: makes ATP, the cell's energy store
nucleolus: makes ribosomes
nuclear envelope: separates nucleus from cytoplasm
lysosome: a vesicle containing protein-digesting enzymes
nucleus: contains chromosomes which control the cell's activities
smooth endoplasmic reticulum: membrane tubes that transport substances within the cell
cell surface membrane: controls what enters and leaves the cell and is important in cell recognition
Golgi apparatus: secretes substances
rough endoplasmic reticulum
mitochondrion
nuclear envelope
cell surface membrane

Figure 1.3 The ultrastructure of an animal cell. On the right is an animal cell as viewed under an electron microscope.

Practical 1.1 To prepare and observe onion epidermal cells

The onion we use as food is the bulb of an onion plant. On the inside of each fleshy leaf is a thin layer of cells called the epidermis (skin). This can easily be removed, mounted on a drop of water on a flat glass slide and viewed using an optical microscope.

Requirements

Plane glass slide and coverslip
Plane white tile
Kitchen knife
Paper towel (or other absorbent paper)
Dropper (Pasteur-type) pipette
Forceps – fine
Mounted needle
Rule, calibrated in mm
Iodine in potassium iodide solution – one or two drops per person
Optical microscope – preferably one per person

1 Use a dropper pipette to put a drop of tap water on a plane glass slide. Leave this on the bench.

2 Use the kitchen knife and plane white tile to cut an onion into four.

3 Take a single piece of fleshy leaf from the cut onion and bend it inwards on itself. Use forceps to remove the thin epidermis that comes away from the inner (concave) surface of the fleshy leaf.

4 Cut the strip of epidermis into a square of 3–5 cm length and place this on the drop of water on the glass slide. (this is called **mounting**). Take care not to fold the strip of epidermis as you do this.

5 Use a mounted needle to lower a glass coverslip over the drop of water containing the strip of epidermis. Figure 1.4 shows you how to do this. If you are successful, you will not trap any air in the water under the coverslip. (If you do trap air, it will appear as circles with heavy black outlines when you look through the microscope.)

6 Use a piece of paper towel to blot up any surplus water from around the coverslip.

7 Put the glass slide on the stage of an optical microscope and use the clips on the microscope stage to hold it in place. Try to position the slide so that the strip of onion epidermis is in the middle of the stage, directly under the objective lens of the microscope.

8 Using the low-power objective lens, look down the microscope at the cells in the onion epidermis. Record what you can see.

9 Now carefully remove the slide from the stage of the microscope and put it on the bench. Use a dropper pipette to put a drop of iodine in potassium iodide solution on the glass slide at one side of the coverslip. Holding a piece of paper towel against the other side of the coverslip, draw the iodine solution under the coverslip until the water appears light yellow. Now clip the slide back on the microscope stage and examine it again.

10 As you look down the microscope, move the slide to your left. Which way do the cells appear to move?

11 As you look down the microscope, move the slide away from you. Which way do the cells appear to move?

12 Which structures can you see in the cells of the onion epidermis?

13 What effect did the iodine in potassium iodide solution have on the onion cells?

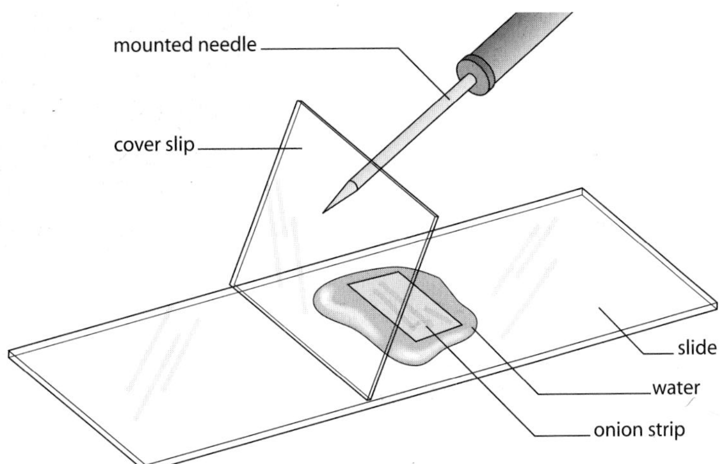

Figure 1.4 Lowering a coverslip onto a slide.

Tissues, organs and organ systems

Most of the cells in our bodies do not look exactly like the ones shown in Figures 1.1, 1.2 and 1.3. This is because cells grow differently (**differentiate**) as they specialise for one particular function. Muscle cells, nerve cells and sperm cells all have a cell surface membrane, nucleus and cytoplasm but their shapes are different from each other (Figure 1.5). If we were to test their chemical composition, we would find that this was different too. These differences are related to the specialised function that each type of cell has. Despite these differences, all these human cells still carry the same genetic information in their nuclei.

Q3: What does this suggest about the activity of the genetic material that controls the activities of human cells?

Specialised cells grow together to form groups of specialised cells. These can be

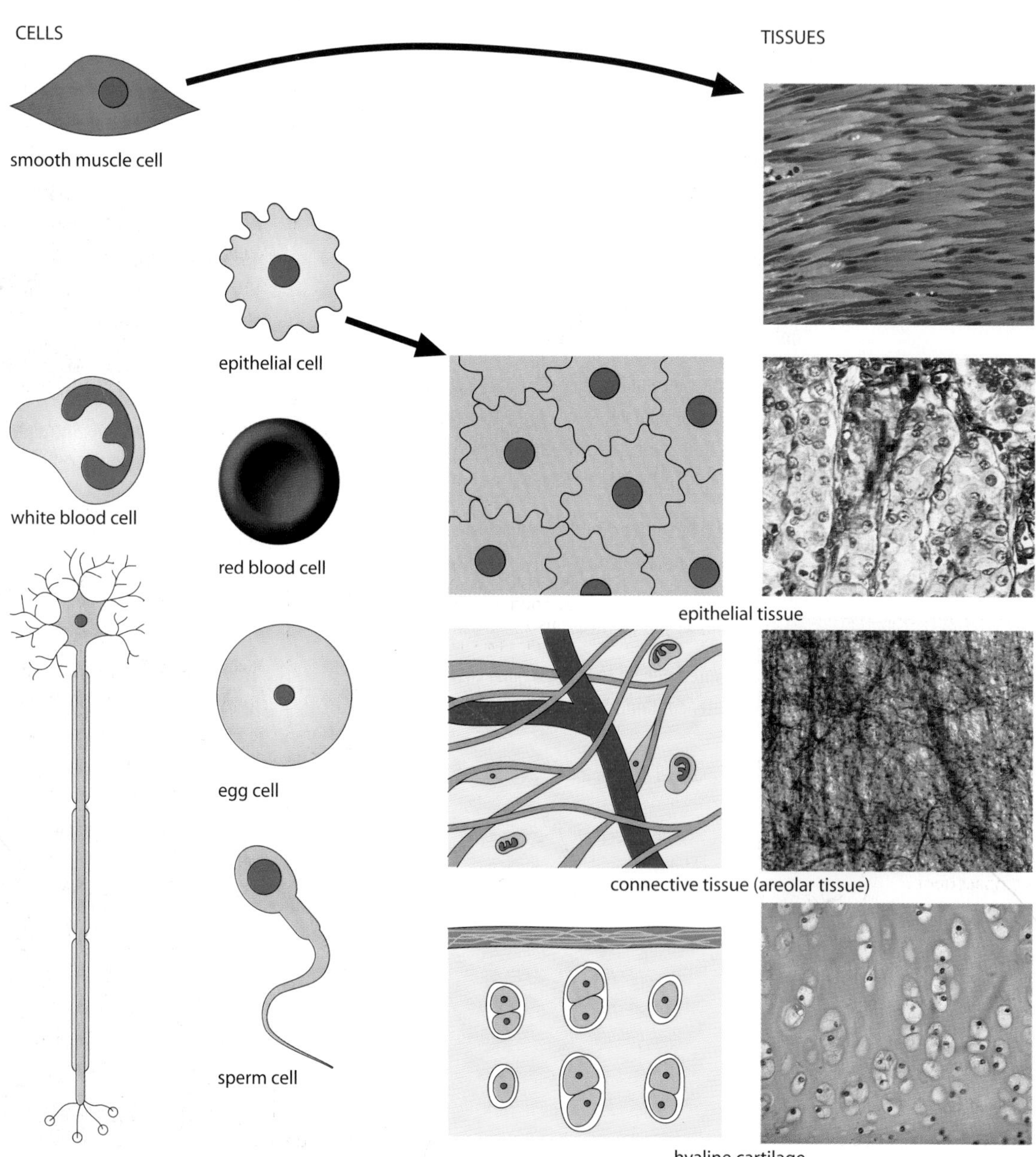

Figure 1.5 Cells, tissues, organs and organ systems.

arranged hierarchically:

- **Cells** – The basic unit of life. You will come across many specialised cell types as you read through this book.
- **Tissues** – A collection of similar cells working together to carry out the same function, e.g. muscle tissue, nervous tissue or epithelial tissue.
- **Organs** – A collection of different tissues working together to carry out one function, e.g. the heart is an organ made of muscle tissue, nervous tissue, connective tissue and epithelial tissue.
- **Organ systems** – A collection of different organs and tissues working together to carry out one function, e.g. the circulatory system is made of the heart (an organ), blood vessels (organs) and blood (a tissue).

Figure 1.5 shows the structure of a number of specialised cells, tissues, organs and of an organ system. You will learn about others as you work through the chapters of this book.

Q4: Which tissues are present in the stomach?

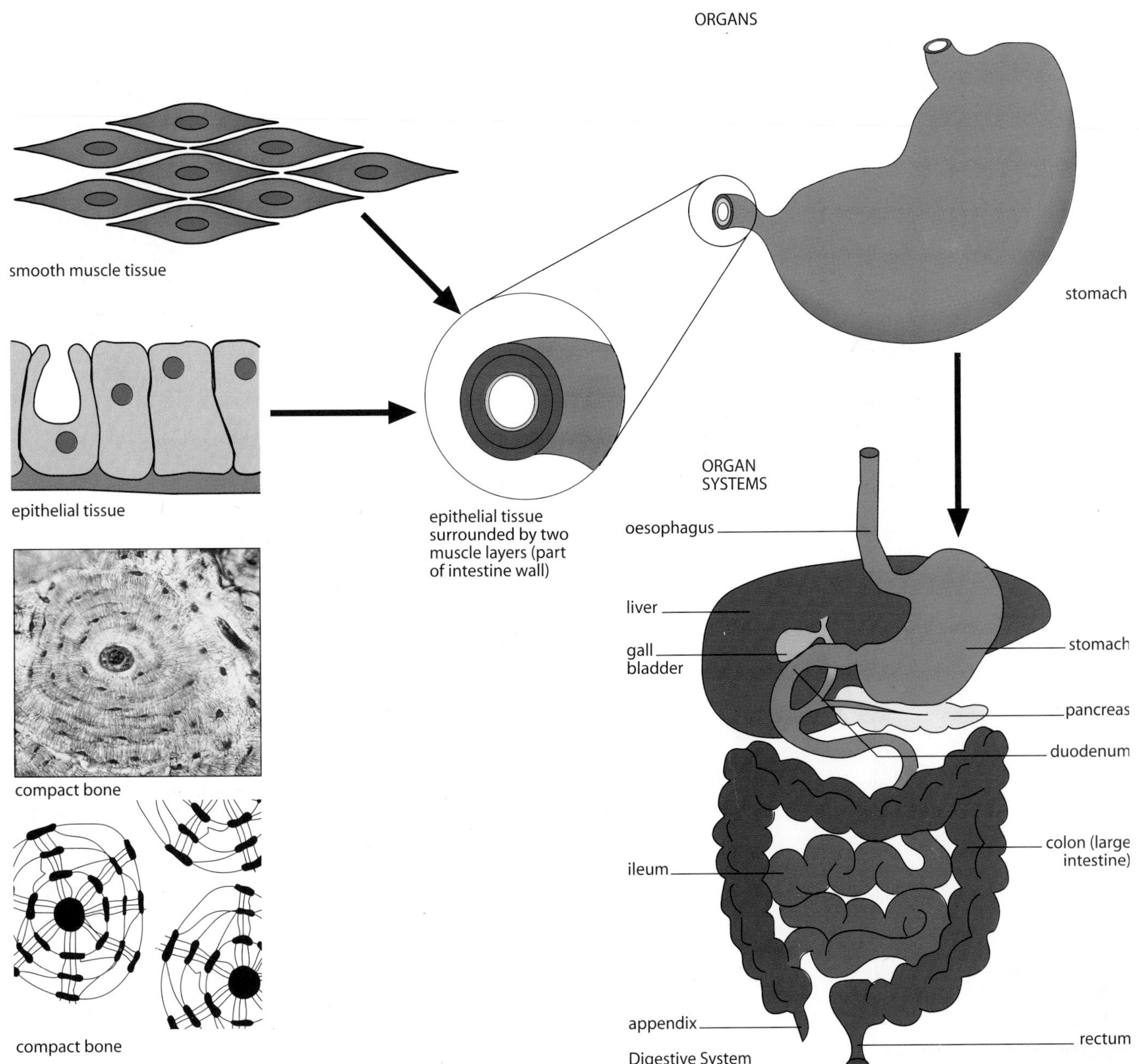

Summary

- Organisms are made of cells.
- Animal and plant cells have an outer cell surface membrane and cytoplasm enclosing a nucleus.
- Plant cells have a cellulose cell wall outside their cell surface membrane and their cytoplasm contains chloroplasts and a large fluid-filled vacuole. Animal cells lack these structures.
- Electron microscopes show more detail of cell structure than do optical (light) microscopes. The additional detail shown by an electron microscope is called cell ultrastructure. Viewed under an electron microscope, it is clear that the cytoplasm is filled with tiny structures, called cell organelles.
- Each cell organelle has a particular function within the cell.
- As cells develop, they grow differently to become specialised for a particular function.
- Specialised cells of one type work together in a tissue.
- Groups of tissues work together to perform one function in an organ.
- Organ systems, such as the circulatory system, contain organs and tissues working together.

Self check
See page 228

CHAPTER 2

Cell metabolism

In this chapter you will learn about matter and energy and use these concepts to learn about some of the activities of cells that involve energy.

Kinetic Theory

The universe is made of matter and energy.

Matter

Matter is made of particles which can be:
- **atoms** – for our purposes, the basic particles
- particles that make up atoms – subatomic particles, such as **electrons**
- particles made when atoms lose or gain electrons – called **ions**
- particles made when atoms chemically join together – called **molecules**.

These particles are constantly moving about. This movement uses energy called **kinetic energy** (meaning literally 'the energy of movement').

Figure 2.1 shows that matter can exist in three states: as a solid, as a liquid and as a gas. Think of a chemical substance such as water. Water is made of particles called water molecules which, in turn, are made of particles (atoms) of hydrogen and oxygen chemically joined together. When you drink a glass of water, you are drinking water in its liquid state. You might cool the water by placing cubes of ice in it. The ice is water in its solid state. When water evaporates, water vapour – a gas – is formed.

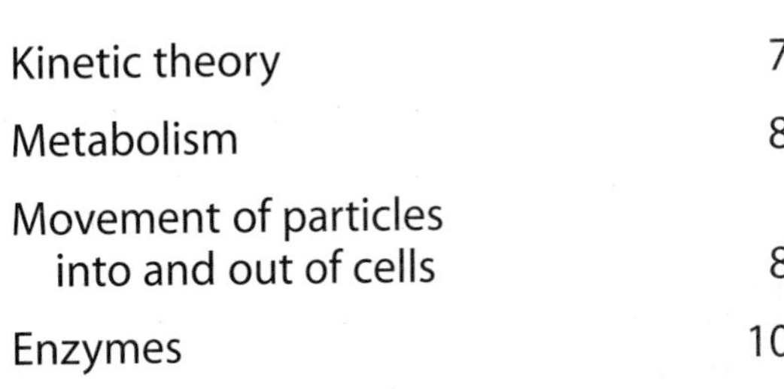

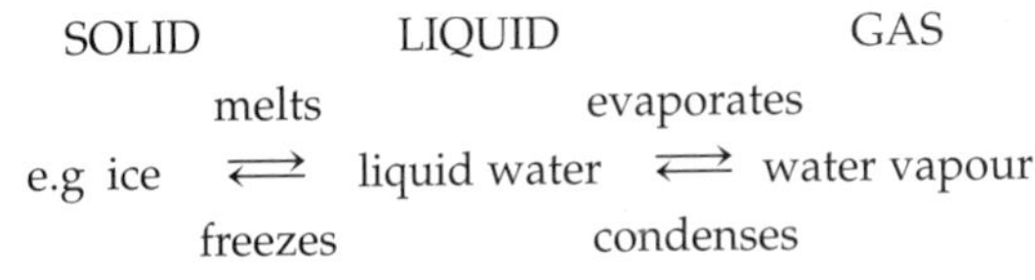

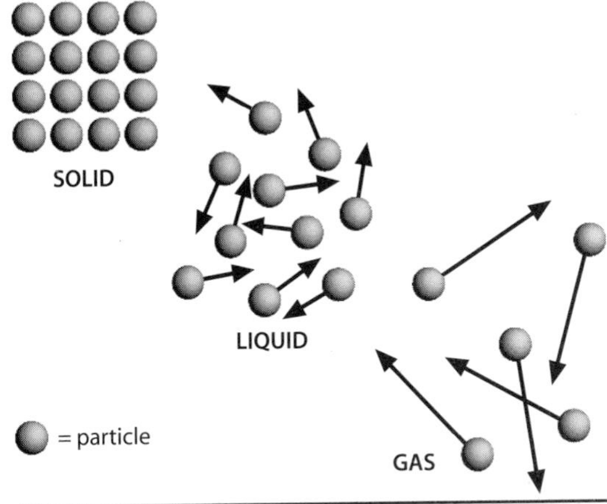

Figure 2.1 The three states of matter.

The particles in a solid move more slowly than those in a liquid which, in turn, move more slowly than those in a gas. To move from one state to another involves adding energy (making particles move faster) or removing energy (making particles move slower).

Q1: Which particles have the most kinetic energy: those in a solid, those in a liquid or those in a gas?

Energy

Although we have used the term energy above, it is difficult to define. It is best defined as the stored ability to do work. The kinetic energy described above is the stored ability of particles to do work as a result of their movement.

Energy exists in many forms. In this book you will learn about:

- heat energy – released as a waste from processes such as cell respiration (see page 37)
- light energy – enabling plants to make food during photosynthesis (see page 191)
- potential chemical energy – energy stored in the food we eat (see page 14) and in cellular stores such as adenosine triphosphate, ATP (see page 37)
- energy transfers – energy used to drive chemical reactions in cells.

Metabolism

Hundreds of chemical reactions occur inside all living cells. Collectively, these are called **metabolism** and can be divided into:

- **anabolism** – reactions in which small molecules combine to form larger ones, e.g. chemicals A + B → chemical AB. These often require energy to make them happen
- **catabolism** – reactions in which large molecules are broken down into smaller ones, e.g. AB → A + B.

These often release energy.

The speed with which the reactions of metabolism occur is called the **metabolic rate**.

Q2: During cell respiration two major reactions occur. In the presence of oxygen, glucose is broken down to form water and carbon dioxide. Energy released from this reaction is used to attach a phosphate group to a molecule of adenosine diphosphate (ADP) to form adenosine triphosphate (ATP). Which reaction is catabolic and which is anabolic?

Movement of particles into and out of cells

All cells are surrounded by a cell surface membrane (see page 1). Any ion or molecule that a cell needs either to use or to get rid of must be able to get through its cell surface membrane.

Diffusion

Diffusion depends on:

- the kinetic energy of ions and molecules – the cell does not have to use its own energy to move them
- the ability of many ions and molecules to get through cell surface membranes.

As a result of their kinetic energy, ions and molecules constantly move about. They move randomly in all directions but will always tend to move from a region where they are in high concentration to one where they are in low concentration. Another way of saying this is that there is a net movement from a high to a low concentration. The distance from the high to the low concentration is called a **concentration gradient**.

Q3: Suggest why diffusion through cell surface membranes is said to be a passive process.

Not all particles can diffuse through cell surface membranes, either because they are too big or because they are chemically incompatible with the membrane. Cell surface membranes will allow the diffusion of glucose molecules and of water molecules, i.e. they are permeable to glucose and to water. Figure 2.2 represents two solutions of glucose separated by a fully permeable membrane.

Q4: Look at Figure 2.2 on page 9: (a) What will happen to the glucose? Give a reason; (b) What will happen to the water? Give a reason; (c) What will eventually happen?

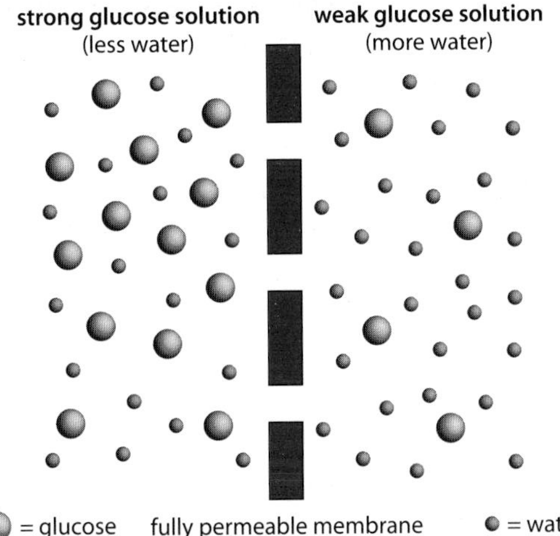

Figure 2.2 Diffusion.

If you cannot answer the questions look at Figure 2.3. You will see that the concentration of glucose and of water is the same on both sides of the membrane, i.e. a **dynamic equilibrium** has been set up. Dynamic means that the molecules are still moving but that there is no *net* movement. (Note that net movement means overall movement, e.g. if 10 molecules move from left to right and 8 move from right to left the net movement is 2 from left to right.)

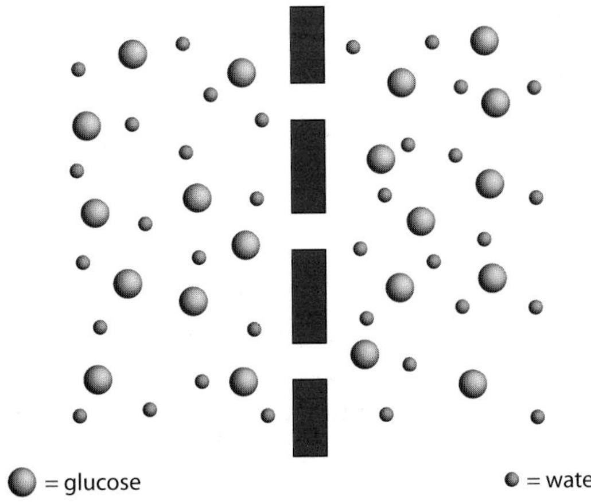

Figure 2.3 Dynamic equilibrium.

Imagine the two glucose solutions in Figure 2.2 separated by a partially permeable membrane. A partially permeable membrane has pores (holes) in it that only allow small molecules through it – in this case water but not glucose.

Q5: What effect would a partially permeable membrane have on the movement of the glucose molecules in Figure 2.2?

Osmosis

Osmosis is a special case of diffusion. It involves:

- solutions in which water is the solvent (the chemical dissolved in it is called the solute)
- diffusion of water molecules from a region where there are lots of them (i.e. a dilute solution) to a region where there are fewer of them (i.e. a concentrated solution)
- a partially permeable membrane – one that will allow free movement of water molecules, but not of the solute molecules, through it.

In Figure 2.4, the net flow of water will therefore be from right to left by the process of diffusion. This movement of water is an example of osmosis.

Definition: Osmosis is the diffusion of water through a partially permeable membrane from a dilute solution to a concentrated solution. It continues until the two concentrations became equal.

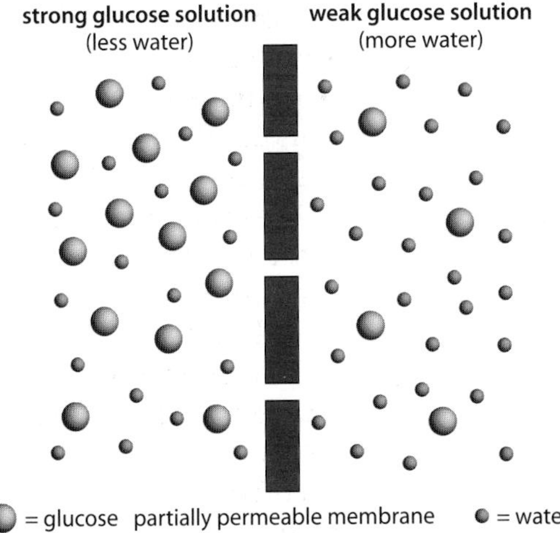

Figure 2.4 Two glucose solutions separated by a partially permeable membrane.

Importance of osmosis to living cells

Cells are surrounded by partially permeable membranes. A red blood cell has a partially permeable cell surface membrane and no cell wall. Figure 2.5 shows what would happen to a red blood cell if it were placed in:

- a solution more concentrated than its own contents (hypertonic) – net flow of water out
- a solution more dilute than its own contents (hypotonic) – net flow of water in.

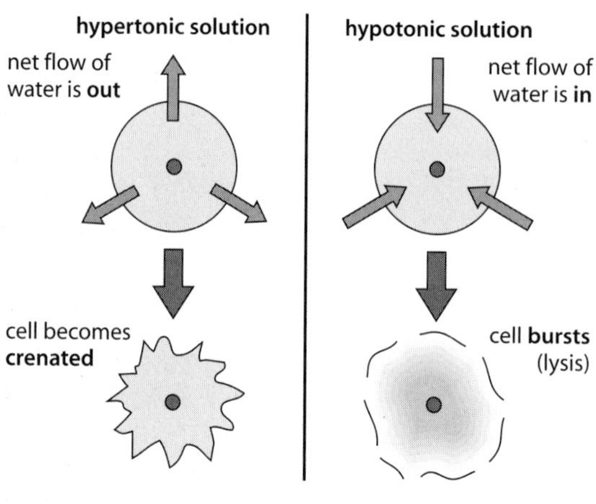

Figure 2.5 Effects of osmosis on red blood cells.

In our bodies we have mechanisms that work to keep our blood plasma at the same concentration as our red blood cells (see page 28).

Q6: Which would be more harmful – our blood plasma becoming more dilute or more concentrated than our red blood cells?

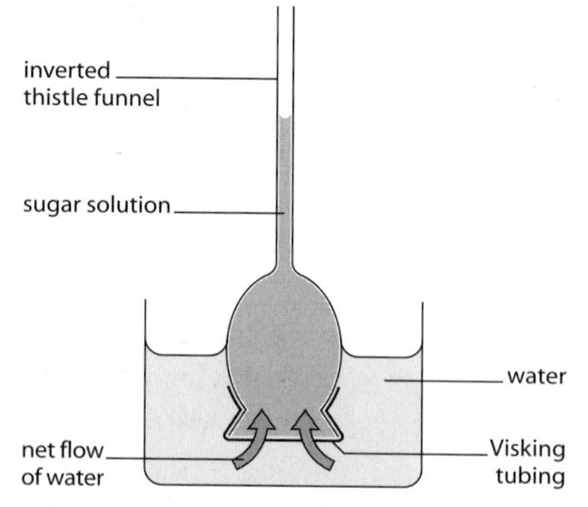

Figure 2.6 Demonstrating osmosis.

Figure 2.6 shows apparatus which can be used to demonstrate osmosis. Like cell surface membranes, Visking tubing is partially permeable.

Active transport

Sometimes cells use their stored energy to move ions or molecules through their surface membranes. This is called active transport and occurs particularly in a cell when:

- substances need to be moved very quickly, e.g. the absorption of glucose in the gut
- substances need to be moved against a concentration gradient, e.g. sodium ions being removed from nerve cells.

Figure 2.7 represents one way in which energy stored in ATP is used to move molecules across membranes via a protein 'pump' in the membrane.

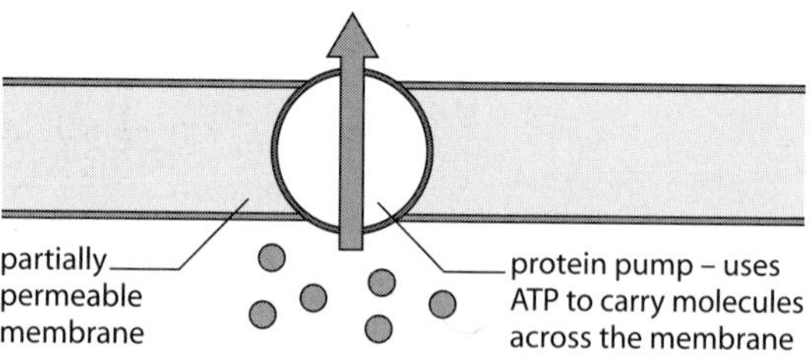

Figure 2.7 Active uptake.

Enzymes

All of the chemical reactions in the body need enzymes. They speed up (catalyse) reactions that would otherwise take too long to allow us to survive. The vast majority are proteins and are unchanged at the end of the reaction. They are named after their substrates, e.g. carbohydrates are digested by carbohydrases and proteins by proteases.

Q7: Suggest the name of an enzyme that breaks down lipids.

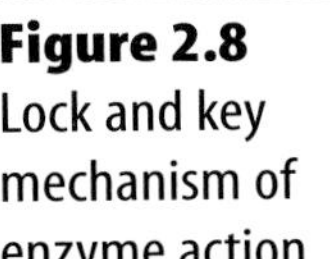

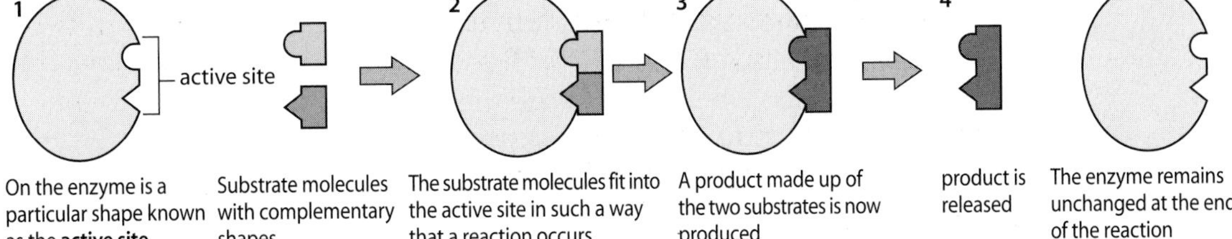

Figure 2.8 Lock and key mechanism of enzyme action.

How enzymes work

Each enzyme is a complex three-dimensional molecule. Part of its structure (the **active site**) has a particular shape that is all important. The mechanism used to explain how the active site works is shown in Figure 2.8 and is called the **lock and key mechanism**.

Properties of enzymes

Enzymes:

- reduce the amount of energy needed for molecules to react together
- are unchanged at the end of the reaction they speed up – look at Figure 2.8
- are specific, i.e. they will only speed up the rate of one reaction. Note in Figure 2.9 how the shape of the substrate molecules must fit into the active site before the reaction will occur. The enzyme will only catalyse (i.e. speed up) the reaction where this occurs

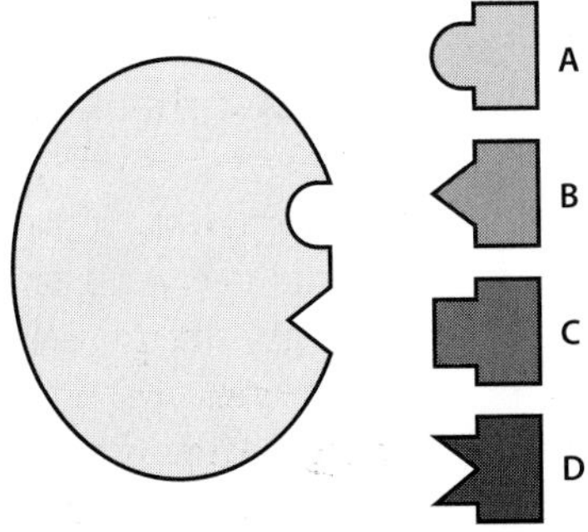

Figure 2.9 Enzyme specificity.

Q8: Imagine two reactions: A + B → AB and C + D → CD. Which of these two reactions will the enzyme shown in Figure 2.9 catalyse?

- are affected by **temperature**. Figure 2.10 shows the effect of temperature on enzyme action. From 0°C to the optimum temperature of the enzyme (usually around 37°C in humans) the rate increases. This can be explained by the kinetic theory, i.e. the enzyme and substrate molecules move around faster as the temperature increases therefore there is a greater chance of them fitting together as they bump into each other more frequently. Above the optimum temperature, the rate rapidly decreases. This is because the higher temperature permanently changes the shape of the enzyme molecules, destroying their active sites (i.e. **denatures** the protein). This change is irreversible

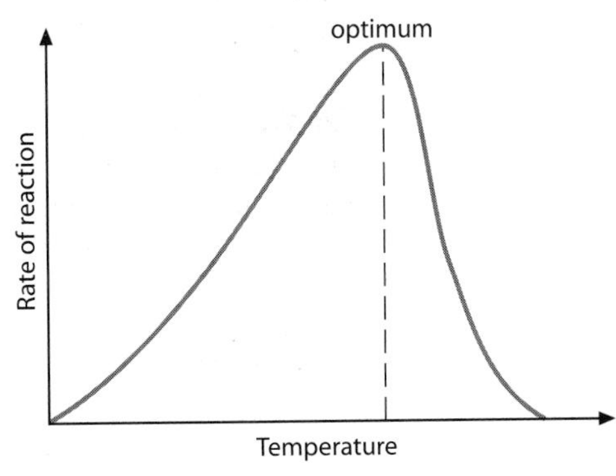

Figure 2.10 The effect of temperature on enzymes.

- are affected by **pH**. Figure 2.11 shows the effect of pH on two different enzymes. As can be seen, both enzymes work over very narrow pH ranges around an optimum value. Either side of the optimum, changes in pH cause a dramatic decrease in the rate of reaction. This is due to the pH affecting the shape of the enzyme which loses its active site. However, the two enzymes shown do not work at the same optimum pH. Pepsin is found in the stomach and the amylase shown in Figure 2.11 is found in the mouth.

Q9: Food decays when bacteria use their own enzymes to digest it. Suggest why placing food in vinegar (ethanoic acid) slows down food decay.

Chapter 3 discusses further the action of enzymes in digestion.

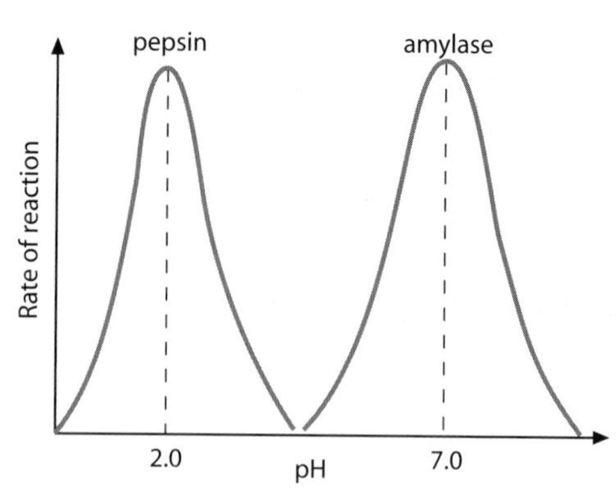

Figure 2.11 The effect of pH on the activity of two enzymes.

Summary

- There are three states of matter – solid, liquid and gas.
- The kinetic theory states that matter is made up of particles that are constantly moving about.
- Metabolism is a name given to the chemical reactions going on inside cells and can be divided into anabolism and catabolism.
- Passive movement of substances does not involve the expenditure of energy by cells.
- Diffusion is the movement of particles from a high to a low concentration, i.e. down a concentration gradient.
- Osmosis is the passive diffusion of water through a partially permeable membrane.
- Active transport of substances involves the expenditure of energy by cells.
- Enzymes are biological catalysts, i.e. they speed up chemical reactions. They are usually proteins and are unchanged at the end of the reaction.
- Enzymes are believed to work by a lock and key mechanism involving the fitting together of the enzyme and its substrate(s). If the shape of the active site is changed, an enzyme loses is catalytic properties. Changes in temperature and in pH change the shape of enzyme molecules, explaining the sensitivity of enzymes to these environmental factors.

Self check
See page 228

CHAPTER 3

Food and nutrition

In this chapter you will learn why humans need food, the types of food that they need in order to stay healthy and how to test for these different types of food. You will learn how food is digested, absorbed and used by the body. Finally you will learn about potential digestive ailments.

The need for food

Unlike plants, humans must have a supply of organic food to provide the raw materials for growth and repair as well as supplying a source of stored energy. Whatever foods you like to eat, your diet must contain:

- proteins
- lipids (fats and oils)
- carbohydrates
- inorganic ions (also called minerals)
- vitamins
- dietary fibre
- water.

Not only does your diet need to contain these substances, it must contain them in the amounts that you need in order to stay healthy. This is called a **balanced diet** and is described more fully in Chapter 14.

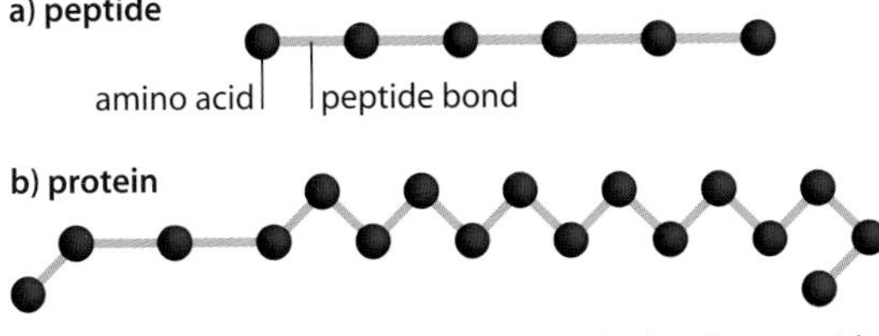

Figure 3.1 A chain of amino acids making up a peptide and a protein.

Types of food

Proteins

Proteins are molecules made of long chains of **amino acids** held together by **peptide bonds** (Figure 3.1). Depending on the amino acids they contain, these chains can be straight (fibrillar), e.g. keratin in hair and skin, or round (globular), e.g. haemoglobin, all enzymes.

Amino acids are:

- the basic building blocks of proteins
- made up of the elements carbon, hydrogen, oxygen and nitrogen – some also contain sulphur
- joined together by peptide bonds
- used inside cells for growth, repair, formation of membranes, formation of enzymes, formation of some hormones and, sometimes, as a source of energy
- of two different types with regard to their usefulness to humans:
  - **essential amino acids** cannot be made by the body so *must* be obtained from the diet
  - **non-essential amino acids** can be made by the body from other amino acids and so need not be in the diet.

Food sources rich in protein include lean meat, fish, eggs, cheese, pulses (peas, beans and lentils), nuts and mycoprotein (see page 171).

Lipids

There is a wide variety of lipid molecules including **triglycerides** (fats and oils), **waxes** (e.g. sebum produced by the skin) and **steroids** (e.g. oestrogen and cholesterol).

Triglycerides are the commonest lipid in our bodies. Triglycerides are:

- made up of the elements carbon, hydrogen and oxygen
- made when one molecule of glycerol combines with three fatty acid molecules (Figure 3.2)
- modified to form **phospholipids** when one of their fatty acids is replaced by a phosphate group. These phospholipids are then used to make cell membranes, including the cell surface membrane, nuclear envelope and cell organelles
- used as a long-term store of energy
- deposited under the skin and around delicate organs where they give protection from knocks and act as a heat insulator.

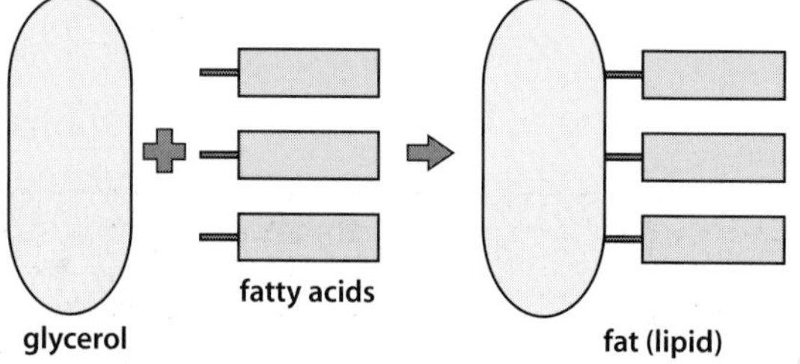

Figure 3.2 Triglyceride formation.

Food sources rich in lipids are butter, margarine, cooking oil, fatty meat, fish. These foods are also important because they contain lipid-soluble vitamins.

Carbohydrates

The simplest carbohydrates are single sugars (**monosaccharides**). These can exist alone or be joined together in chains. Figure 3.3 represents different types of carbohydrate molecules.

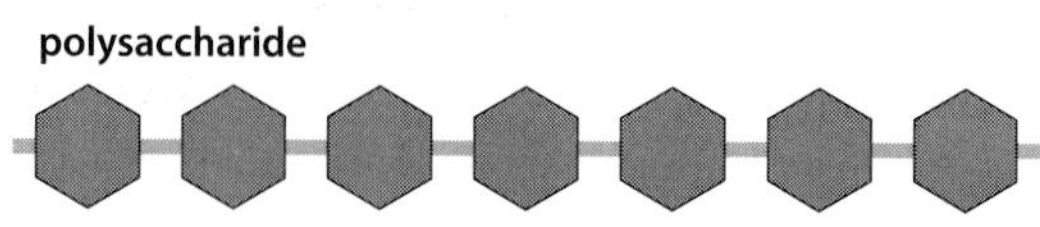

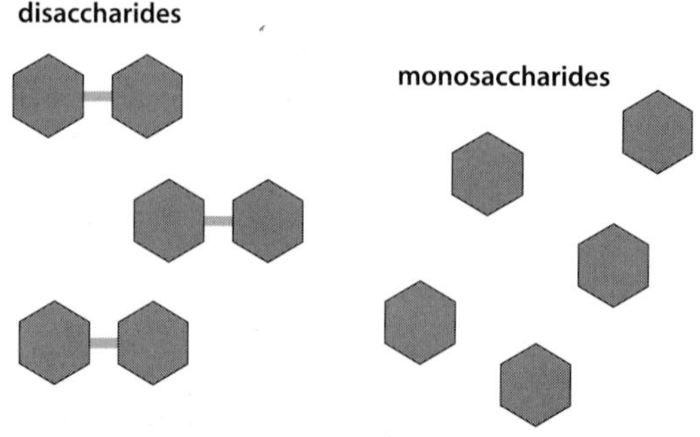

Figure 3.3 Polysaccharides, dissacharides and monosaccharides.

Monosaccharides

These are sometimes called simple sugars since they are made up from one (*mono*) sugar unit (*saccharide*). Monosaccharides:

- are made up of the elements carbon, hydrogen and oxygen with the ratio of hydrogen to oxygen being two: one
- are made up of a single sugar unit (saccharide)
- are soluble and sweet
- are used to supply cells with the energy they need to make ATP (page 37)
- include glucose, fructose and galactose.

Food sources rich in monosaccharides include biscuits, cakes and honey.

Disaccharides

These carbohydrates:

- are made when two monosaccharides are joined together by a glycosidic bond
- are soluble and sweet
- are used as sources of energy
- include maltose (malt sugar), sucrose (cane sugar or beet sugar) and lactose (milk sugar).

Food sources rich in disaccharides include cane (or beet) sugar, fruit and milk.

Polysaccharides

These carbohydrates are relatively large chains. Polysaccharides:

- are made up of many (*poly*) sugar units (*saccharides*) joined together by glycosidic bonds
- are insoluble
- are used as energy storage compounds
- include starch and cellulose (in plants) and glycogen (in fungi and in animals, including humans).

Food sources rich in starch include bread, pasta, potatoes, cassava and yams.

Q1: Where is cellulose found in nature?

Inorganic ions (minerals)

Inorganic ions are relatively simple structures. They are:

- all soluble in water
- put to specific use in the body (Table 3.1).

Vitamins

Vitamins are substances that are needed in order to keep us healthy. Like inorganic ions, each vitamin plays a different role in the body.

Vitamins are:

- needed in tiny amounts in the diet
- water-soluble (B-group vitamins and vitamin C) or lipid-soluble (vitamins A, D and K). This affects the type of food in which they are likely to be found
- put to specific use in the body (Table 3.2 on page 16) so that you cannot compensate for the lack of one vitamin by eating more of another.

Dietary fibre

This is made up mainly of cellulose from the walls of plants. It provides bulk to the faeces to stimulate peristalsis and therefore prevents constipation. By regularly removing faeces, inflammation of the colon (diverticulitis) and bowel cancer are less likely to occur.

Water

Water is present:

- in blood plasma, which makes up about 55% of our blood volume
- around all the cells in our bodies, forming tissue fluid
- inside cells – many cells contain approximately 70% water

Table 3.1 Roles of minerals in the body

Mineral	Sources	Use in the body	Deficiency
Iron	Liver, eggs, green vegetables, e.g. spinach	Production of haemoglobin in red blood cells	Anaemia – reduction in red blood cell count
Iodine	Water, table salt	Production of thyroxine which controls the metabolic rate	Reduction in metabolic rate therefore person is very sluggish in adult; causes cretinism in the young
Calcium	Cheese, milk, water, tinned tuna/salmon	Healthy bones and teeth; blood clotting; muscle contraction	Weak bones; poor blood clotting
Fluoride	Water; some toothpastes	Strengthens enamel in teeth	Tooth decay
Phosphate	Water, fresh vegetables, dairy products, milk, liver	ATP production; bones and teeth; nucleic acids (DNA and RNA)	Rarely deficient
Sodium and potassium	Water, fresh vegetables, milk, liver	Nerve impulse conduction	Rarely deficient

Table 3.2 Roles of vitamins in the body

Vitamin	Source	Use in the body	Deficiency
A	Milk, butter, liver, fresh vegetables, eg. carrots	Manufacture of rhodopsin in the rods in the eye	Nightblindness
B group	Yeast extract, liver, eggs and vegetables	Many uses, particularly in respiration	Many, e.g. nervous and muscle systems are affected
C	Fresh fruit, particularly citrus fruits, eg. oranges	Healing of wounds, connective tissue formation, uptake of iron from gut	Scurvy – bleeding gums, teeth fall out; can lead to anaemia
D	Liver, butter, cheese; also action of sunlight on skin	Absorption of calcium and phosphate from food therefore important in bone formation	Rickets – weakened bones
K	Green vegetables; gut bacteria produce this in the colon	Clotting of blood	Poor clotting of blood

Gut microbes

Present in the colon are a large range of microbes, particularly the bacterium *Escherichia coli*. This acts on the cellulose in food and produces vitamin K and vitamins of the B group. These are absorbed through the colon and used by the body.

Practical 3.1 Food tests

SAFETY PRECAUTIONS: *always work to your teacher's/lecturer's instructions.*

1 Never taste any chemicals or foods to be tested.
2 Wear eye protection when indicated.
3 Tie long hair back.
4 When heating chemicals, use a water bath whenever possible.
5 When heating, never point test tubes at one another.
6 When heating, never look down a test tube.
7 Always report any spillages.

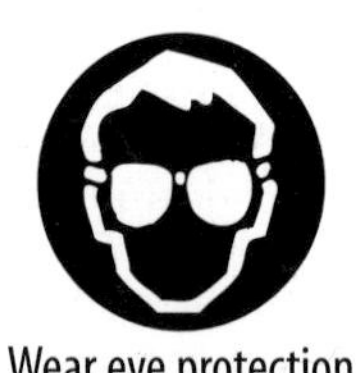
Wear eye protection

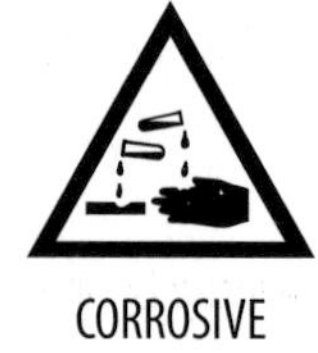
CORROSIVE
Sodium hydroxide

A: To test for proteins using the Biuret test

Requirements

Test tubes
Test tube rack
Food containing protein
Dilute sodium hydroxide solution
1% copper sulphate solution

1 Make a suspension of food by mixing it with water.

2 Add 2 cm^3 of sodium hydroxide (dilute) to 2 cm^3 of this suspension.

3 Add fresh 1% copper sulphate solution drop by drop.

4 A positive result will be indicated by a violet colour.

B: To test for lipids

Requirements
Fat or oil
Filter paper

1 Place a drop of oil or rub a sample of food onto a piece of filter paper.

2 Allow to dry.

3 A positive test will be indicated by a translucent stain.

C: To test for carbohydrates

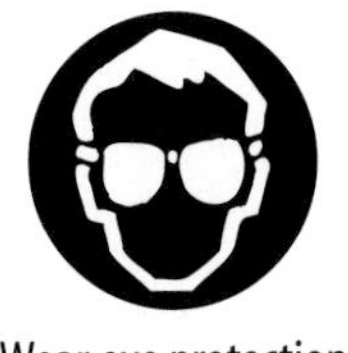

Wear eye protection

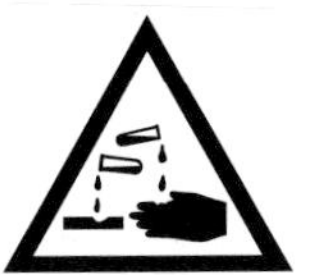

CORROSIVE
Hydrochloric acid

Requirements
Test tubes
Test tube racks
Water baths for boiling
Dilute sodium hydroxide solution
Dilute hydrochloric acid
Benedict's reagent
Iodine in potassium iodide solution
Sucrose solution
Glucose solution

NB: Always make up a fresh sucrose solution. Bacterial decay may convert it into glucose and fructose.

Starch

1 Make a suspension of the food by mixing it with water.

2 Add two or three drops of iodine dissolved in potassium iodide solution.

3 A positive test will be indicated by a blue-black colour.

Reducing sugars, e.g. glucose

1 Add 2 cm^3 of Benedict's solution to 2 cm^3 of the food suspension.

2 Boil gently using a water bath.

3 A positive test is seen by an orange or reddy brown precipitate.

NB: All monosaccharides and all disaccharides apart from sucrose are reducing sugars.

Non-reducing sugars, e.g. sucrose

To identify these, two tests must be performed.

a)

1 Add 2 cm^3 of Benedict's solution to 2 cm^3 of the sucrose solution.

2 Boil.

3 Note that the solution stays blue.

b)

1 Take a second sample of 2 cm^3 of sucrose solution.

2 Add 2 drops of hydrochloric acid.

3 Boil this mixture for 2 to 3 minutes.

4 Cool and neutralise with 1 cm^3 of dilute sodium hydroxide solution.

5 Add 2 cm^3 of Benedict's solution.

6 Boil.

7 A positive result will be seen by a orange or reddy brown precipitate.

NB: By boiling with dilute hydrochloric acid, the sucrose is broken down into glucose and fructose, both of which are reducing sugars.

Practical 3.2 To identify four unknown solutions using food tests

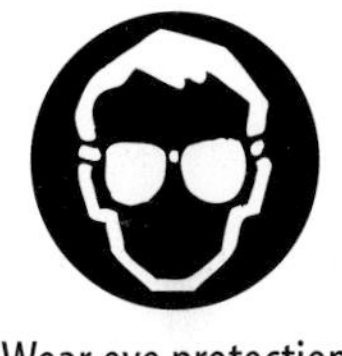

Wear eye protection

Requirements
Test tubes
Test tube racks
Water baths for boiling
Iodine in potassium iodide solution
Dilute sodium hydroxide solution
1% copper sulphate solution
Benedict's reagent
Four solutions labelled A, B, C and D

You are given four unknown solutions labelled A, B, C and D and are told that they are glucose, sucrose, starch and protein, though not necessarily in that order. The aim is to identify which is which in a logical manner.

1 Add 1 cm^3 of each solution to a separate test tube and label.

2 To each add 2 drops of iodine in potassium iodide solution.

3 The solution that goes blue-black is starch.

4 Add 1 cm^3 of the three remaining solutions to separate test tubes and label.

5 Perform the Biuret test (see above for details).

6 The solution turning violet is protein.

7 Add 1 cm^3 of the two remaining solutions to two test tubes and label.

8 Perform the Benedict's test.

9 The solution giving a red/brown precipitate is glucose.

10 The solution left over must therefore be sucrose.

Practical 3.3 To identify four unknown solutions using food tests plus your knowledge of enzymes

You are given four unknown solutions labelled A, B, C and D and are told that these are glucose, sucrose, sucrase (invertase) and starch, though not in that order. You are only allowed Benedict's solution and iodine in potassium iodide solution as reagents. You know that sucrase is an enzyme which converts sucrose to glucose and fructose. The aim is to identify each solution.

Requirements
- Test tubes
- Test tube racks
- Pipettes
- Pipette fillers
- Water bath
- Benedict's reagent
- Four unknown solutions labelled A, B, C and D
- Iodine in potassium iodide solution

Wear eye protection

1 Place 1 cm^3 of each solution into separate test tubes and label.

2 Add two drops of iodine in potassium iodide to each.

3 The solution which goes blue-black is starch.

4 Place 1 cm^3 of the three remaining solutions into separate test tubes and label.

5 Perform Benedict's test on each.

6 The one that gives the orange or reddy-brown precipitate is glucose.

7 The remaining two solutions are sucrose and sucrase.

What does boiling do to enzymes? (see page 11)

This fact is needed in order to identify which of the remaining two solutions is which. Imagine that the two solutions are B and C. Two experiments must now be performed:

a)

1 Place 1 cm^3 of B in a test tube and boil for 5 minutes.

2 Cool.

3 Add to C and leave for 3 minutes.

4 Perform Benedict's test.

b)

1 Place 1 cm^3 of C in a test tube and boil for 5 minutes as in a).

2 Cool.

3 Add to B and leave for 3 minutes.

4 Perform Benedict's test.

5 What does sucrase do?

6 If an orange or reddy-brown precipitate was produced in experiment a) which solution is which?

7 If an orange or reddy-brown precipitate was produced in experiment b) which solution is which?

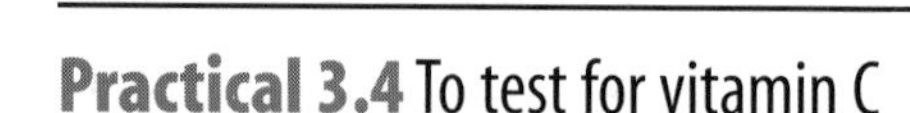

Practical 3.4 To test for vitamin C

Requirements
- Test tubes
- Test tube racks
- 1 cm^3 syringes
- Beakers
- Several foods, e.g. lemons, etc.
- DCPIP solution

1 Pipette 1 cm^3 of DCPIP into a test tube.

2 Extract the juice from e.g. a lemon or an orange.

3 Using a syringe, add the juice to the DCPIP a drop at a time.

4 The blue DCPIP will turn colourless/pale if vitamin C is present.

Practical 3.5 To determine the percentage of vitamin C in various foods

Requirements

As for Practical 3.4 plus 0.1% ascorbic acid (vitamin C) solution

1 Extract the juice from several foods, e.g. lemons, oranges, grapes, potatoes, etc.

2 Place 1 cm^3 of DCPIP into a test tube.

3 Using a syringe, add 0.1% vitamin C solution drop by drop until the blue colour goes colourless.

4 Record the volume of the ascorbic acid added.

5 Repeat instructions 1 to 4 with each food extract in turn.

Calculation: Suppose that it took 6 drops of 0.1% ascorbic acid solution to decolourise the DCPIP. If the lemon took 3 drops to decolourise the DCPIP, there must be double the vitamin C content in lemons as in the 0.1% ascorbic acid solution (as it took half the number of drops). Therefore the percentage of vitamin C is 0.2%.

General formula: (number of drops of 0.1% vitamin C $\div$ number of drops of extract) $\times$ 0.1%

6 Calculate the following using the assumed values for the decolourisation of the DCPIP: a) orange = 2 drops; b) grapes = 8 drops; c) potato = 36 drops.

Structure of the alimentary canal and digestion

Our alimentary canal (gut) is adapted to enable us to:

- take food into our bodies (**ingestion**)
- break food down into smaller pieces with a large surface area for enzymes to act on (**physical digestion**)
- break down large molecules into smaller, soluble molecules (**chemical digestion**)
- absorb small, soluble molecules (**absorption**)
- get rid of the undigested remains of the food we have eaten (**egestion**, or **defecation**).

Figure 3.4 represents the alimentary canal as a simple tube and shows the key terms used in nutrition. Figure 3.5 shows the alimentary canal and associated organs.

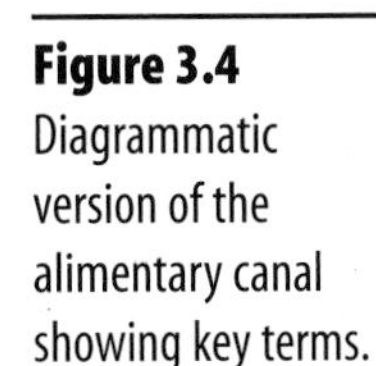

Figure 3.4 Diagrammatic version of the alimentary canal showing key terms.

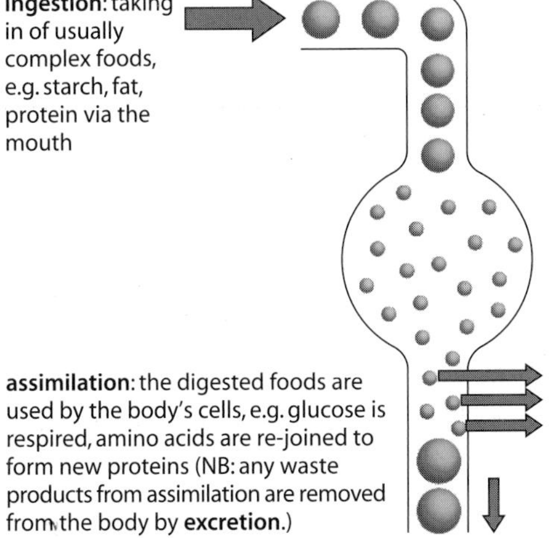

digestion: the large molecules are broken down by enzymes into smaller molecules

absorption: as the molecules are small they can be absorbed into the blood stream and lymph

egestion (defecation): removal of the **undigested** material

mouth cavity (buccal cavity)
mouth
tongue
salivary gland
gullet (oesophagus)
liver
gall bladder
bile duct
pancreas
abdominal cavity
soft palate
throat (pharynx)
epiglottis
diaphragm
ring of muscle (pyloric sphincter)
stomach
duodenum
ileum
small intestine
colon
caecum
appendix
rectum
large intestine
anus
ring of muscle around anus

Figure 3.5 Human alimentary canal and its associated organs.

Mouth

Digestion begins here by:

- **physical means** where the food is broken down into smaller pieces by the teeth (**mastication**)
- **chemical means** which begins the conversion of starch to maltose. The saliva has a pH of about 7.0 – the pH at which salivary amylase works best. Saliva is also a fluid which makes it easier for food to be swallowed.

Practical 3.6 To demonstrate the affect of temperature on amylase

Amylase converts starch to sugar. This change can be detected by the absence of a blue-black colour when a sample of the reaction mixture is added to iodine in potassium iodide. By timing this change at different temperatures, the effect of temperature on the enzyme can be shown.

Requirements

Test tubes
Test tube racks
Chinagraph pencil
Pipettes (1 cm^3 and 5 cm^3)
Pipette filters
Water baths (use a beaker with cold water for 20°C)
Dimple trays
Teat pipettes
Glass rods
Stop clocks
De-ionised water
1% starch solution
1% amylase solution
Iodine in potassium iodide solution

1 Pipette 1 cm^3 of amylase into a test tube and label.

2 Pipette 3 cm^3 of starch into another test tube and label.

3 Place each test tube into a water bath at 30°C for 15 minutes to allow each solution to reach this temperature.

4 During this time place a drop of iodine in potassium iodide solution into the dimples of a dimple tray using a teat pipette.

5 After 15 minutes mix the two solutions, start a stop clock and take a sample of the reaction mixture using a clean glass rod. Place this into an iodine drop (this should turn blue-black).

6 Clean the glass rod, take another sample after 30 seconds and test for the presence/absence of starch.

7 Repeat until there is no blue-black colour and record the time in minutes.

8 Repeat the whole experiment using water baths at 10°C, 20°C, 40°C and 70°C.

9 Controls should be set up at each temperature of:

a) 1 cm^3 de-ionised water and 3 cm^3 starch.

b) 1 cm^3 amylase and 3 cm^3 de-ionised water.

10 Record the results as a table:

Temperature /°C	Time for the blue-black colour to disappear /mins	Rate = 1/time

11 Graph the results.

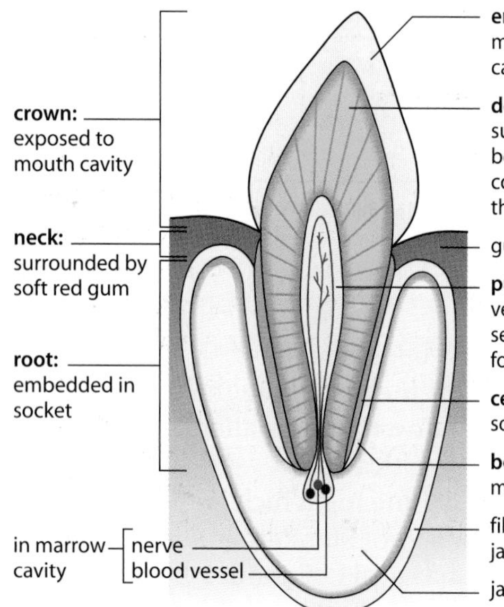

Figure 3.6 Structure of a canine tooth.

Teeth

We have two sets of teeth in our lifetime:
- milk (deciduous) teeth in childhood
- permanent teeth – replace the milk teeth from the age of about six years onwards.

There are four types of teeth:
- **incisors** – chisel-like for biting
- **canines** – pointed – no particular function in humans (Figure 3.6)
- **premolars** – cheek teeth – ridged for grinding
- **molars** – cheek teeth – ridged for grinding.

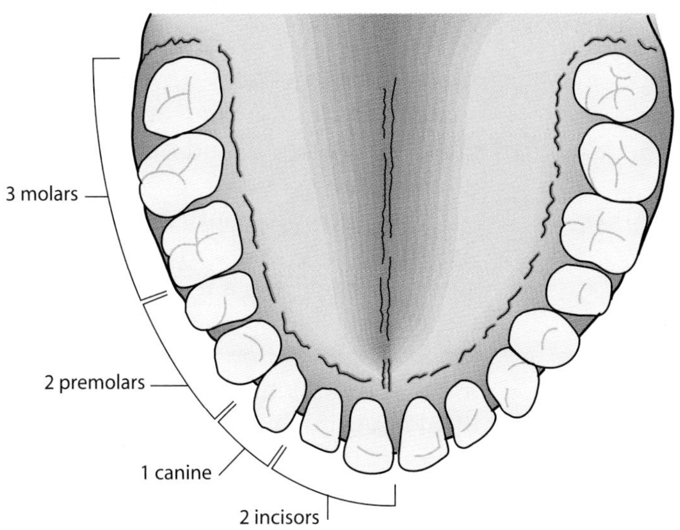

Figure 3.7 Human dentition.

In humans the upper and lower jaws have the same number and type of teeth (i.e. dentition) as seen in Figure 3.7. Instead of using a diagram like Figure 3.7, dentition can be represented using a **dental formula**. To work out the dental formula, an imaginary line is drawn down the middle of the upper and lower jaw. Then, the number of incisors on the upper and lower jaw to one side of this line is counted and represented (i 2/2). This is repeated for the canines (c), premolars (pm) and molars (m), giving:

i 2/2 c 1/1 pm 2/2 m 3/3

Q2: What is the maximum number of teeth in the adult human dentition?

Care of the teeth

Plaque is a mixture of saliva, food and bacteria which forms naturally on the teeth. Bacteria in the plaque produce acids and toxins (poisons) from the food, particularly if the food is sugary.

Dental caries are caused by the acid dissolving the enamel and the dentine of the tooth. This leads to a cavity in the tooth which may become infected, leading to toothache.

Periodontal disease is caused by the bacterial toxins. These cause inflammation of the gum at the point where the tooth and gum meet. Eventually the gum may pull back from the tooth and the tooth may fall out later in life.

Prevention:

1 Brush teeth thoroughly at least twice every day to remove plaque. Disclosing tablets can be chewed which stain plaque and therefore can be used as a check on the thoroughness of brushing. Use dental floss at least once a week. Change your tooth-brush every two months.
2 Diet – try to avoid sugary foods on which the bacteria thrive. Do not eat between meals.
3 Tooth paste – use the types with fluoride as this strengthens the enamel.
4 Visit the dentist regularly – this ensures that any problems are resolved. Ideally this should be every six months.

Swallowing

Swallowing is a complex series of actions which occur when you use your tongue to push food to the back of your mouth (Figure 3.8). Apart from the conscious act of pushing the tongue backwards, the other actions of swallowing are controlled involuntarily, i.e. they occur automatically. The role of the tongue is very important in that it possesses taste buds and also rolls the food into a ball (**bolus**) just before swallowing.

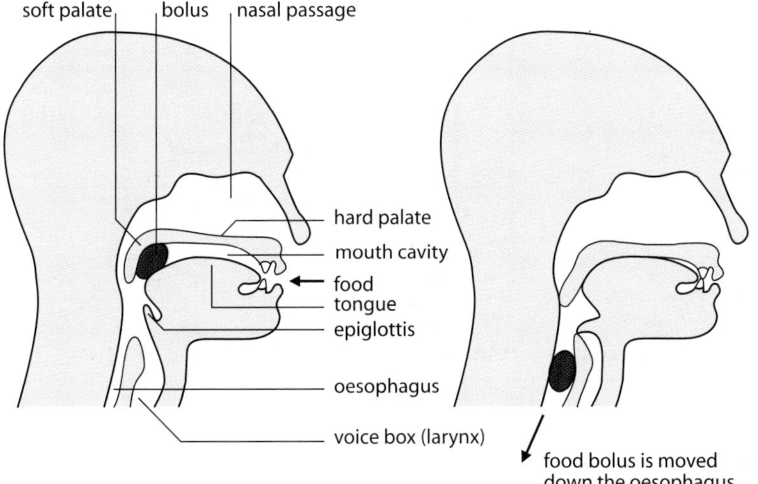

Figure 3.8 Swallowing.

Q3: Use Figure 3.8 to describe in words the functions during swallowing of: (a) the epiglottis; (b) the soft palate.

Oesophagus

After swallowing, a food bolus travels down the oesophagus by:

- gravity if you are standing or sitting vertically
- **peristalsis** – a wave-like contraction and relaxation of the circular muscles in the oesophagus that pushes the bolus along (Figure 3.9).

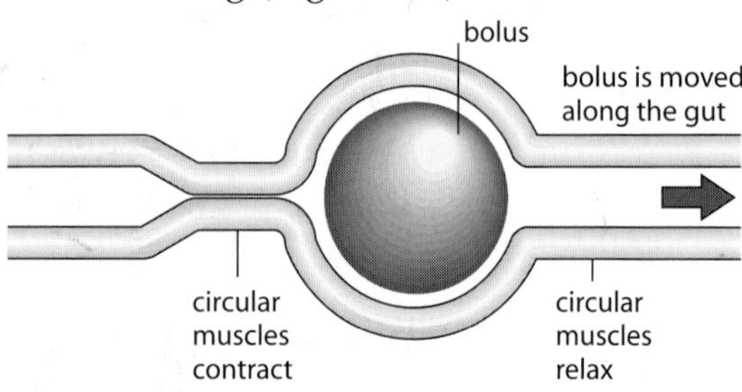

Figure 3.9 Peristalsis.

Stomach

The stomach is a highly muscular sac with sphincter muscles surrounding both openings. By its churning action the food is made into a semi-solid mass known as **chyme**. In the stomach:

- the pH drops to about 1.5 due to the secretion of hydrochloric acid by the stomach lining. As a result: many bacteria taken in with the food are killed; the breakdown of starch to maltose by salivary amylase stops; the ideal environment for stomach enzymes is produced
- the protease, pepsin, breaks down protein to smaller chains of amino acids called **polypeptides**
- some substances, e.g. alcohol, are absorbed.

Q4: Can you think of any advantage to the body of having the stomach contents highly acidic?

Practical 3.7 To demonstrate the effect of pH on a protease, e.g. pepsin

Pepsin acts on proteins, e.g. albumen, turning it clear from a cloudy suspension. By using buffers (chemicals which keep a solution at a certain pH) we can see the effect of pH on the enzyme.

Requirements

Test tubes
Test tube racks
Chinagraph pencils
Stop clocks
Pipettes (1 cm^3 and 5 cm^3)
Pipette filters
De-ionised water
Water bath at 30°C
1% pepsin solution
1% albumen suspension
Range of pH buffers

1 Pipette 1 cm^3 of pepsin and 1 cm^3 of pH buffer 7.0 into a test tube and label.

2 Pipette 3 cm^3 of albumen solution into another test tube and label.

3 Place these in a water bath at 30°C for fifteen minutes so that the solutions reach this temperature.

4 After this time mix the two solutions and time how long it takes for the cloudy suspension to clear. Record this time in minutes.

5 Repeat the experiment using pH buffers 4.0, 5.0, 6.0, 8.0 and 9.0.

6 Record the results as a table:

pH	Time for the suspension to clear /mins	Rate = 1/time

7 Graph the results.

8 Controls should be set up at each pH of 1 cm^3 de-ionised water, 1 cm^3 buffer and 3 cm^3 albumen.

Duodenum

Periodically the pyloric sphincter muscle relaxes and chyme is released into the duodenum. Here it receives secretions from the liver (bile) and pancreas (pancreatic juice).

Bile

Bile:

- is produced by the liver and stored in the gall bladder
- is alkaline therefore contributes to the pH rise to about 8.0 in the duodenum
- emulsifies lipids, i.e. changes large lipid drops into many smaller lipid droplets that can mix with water (Figure 3.10).

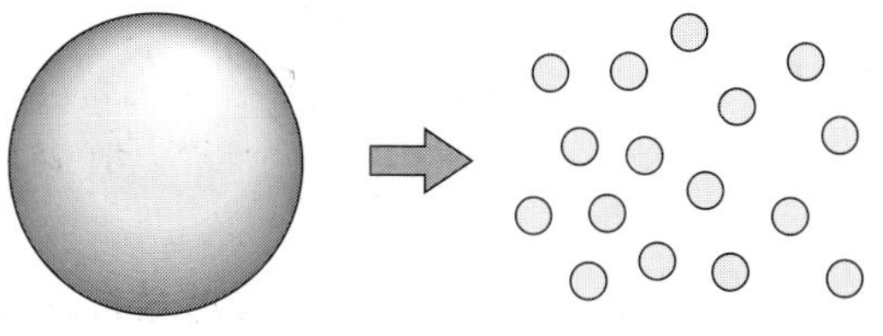

Figure 3.10 Emulsification.

Q5: (a) What has happened to the surface area of the lipid in Figure 3.10? (b) What will therefore happen to the speed of their digestion?

Pancreatic juice

Pancreatic juice:

- is produced by the pancreas
- is alkaline therefore contributes to the pH rise to about 8.0 in the duodenum
- contains enzymes:
  - amylase which converts any remaining starch to maltose
  - proteases, e.g. trypsin, which convert polypeptides to peptides
  - lipases which convert the emulsified lipids to fatty acids and glycerol.

Figure 3.11 shows the duodenum and its relationship to the liver and pancreas.

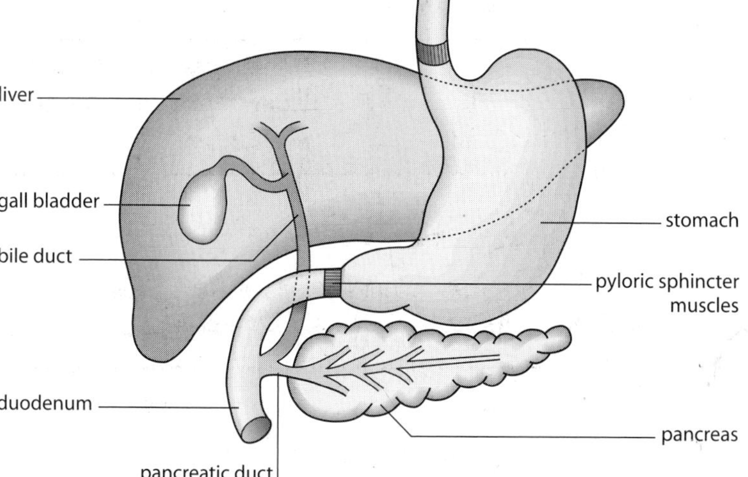

Figure 3.11 Duodenum showing associated structures.

Ileum

Digestion is completed here by enzymes that work either on the surface membrane or in the cytoplasm of cells lining the ileum.

- Maltase converts maltose to glucose.
- Sucrase (also called invertase) converts sucrose to glucose and fructose.
- Lactase converts lactose to glucose and galactose.
- Dipeptidases convert dipeptides into individual amino acids.
- All these enzymes require a neutral/alkaline pH.

Absorption can now occur and the ileum is very well adapted for this purpose as can be seen in Figure 3.12. Table 3.3 shows what happens to the end products of digestion once they have been absorbed.

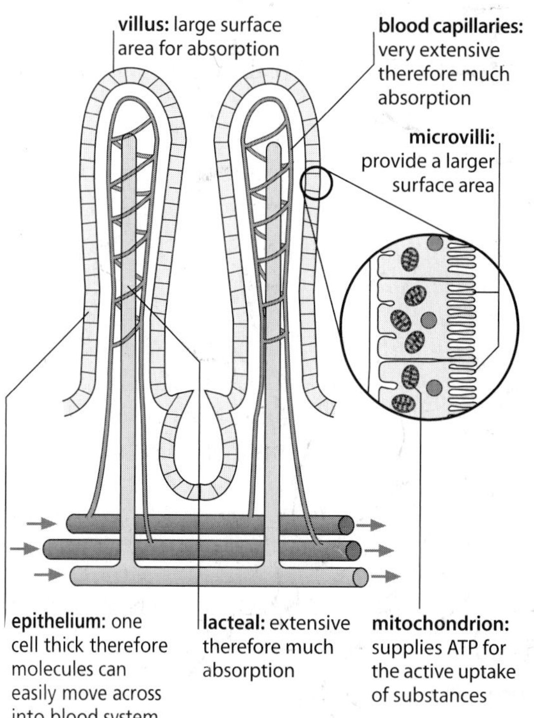

Figure 3.12 Villi in the small intestine.

Table 3.3 Fate of absorbed foods

End product of digestion	Fate(s)
Amino acids	• Absorbed into the hepatic portal vein by diffusion and active transport and travel to the liver • Some pass through the liver and go to all body cells where they are made into new proteins for, e.g. growth, repair, enzymes • Excess amino acids are deaminated in the liver to form urea which is excreted by the kidneys
Glucose	• Absorbed into the hepatic portal vein by diffusion and active transport and travels to the liver • Some passes through the liver and travels to all cells for use in respiration • Excess glucose is converted to glycogen and stored in the liver and muscles
Fatty acids and glycerol	• Absorbed into the lacteal, which is part of the lymph system, by diffusion • Eventually this drains into the blood stream • Excess is stored around vital organs for, e.g. insulation, protection

Large intestine (appendix, caecum, colon and rectum)

- The caecum and appendix have no specific function in humans
- The colon absorbs water so that the faeces become drier
- The colon is inhabited by many mutualistic bacteria which
  - digest the remaining food, producing vitamin K and the B-group vitamins (see page 16)
  - prevent other harmful bacteria from growing and causing discomfort or disease
- The dry faeces are stored in the rectum and periodically released (egestion, also called defecation).

Liver

The liver is the largest organ in the human body and has many different functions:

- control of blood sugar level (under the control of insulin and glucagon – see page 55)
- removal of the nitrogen-containing part of excess amino acids (**deamination**) so that the rest of the molecule can be used as an energy source
- production of urea which contains the nitrogen-containing part of excess amino acid molecules
- production of blood proteins, including haemoglobin and fibrinogen (used in blood clotting)
- generation of heat, therefore very important in temperature regulation
- destruction of old red blood cells
- production of bile
- breakdown of toxins (poisons), e.g. alcohol and drugs, into non-toxic compounds
- storage of vitamins, e.g. A, D, K; minerals, e.g. iron; carbohydrate, e.g. glycogen.

Q 6: One of the most difficult parts of this topic is learning what each enzyme does and where it is found. To help with this make a table with the various regions, pH, etc. An example has been given on page 25 to help you start. You will need to use your notes carefully.

Some digestive ailments

Gastric ulcers

The stomach is lined with a very thick layer of mucus. This prevents its own hydrochloric acid and pepsin from harming it. However, sometimes this layer of mucus becomes thinner or non-existent and the stomach's resistance is reduced. The hydrochloric acid burns the

Table 3.4 Table for Question 6

Region	pH	Secretion	Activities
1 Mouth	7.0	Saliva	(i) Teeth – allows mastication therefore achieves a large surface area for enzyme activity and helps swallowing. Four types: incisors, canines, pre-molars, molars. Two dentitions: milk and permanent. (ii) Tongue – helps with taste and rolling the food into a bolus. (iii) Saliva – contains amylase which converts starch to maltose. A fluid, therefore helps with swallowing.
2 Oesophagus	7.0	Mucus	(i) Digestion of starch to maltose still occurs. (ii) Food moved down by gravity and peristalsis (contraction and relaxation of the circular muscles)
3 Stomach	2.0	Hydrochloric acid and enzymes	

stomach lining followed by the pepsin which begins to digest it. This leads to gastric ulcers, i.e. inflammation of the stomach. The cause of these is unclear but they are known to be influenced by:

- stress
- alcohol consumption.

At the moment, expensive drugs that reduce acid secretion or surgical removal of part of the stomach are the standard treatments for gastric ulcers.

Recently a new possible explanation has been put forward. This is that a bacterial infection might stimulate excess acid release. If this is true then treatments of the condition will become a lot less expensive through the use of antibiotics.

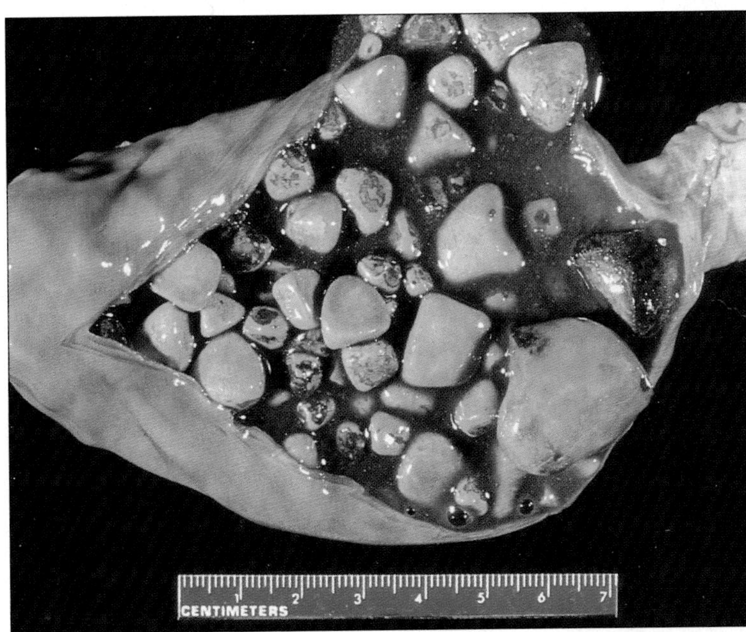

Figure 3.13 Gall stones.

Pancreatitis

This is an inflammation of the pancreas due to either or both:

- alcohol consumption
- gall stones, which block the pancreatic duct connecting the pancreas to the duodenum.

Eventually the enzymes in the pancreatic juice digest the pancreas and even leak into the body cavity where they can digest other organs.

Gall stones

These form in the gall bladder due to cholesterol becoming solid (Figure 3.13). This can produce a number of small stones or one large one that can fill the entire gall bladder.

Treatments vary but include:

- surgery – to remove the gall stone or even the entire gall bladder
- use of chemicals to dissolve the gall stone gradually.
- ultra sound to break up the gall stone.

Summary

- The seven constituents of a balanced diet are proteins, lipids, carbohydrates, inorganic ions (minerals), vitamins, dietary fibre and water.
- The basic unit of a protein is the amino acid. Amino acids are needed to make new proteins for growth, repair, some hormones and most enzymes.
- The most common lipids are triglycerides. These are made up of fatty acids and glycerol.
- Carbohydrates can be polysaccharides, disaccharides and monosaccharides.
- Vitamins are substances that are essential for the correct working of the body and are needed in very small amounts.
- Biuret test is a test for protein.
- Benedict's reagent is a test for reducing sugar.
- Iodine in potassium iodide is a test for starch.
- DCPIP is a test for vitamin C.
- The formation of a translucent stain will show the presence of a lipid.
- Digestion of complex foods is necessary before absorption and assimilation can occur.
- The main enzymes dealt with are:
  - amylases, which convert starch to sugars;
  - proteases, e.g. pepsin, which convert proteins to amino acids;
  - lipases, which convert lipids to fatty acids and glycerol.
- There are four types of teeth in the adult dentition: incisors, canines, premolars and molars.
- Dental care is very important and involves several essential activities.
- Absorption in the small intestine is aided by villi, microvilli and a very rich blood supply.
- The liver is the largest organ in the body and has numerous functions.
- Microbes in the gut produce vitamin K and the B-group vitamins.
- There are several potential problems in the alimentary canal, e.g. ulcers and gall stones.

Self check
See page 229

CHAPTER 4

Circulation

In this chapter you will learn why a circulatory system is necessary and about the structure and functioning of our own circulatory system. You will also learn about the structure and functions of blood and about blood groups. Finally, you will learn how materials leave the blood to bathe body cells and about the lymph system that helps to return some of these materials to the circulatory system.

Why have a circulatory system?

Single-celled organisms do not need a circulatory system. Since they are small and have a relatively large surface area, diffusion is efficient enough to carry in the substances they need and to carry out their wastes. However, in larger organisms a circulatory system is essential to supply their billions of cells as diffusion alone is too slow.

The human circulatory system consists of:

- **blood** – a fluid that transports dissolved substances around the body. It also carries **blood cells** that have a variety of functions
- **blood vessels** – tubes that carry the blood to all parts of the body. The smallest of these tubes 'leak' fluids out to body cells
- **heart** – a muscular pump that moves the blood around the body.

Functions of the blood

These include:

- **transport** – of substances (e.g. glucose, amino acids, carbon dioxide), of antibodies and of heat
- **temperature regulation** – see Chapter 7
- **defence against disease** – through the action of white blood cells
- **reproduction** – e.g. the penis is made erect by the use of blood (see Chapter 11).

Blood structure

The composition of human blood can be represented as a chart:

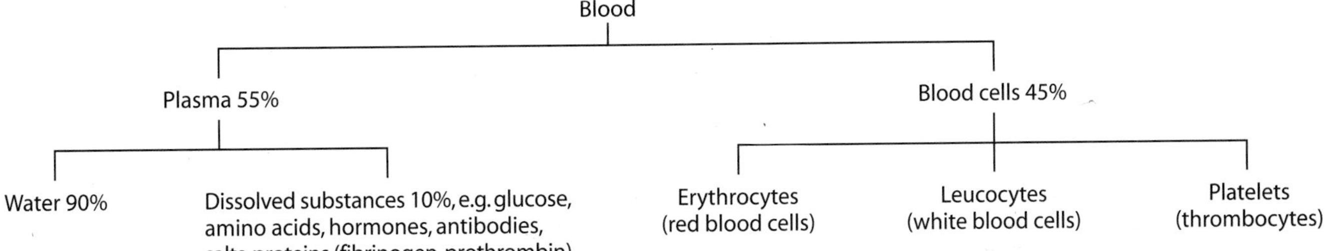

Although blood is fluid, notice that almost half of it is made from cells. These cells have important, but specific, functions that are described below.

As well as carrying the blood cells, the blood plasma carries dissolved metabolites (such as glucose, amino acids and carbon dioxide) and suspended antibodies.

Roles of the blood cells

Red blood cells

Red blood cells (or **erythrocytes**) are the most numerous of our blood cells. In a healthy human, each mm^3 of blood (about one drop) contains about 5 million red blood cells. They are so numerous that if they clumped together they would block all but the widest blood vessels.

Figure 4.1 shows a single red blood cell. It is unique among human cells in that it does not contain a nucleus. Instead its cytoplasm is full of haemoglobin, the pigment which makes these cells (and our blood) appear red.

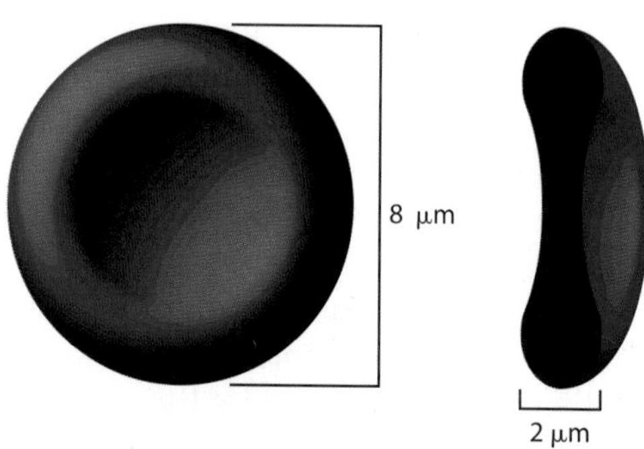

Biconcave or ring doughnut shape. Best surface area to volume ratio for gaseous exchange. No nucleus so can pack in more haemoglobin. Elastic partially permeable membrane to allow them to squeeze through capillaries.

Produced in the marrow of some bones. Live for approximately 17 weeks then are destroyed in the liver and spleen. Usually between 4 to 6 million per mm^3 blood. Function is to transport O_2 and some CO_2.

Figure 4.1 Red blood cell or erythrocyte.

As Figure 4.2 shows, the role of haemoglobin is to transport oxygen from our lungs to the cells of our body. Our ability to transport oxygen is affected by:

- **anaemia** – caused either by too few red blood cells or by red blood cells having too little haemoglobin in their cytoplasm. One of the most common reasons for the latter is a lack of iron in the diet (simple anaemia)
- **carbon monoxide** – a gas that is taken up by haemoglobin in preference to oxygen, forming **carboxyhaemoglobin**. This leads to lack of oxygen in the blood, causing drowsiness and even death. **NB:** It is for this reason that gas fires should be serviced regularly
- **high altitudes** – since there is less oxygen in the air at high altitudes, people eventually acclimatise by forming more red blood cells.

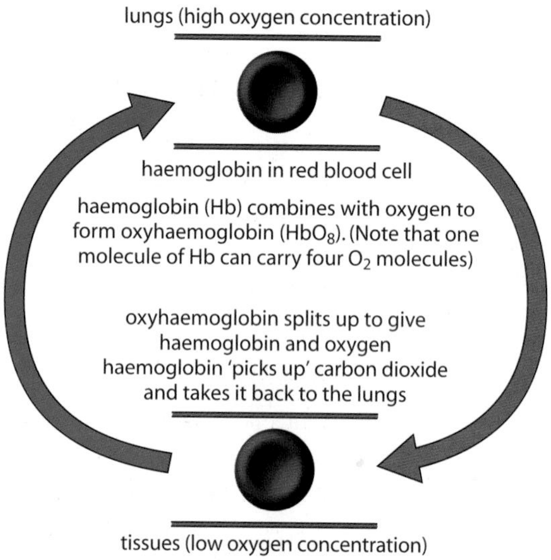

lungs (high oxygen concentration)

haemoglobin in red blood cell

haemoglobin (Hb) combines with oxygen to form oxyhaemoglobin (HbO_8). (Note that one molecule of Hb can carry four O_2 molecules)

oxyhaemoglobin splits up to give haemoglobin and oxygen
haemoglobin 'picks up' carbon dioxide and takes it back to the lungs

tissues (low oxygen concentration)

Figure 4.2 Role of haemoglobin.

Q1: By which process will the oxygen move from the lungs to the red blood cells?

Q2: How is (a) glucose; (b) oxygen carried in the blood?

White blood cells

White blood cells (or **leucocytes**) come in many different shapes and sizes. Figure 4.3 shows the three types of white cell:

- **monocytes** – wander around the body engulfing cells and cell debris by a process known as phagocytosis (Figure 4.4)
- **neutrophils** – wander around the body engulfing cells and cell debris by phagocytosis
- **lymphocytes** – one type of which produces antibodies.

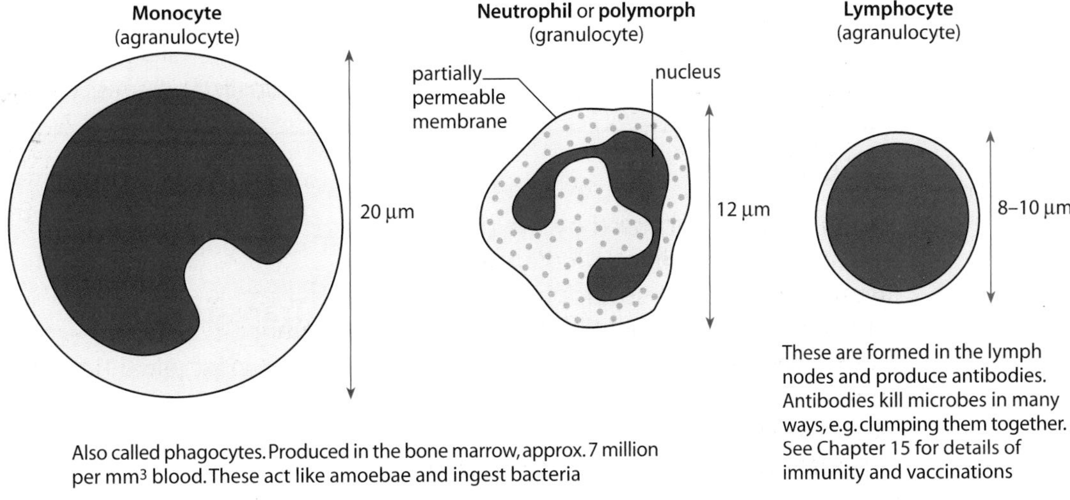

Figure 4.3 Types of leucocyte.

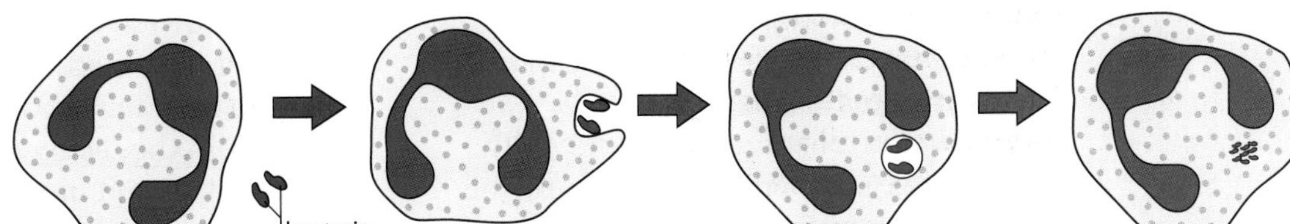

Figure 4.4 Phagocytosis.

Platelets

Platelets (or **thrombocytes**) are non-nucleated cell fragments formed in the bone marrow. In a healthy human, there are approximately 250 000 per mm^3 of blood. They are involved in blood clotting, a vital process which:

- prevents excessive blood loss from damaged blood vessels
- prevents entry of pathogens through damaged skin.

Figure 4.5 shows the major stages in the clotting process. The clot itself is formed when a mesh of protein strands traps red blood cells, to make an impenetrable barrier. The platelets (along with the walls of damaged blood vessels) release an enzyme, **thrombokinase** (thromboplastin), that starts this process. **NB:** Serum is plasma without fibrinogen.

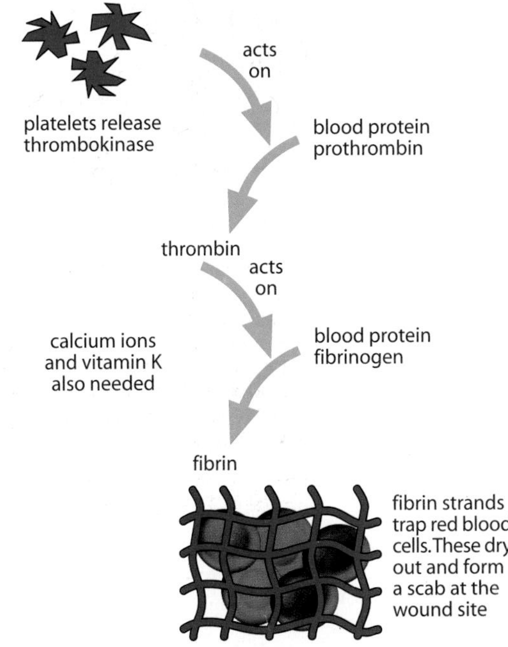

Figure 4.5 Stages in clotting of blood.

Practical 4.1 To observe blood cells from a prepared slide

For health and safety reasons, you are not allowed to make blood smears in the laboratory of your college or school. Prepared slides of human blood are quite safe to use.

Requirements
Microscope
Blood smear slide (prepared).

1 Clip a prepared slide of a human blood smear on the stage of a microscope.

2 Focus the slide using the low power objective of the microscope.

3 Switch to the high power objective and refocus if necessary.

4 Identify the blood cells you can see, using Figure 4.6.

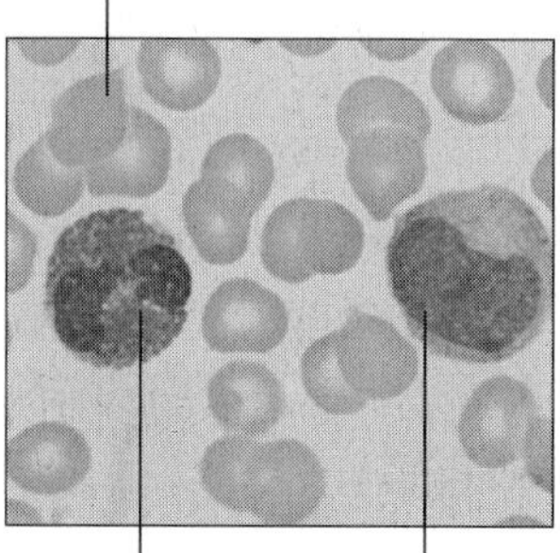

Figure 4.6 A blood smear.

Blood groups

Blood groups are caused by the presence of particular proteins (called **antigens**, or **agglutinins**) on the surface membrane of red blood cells. People without a particular antigen are capable of producing an **antibody** that will attack the antigen if blood cells carrying it ever leak into their blood. If this were to happen, the foreign blood cells would stick together (clumping, or **agglutination**), blocking blood vessels and leading to death in extreme cases.

One of the blood groups is the **ABO** system (see Chapter 19 to learn how this blood group system is inherited). People are born with a combination of antigens on the surface membrane of their red blood cells (see Table 4.1). People who are blood group A have red blood cells with a protein called antigen A on the surface membrane of their red blood cells. Always present in their plasma is an antibody that will attack antigen B, called anti-B (sometimes also called β). The reverse is true for people who are blood group B. Notice that people always produce an antibody that attacks the antigen they lack: otherwise we would clump our own red blood cells!

Table 4.1 Blood groups

Blood group name	Antigen on red blood cell	Antibody in plasma
A	A	β (anti-B)
B	B	α (anti-A)
AB	AB	none
0	none	α and β

Transfusions

The most usual time our ABO blood group becomes important to us is during blood transfusions, e.g. following an accident or during an operation. To prevent harm, we need to know the ABO group of the recipient (the person receiving the blood) and of the donor (the blood to be transfused).

To avoid the recipient's antibodies clumping the red blood cells from the donor's blood we need to ensure the recipient's plasma does not contain the antibody against an antigen carried by the donor's red blood cells. Table 4.2 shows which blood transfusions can be performed safely.

Key points:

- need only worry about the *donor's antigens* and the *recipient's antibodies*
- a small amount of clumping of the recipient's red blood cells can be tolerated by the body.

Table 4.2 Transfusions

Donor group	Recipient group			
	A β	B α	AB	0 αβ
A β	✓	✗	✓	✗
B α	✗	✓	✓	✗
AB	✗	✗	✓	✗
0 αβ	✓	✓	✓	✓

✓ = Safe ✗ = Unsafe

Rhesus blood system and haemolytic disease of the newborn

About 85% of the British population have a **rhesus** antigen on their red blood cells: they are called rhesus positive (Rh^+). The remaining 15% do not have this rhesus antigen and are called rhesus negative (Rh^-).

A problem might arise when a Rh^+ child is born to a Rh^- mother:

- In late pregnancy, some fragments of fetal cells containing the rhesus antigen get across the placenta and into the mother's blood.
- She responds by producing the rhesus antibodies. Unlike the ABO system, she did not already have these antibodies.
- These maternal rhesus antibodies move across the placenta and clump the fetal red blood cells.
- This is not a problem with the first child because it occurs so late during pregnancy, but it is with any other Rh^+ babies the mother might carry. In later pregnancies, the mother makes the rhesus antibodies much earlier. They reach high concentrations in the blood of the fetus, clumping its cells and causing either haemolytic disease or death.

Treatment can be either:

- transfusion of Rh^- blood in the womb or
- giving the mother a protein which coats the fetal cells, so stopping the rhesus antibodies from functioning.

Q3: (a) Group O is called a universal donor. Why? (b) Group AB is called a universal recipient. Why?

Structure of the heart

The heart is a muscular pump that pushes blood around the body. It is made of a type of muscle, called **cardiac muscle**, that is found only here. Cardiac muscle tissue is shown in Figure 4.7. Notice the striations in the muscle cells: these are protein fibres that enable the cell to contract. Also notice that the cells are stacked in columns with cross-bridges between them. This arrangement allows the cells to communicate so that they contract at the same time.

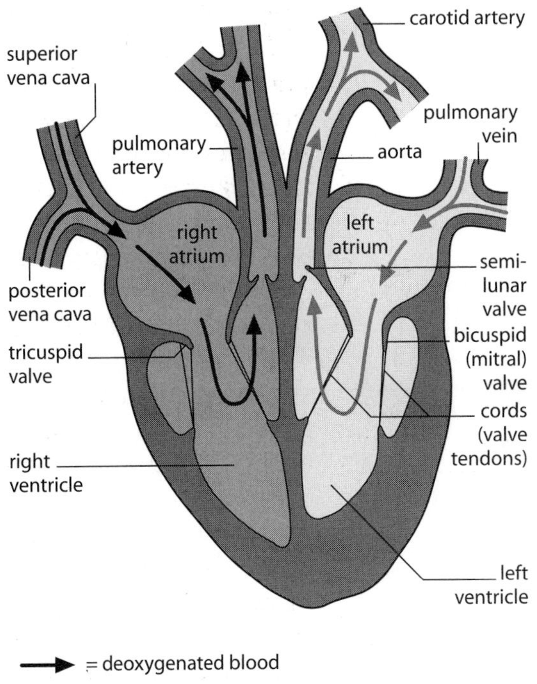

Figure 4.8 Structure of the heart and associated blood vessels.

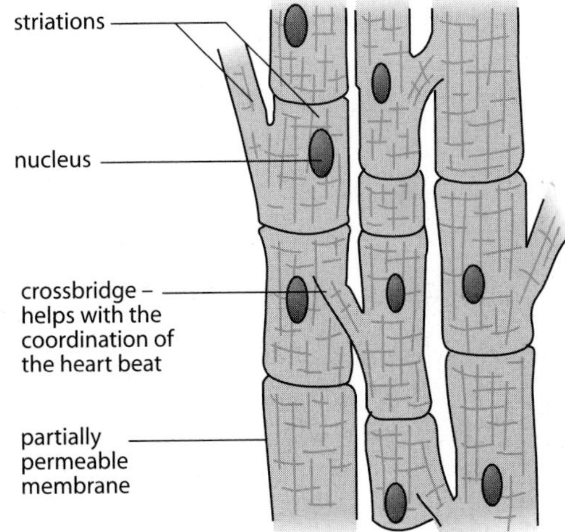

Figure 4.7 Cardiac muscle tissue.

The heart itself is actually two pumps lying side by side (Figure 4.8). Each side receives blood from the veins into an **atrium**. Blood from this atrium flows into a **ventricle** whose contraction forces the blood into an artery. Valves between the atrium and ventricle on each side prevent the backflow of blood during a heartbeat.

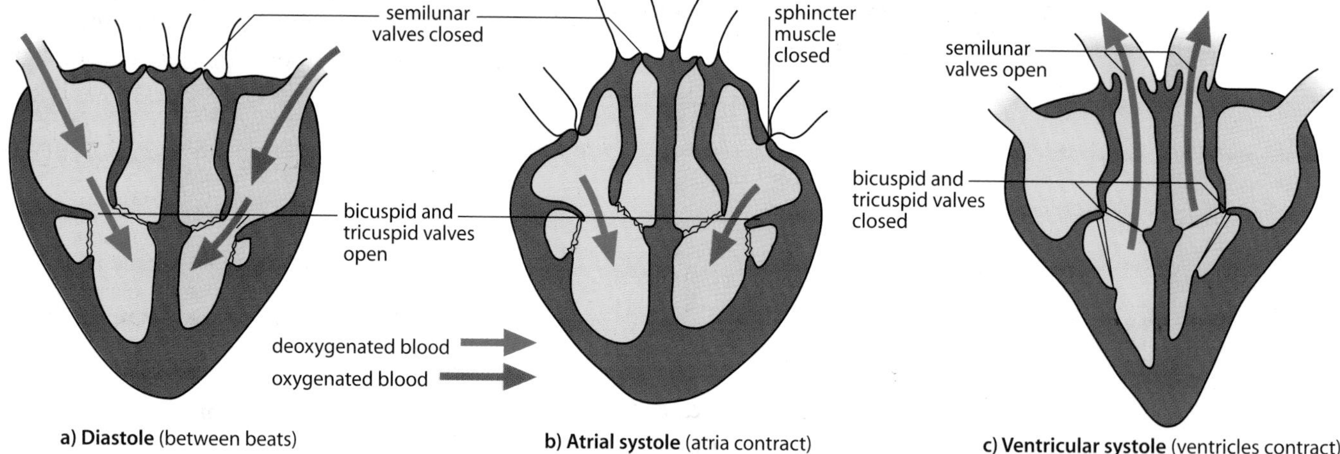

Figure 4.9 Blood flow through the heart.

Flow of blood through the heart

Contraction of a chamber of the heart is called **systole**. The resting state, when the cardiac muscle is relaxed, is called **diastole**. The two atria on each side of the heart contract and relax at the same time. The two ventricles relax and contract at a different time from the atria but at the same time as each other. One complete heartbeart involves the following stages.

- **Diastole**: atria and ventricles relax and blood enters the heart from the vena cavae and pulmonary veins. Semilunar valves prevent any backflow of blood from the pulmonary artery and aorta into the ventricles (Figure 4.9a).
- **Atrial systole**: Both atria contract together. As a consequence, their volume will decrease so that the blood pressure within them increases. Blood at high pressure will flow through the bicuspid and tricuspid valves into the ventricles (Figure 4.9b). At this stage, the muscles around the pulmonary veins and vena cavae constrict so that blood is forced one way into the ventricles.
- **Ventricular systole**: Both ventricles contract together. At the same time, the atria begin to relax. As the ventricles contract, their volume decreases so that their pressure increases. Eventually the pressure in the ventricles is greater than that in the atria, so the bicuspid and tricuspid valves are pushed closed. As the pressure in the ventricles also becomes higher than that in the arteries, the semilunar valves are pushed open and blood flows into these vessels (Figure 4.9c).

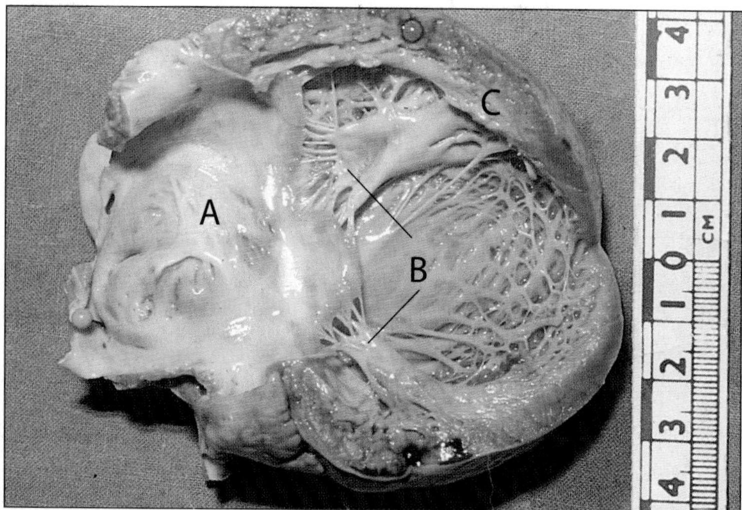

Figure 4.10 Human heart (dissection of left side with top of heart to the left of the photograph).

Q4: What happens to (a) the volume and (b) the pressure in the ventricles when the ventricles contract and the atria relax, i.e. during ventricular systole?

Q5: What is the role of the bicuspid and tricuspid valves?

Q6: What is the role of the semilunar valves?

Q7: Suggest a role for the tendons shown in Figure 4.8.

Q8: Suggest why the left ventricle is thicker than the right ventricle.

Q9: Suggest why the walls of the atria are much thinner than those of the ventricles.

Q10: Name the structures labelled A, B and C in Figure 4.10.

Heart sounds

The 'lubb-dupp' sounds that can be detected through the chest wall using a stethoscope are caused by the closure of the heart valves:

- 'lubb' – closure of the bicuspid and tricuspid valves (louder sound)
- 'dupp' – closure of the semilunar valves (softer sound).

Blood pressure

The pumping action of the heart builds up a high pressure that enables blood to be pumped around the circulatory system. The key points are:

- contraction of the ventricles is the main source of the blood pressure
- the pressures in the aorta and pulmonary artery remain relatively constant as they contain elastic tissue. As the ventricles contract, the aorta and pulmonary artery are stretched and expand. As the ventricles relax, these vessels move back to their original diameter. This recoil is very important in helping to push the blood along the arteries
- as the blood travels along the circulatory system, friction between the blood and the walls of the blood vessels causes a fall in blood pressure.

Q11: Figure 4.11 represents the pressure of blood as it travels from arteries through capillaries to veins. (a) Explain the wavy nature of the curve in the arteries and arterioles; (b) In which part of the blood system does the greatest fall in pressure occur?

Pulse

The arteries expand when the ventricles contract, and recoil when they relax. This movement of the walls out then in is the pulse and can be felt when an artery near to the skin passes over something hard, such as a bone. The most common places for the pulse to be felt are in the neck (where the carotid artery passes over thick muscle) and on the inside of the wrist (where the artery passes over the wrist bones).

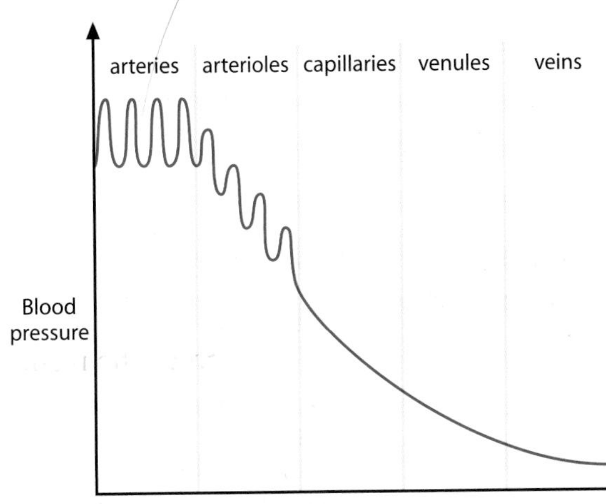

Figure 4.11 Blood pressure in different parts of the circulatory system.

Circulatory system

Like all mammals, humans have a **double** circulation (Figure 4.12). This means that for each circuit of the body, a red blood cell will pass through the heart twice.

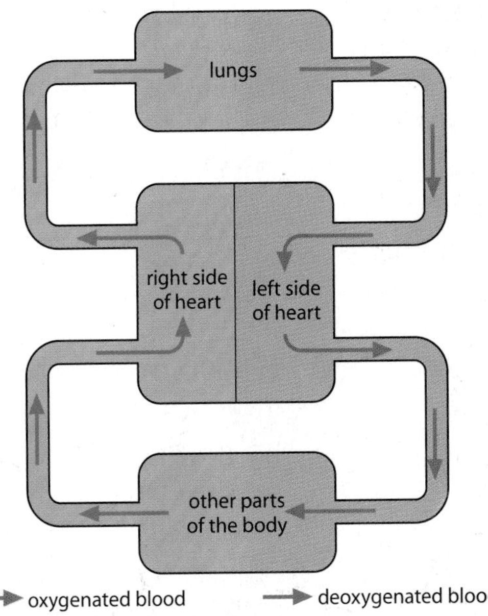

Figure 4.12 Double circulation.

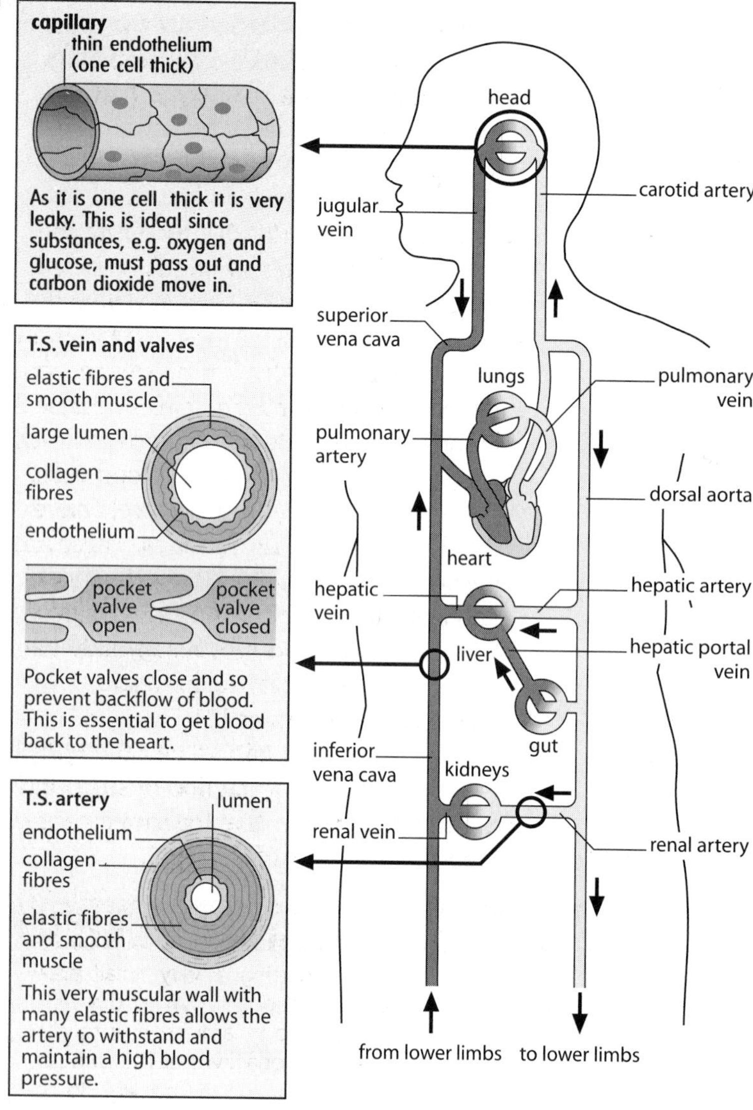

Figure 4.13 Circulatory system and types of blood vessels.

Figure 4.13 shows a simple summary of the circulatory system and types of blood vessel.

Q12: Use Figure 4.13 to identify three differences between an artery and a vein.

How blood gets back to the heart

Veins carry blood at low pressure back to the heart. The pressure in the veins is so low that it is not sufficient to push the blood back to the heart. The following processes are essential in helping blood to get back to the heart:

- **gravity** – from the head region if we are standing or sitting erect
- **skeletal muscle** – veins are surrounded by skeletal muscle, particularly in the calf. As these muscles contract they squeeze the veins, pushing against the blood they contain
- **valves** – prevent backflow of blood when the muscle squeezes the vein (Figure 4.14). As a result, the blood must flow in a single direction back to the heart

a) muscle relaxed
b) muscle contracted
vein
valves
blood pushed through open valve
closed valve prevents back flow

Figure 4.14 Veins and valves.

- **partial vacuum in chest** – we breathe in by causing a partial vacuum in our chest cavity (see page 41). This partial vacuum not only causes atmospheric air to be pushed into our lungs, it also causes blood to be pushed into the major veins leading to the heart.

Tissue fluid

If blood never left the blood vessels, it would not be able to supply body cells with the nutrients they need. Blood cannot leave the arteries and veins, but the capillaries do let small molecules through their walls. The small molecules that leave capillaries and bathe the body cells form the **tissue fluid**.

Q13: Suggest four molecules that are small enough to pass out of the blood through the capillary wall.

Figure 4.15 shows a capillary network surrounded by a group of body cells. Note that, in the formation of tissue fluid:

- there is a relatively high blood pressure at

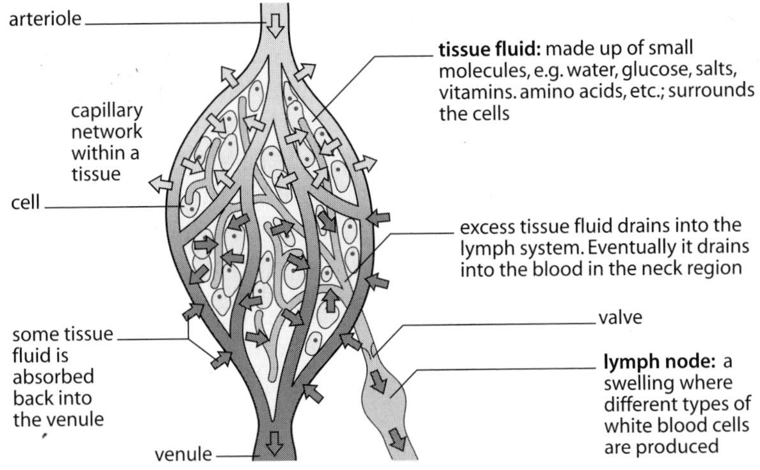

Figure 4.15 Formation of tissue fluid.

the arterial end of the capillaries which forces small molecules from the blood through the capillary wall

- large molecules, e.g. proteins, and red blood cells, stay inside the capillary
- the tissues are therefore surrounded by a fluid from which they obtain their nutrients and into which they pass wastes
- at the venous end of the capillary, the loss of molecules from the blood has caused the blood pressure to fall. As a result, it is now less than the pressure of the tissue fluid so that much of the tissue fluid is reabsorbed into the capillaries that lead to the venule.

Lymph system

Not all tissue fluid is reabsorbed into the capillaries. Some drains into blind-ended capillaries of the lymph system where it becomes **lymph**. One of these is shown in Figure 4.15. Eventually, lymph returns to the blood system through veins in the neck.

- Lymph is a colourless fluid, rich in lipids and containing many white blood cells.
- Along their length, lymph vessels have swellings called **lymph nodes**. These are particularly common in the groin, neck and armpits. Lymphocytes, which are a type of white blood cell, accumulate here and are important in the immune response (see Chapter 15).
- Lymph vessels contain valves; the lymph is moved by the contraction of surrounding muscles (rather like the movement of blood in the veins of the legs).

Heart disease

Coronary heart disease is one of the commonest causes of death in the UK. Included in this category of illness are:

- **angina** – pain across the chest, left arm and shoulder caused by insufficient blood getting to the heart muscle. This can be controlled by drugs.
- **heart attack** (coronary thrombosis) – a blockage occurs in a coronary artery so that some cardiac muscle is starved of blood (Figure 4.16). These muscle cells die (myocardial infarction) and the heart becomes progressively weaker. One of the most common causes of this blockage is **atherosclerosis** where fatty material, particularly cholesterol, is deposited on the inner wall of the coronary arteries (Figure 4.17). These deposits are called **atheromas**.

There is a strong genetic component making some people more likely to suffer heart attacks than others. Among other factors that contribute to coronary heart disease are:

- dietary intake that is high in fats
- smoking – causes fat deposits in the arteries
- high blood pressure – increases the risk of fatty deposits in the arteries
- lack of regular exercise.

Treatment of heart disease can be by:

- **balloon inflation** – this procedure involves putting a very small tube (catheter) about 1 mm in diameter with a balloon around it into the diseased coronary vessel. The catheter is pushed through the partially closed vessel until the balloon portion of the catheter straddles the part that is nearly blocked. The balloon is inflated, stretching the diseased vessel so that it opens out. Blood flow is thus increased.
- **heart bypass** – this procedure is used during surgery to the heart. During surgery, a mechanical pump is used to make the blood flow through the body. This allows surgeons to deal with the heart problem, e.g. replacement of a new heart valve, without disrupting blood flow.

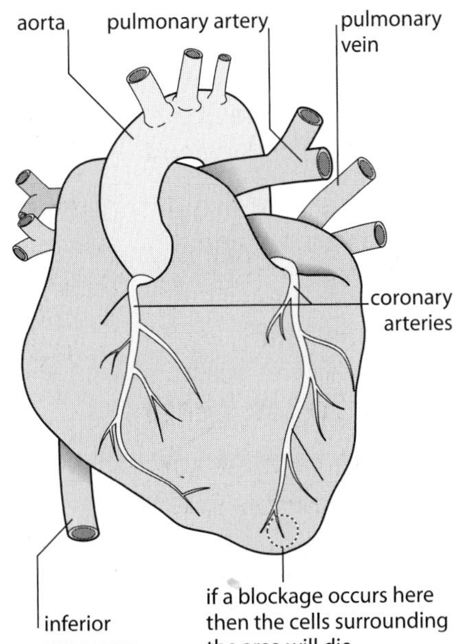

Figure 4.16 The heart showing coronary arteries.

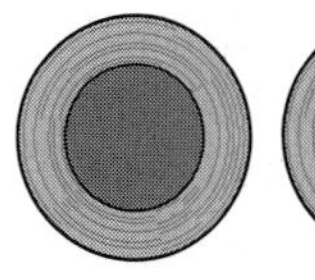

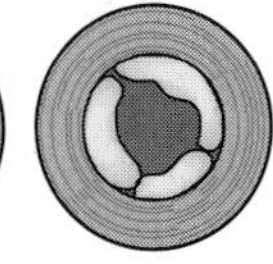

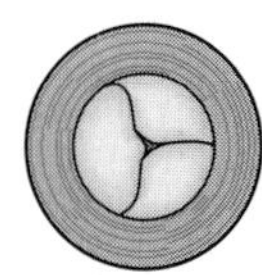

Figure 4.17 Atherosclerosis.

Summary

- A circulatory system ensures that metabolites are distributed around the body of large animals fast enough to keep them alive.
- Functions of the blood include transport, temperature regulation and protection against disease.
- Red blood cells (erythrocytes) are used in the transport of oxygen. Their adaptations for this role include the absence of a nucleus, an elastic partially permeable surface membrane, cytoplasm rich in haemoglobin and a biconcave shape.
- Factors affecting oxygen transport include altitude and diet, e.g. lack of iron.
- White blood cells (leucocytes) perform a protective role either by engulfing cells and cell debris (phagocytosis) or by producing antibodies.
- Platelets begin the process of blood clotting, preventing blood loss and infection by pathogens.
- There are four blood groups in the human ABO system: groups A, B, AB and O. Knowledge of these is very important when giving blood transfusions.
- Another type of blood grouping is the rhesus system. This can cause problems during pregnancy if a rhesus negative mother has more than one rhesus positive child.
- The heart is two muscular pumps combined in one organ. There are two chambers on each side, an atrium and a ventricle, separated by valves.
- Regular contraction (systole) and relaxation (diastole) occurs in the heart, resulting in a one-way flow of blood.
- Due to the sudden closure of the bicuspid and tricuspid valves, the heart makes a 'lubb' sound. Due to the sudden closure of the semilunar valves the heart makes a softer 'dupp' sound.
- Blood leaves the heart in arteries. These divide into smaller arterioles which, in turn, divide into thin-walled capillaries. Venules emerge from capillaries and lead into veins which take blood back to the heart.
- Friction between blood and the walls of the blood vessels causes a drop in blood pressure as it flows from the heart. The greatest pressure drop in the circulatory system occurs in the arterioles.
- Humans have a double circulation. For each circuit of the body a red blood cell makes, it will pass through the heart twice.
- A pulse is the outward and inward movement of an artery close to the surface of the body.
- Return of blood to the heart is helped by gravity, contraction of skeletal muscle around the veins and by the pressure in the chest during breathing.
- Tissue fluid is forced out of the capillaries and bathes the cells that they supply.
- Lymph is formed from excess tissue fluid. It carries a lot of lipid and white blood cells.
- Coronary heart disease concerns disorders of the coronary blood vessels, e.g. atherosclerosis.

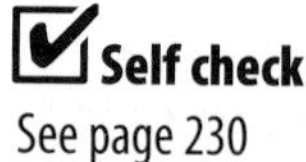

See page 230

CHAPTER 5

Cell respiration and gas exchange

In this chapter you will learn about the processes of aerobic and anaerobic respiration and the economic uses of these processes. You will learn the structure of the breathing system and see how it is involved in exchanging the gases involved in cell respiration. Finally, you will look at the control of breathing, the effects of exercise on the system and artificial resuscitation.

Cell respiration

Energy was defined on page 8 as the stored ability to do work. Cells in our bodies do work when, for example, muscle cells contract or nerve cells pass impulses. The energy to do this work comes from one energy store present in all cells, i.e. adenosine triphosphate (**ATP**). This releases its energy when it breaks down:

adenosine triphosphate (ATP) → adenosine diphosphate (ADP) + phosphate (P) + energy

If they are to continue to do work, and therefore to stay alive, all cells must have a supply of ATP in their cells. Cell respiration is the process by which this ATP is made. It involves:

- the breakdown of food (mainly glucose and lipid) to release the energy stored in their molecules
- some of this energy being used to rebuild ATP from ADP and phosphate: adenosine diphosphate + phosphate + energy from food → ATP
- the rest of the energy being lost from cells as heat.

Q1: What would happen to a cell if it had no store of ATP?

There are two types of respiration: **aerobic respiration** and **anaerobic respiration.**

Aerobic respiration

In this process the breakdown of food involves the use of oxygen. Carbon dioxide and water are always produced as waste-products and energy to rebuild ATP is released. The most commonly used food (and the only one that cells in our brains can use) is glucose. Aerobic respiration of glucose can be represented by the chemical equation:

glucose + oxygen → carbon dioxide + water + energy

Aerobic respiration occurs inside the mitochondria of our cells (page 2) and releases a great deal of energy (enough to rebuild up to 38 molecules of ATP).

Anaerobic respiration

In this process the breakdown of food does not involve oxygen. Instead of carbon dioxide and water, other waste-products are produced:

- in bacteria and in animals (including humans), lactate is produced as a waste-product (glucose → lactate + energy)
- in fungi and in plants, ethanol and carbon dioxide are produced as waste-products (glucose → ethanol + carbon dioxide + energy).

Anaerobic respiration occurs in the cytoplasm of cells (i.e. not inside mitochondria) and releases much less energy than aerobic respiration.

Q2: Copy out Table 5.1 below and, using the information given above, fill in the blanks.

Oxygen debt

Humans must respire aerobically: without oxygen we die. However, during vigorous exercise, oxygen cannot be delivered to active muscle cells quickly enough so that some respire anaerobically. Lactate is produced as a waste-product and builds up in the muscle cells that are short of oxygen, leading to muscle fatigue and soreness.

When exercise stops the lactate is removed in two stages:

- **Stage 1**: oxygen is used to convert about 20% of the lactate into carbon dioxide, water and energy
- **Stage 2**: the energy released from lactate in Stage 1 is used to convert the remaining lactate into glycogen (page 55) which can be stored in cells in the muscle or in the liver.

The oxygen needed in Stage 1 is referred to as the **oxygen debt**. Once all the lactate has been removed, the oxygen debt has been repaid.

Economic uses of cell respiration

Yeast is a single-celled fungus (page 147) that can respire both aerobically and anaerobically. Even when there is plenty of oxygen, yeast cells break down glucose anaerobically to form ethanol and carbon dioxide. Only when its glucose supply is nearly used up will the yeast use oxygen to break down the ethanol and produce carbon dioxide and water by aerobic respiration. For centuries humans have exploited this behaviour of yeast in brewing and bread-making.

Brewing

The production of beer and wine are major, world-wide industries. When yeast is used to ferment the sugars from germinating grain, ales and beers are formed. When yeast is used to ferment the sugars in fruit (usually grapes), wines are formed. At the end of both processes, the spent yeast can be eaten since it is a rich source of vitamins (especially B-group vitamins).

Table 5.1 Comparison of aerobic and anaerobic respiration

		Type of respiration	
		Aerobic	Anaerobic
1	Is oxygen required?		
2	How much energy is produced?		
3	What are the waste-products?		
4	Where does it occur in the cell?		

Q3: Alcohol abuse can cause serious problems to people. List any three problems that heavy drinkers may encounter. If you have trouble with this question refer to Chapter 14.

Bread-making

By mixing flour, water, sugar and yeast a dough is produced. Gentle warming will allow the yeast to break down the sugar, producing ethanol and carbon dioxide. The carbon dioxide causes the dough to rise (increase in volume). On baking, the yeast cells are killed and the alcohol evaporates (see also Chapter 20).

Structure of the respiratory (breathing) system

For cell respiration to occur efficiently it is essential to get adequate supplies of oxygen to the cells and remove the carbon dioxide they produce. This is called **gas exchange** and occurs through permeable gas-exchange surfaces. In humans, the gas-exchange surface is the lining of our lungs and respiratory gases are carried between respiring cells and our gas-exchange surface in our blood. The lungs are part of a respiratory (breathing) system which ensures that fresh, oxygen-rich air is brought into our lungs and stale air, rich in carbon dioxide, is removed from our lungs.

The terms respiration and breathing are often confused. You should remember that:

- respiration is the process occurring inside cells whereby food molecules such as glucose are broken down and the stored energy they release is used to build up ATP
- breathing is drawing air into, and expelling it from, the lungs using muscles in the diaphragm and between the ribs (intercostal muscles).

Figures 5.1 and 5.2 show the structures inside a human head and thorax (chest) that are involved in breathing. Use these figures and Table 5.2 to learn the names and functions of these structures.

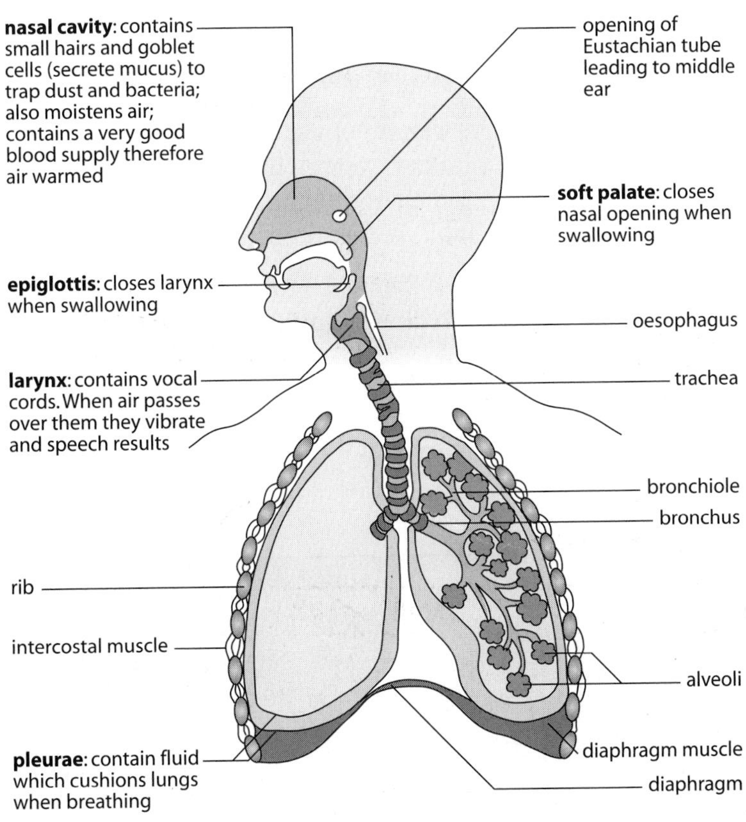
nasal cavity: contains small hairs and goblet cells (secrete mucus) to trap dust and bacteria; also moistens air; contains a very good blood supply therefore air warmed
opening of Eustachian tube leading to middle ear
soft palate: closes nasal opening when swallowing
epiglottis: closes larynx when swallowing
oesophagus
larynx: contains vocal cords. When air passes over them they vibrate and speech results
trachea
bronchiole
bronchus
rib
intercostal muscle
alveoli
pleurae: contain fluid which cushions lungs when breathing
diaphragm muscle
diaphragm

Figure 5.1 Section through the head and thorax showing the breathing system.

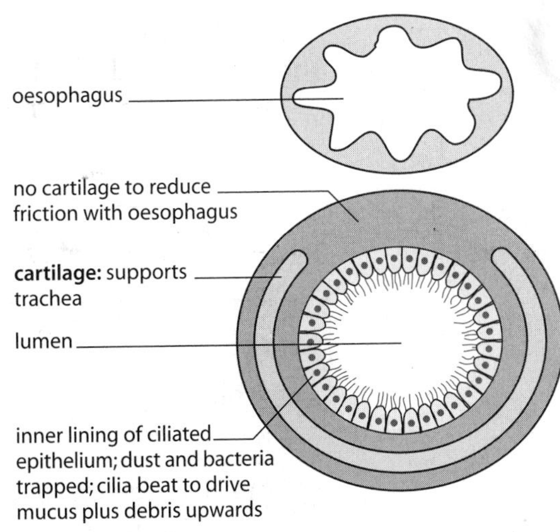
oesophagus
no cartilage to reduce friction with oesophagus
cartilage: supports trachea
lumen
inner lining of ciliated epithelium; dust and bacteria trapped; cilia beat to drive mucus plus debris upwards

Figure 5.2 Transverse section through the trachea and oesophagus.

Table 5.2 Structure and functions of the human breathing system

Name of part	Structure	Function(s)
Larynx	Top of the trachea. Contains vocal cords	Vocal cords vibrate and produce sound
Trachea	A tube stiffened by C-shaped rings of cartilage	Carries air in and out of lungs. Cartilage holds the tube open. C-shaped ring allows the oesophagus behind it to expand when it carries food (Figure 5.2)
Bronchi	Two branches of the trachea	Carry air in and out of each lung
Bronchioles	Very thin tubes branching from each bronchus. Only larger bronchioles contain cartilage	Carry air to and from the alveoli
Alveoli	Blind-ended air sacs. Their walls are one cell thick and are surrounded by blood capillaries	Gas exchange occurs here

Gas exchange

During this process oxygen diffuses from the air in the alveolus into the blood capillaries around the alveolus and carbon dioxide diffuses in the opposite direction. Figure 5.3 summarises the steps in this process and Figure 5.4 shows a photomicrograph of lung tissue.

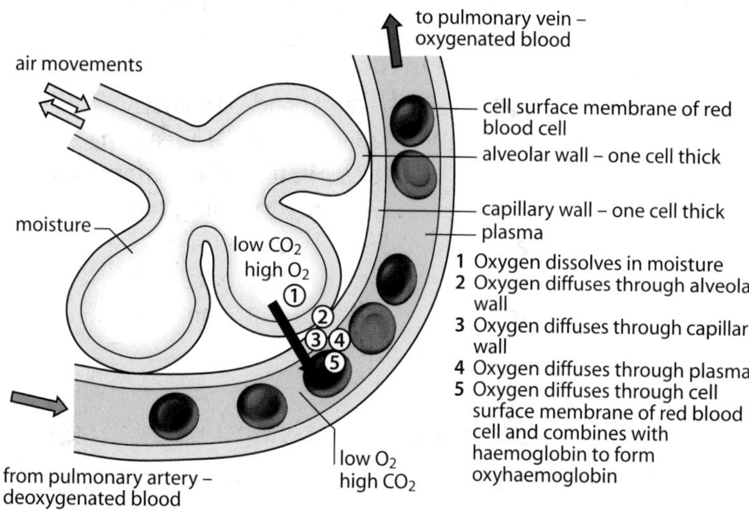

Figure 5.3 Gaseous exchange.

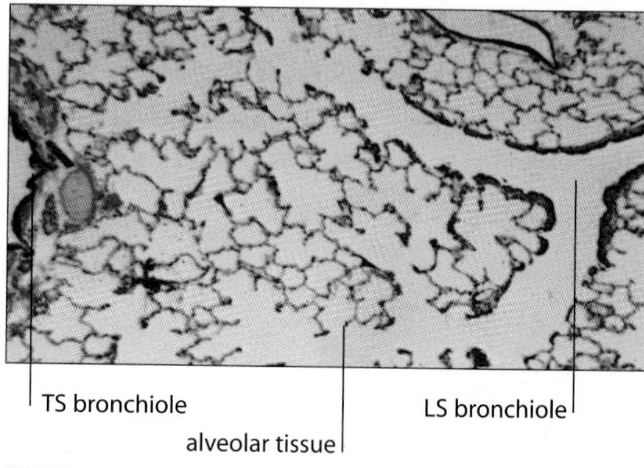

Figure 5.4 Photomicrograph of lung tissue showing alveolar tissue and a transverse section through a bronchiole.

As a result of its treatment in the respiratory system, the composition of expired air is different from that of inspired air. Table 5.3 shows these differences.

Q4: Use Figure 5.3 to list the route of carbon dioxide during gas exchange.

Q5: Use Figures 5.3 and 5.4 to list three ways in which alveoli are well adapted for gas exchange.

Table 5.3 Comparison of inspired and expired air

Component	Inspired air	Expired air
Oxygen	21%	16%
Carbon dioxide	0.04%	4%
Nitrogen	79%	79%
Water vapour	Variable	Saturated
Temperature	Variable	Warm
Purity	Variable	Most dust particles removed

Mechanism of breathing

Exchange of gases will only continue efficiently if the air inside the alveoli is replaced. This is what our breathing mechanism does.

Movement of air during breathing depends on the fact that air will move from a high pressure region to a low pressure region.

- Air is breathed in (**inspiration**) when we expand our chest. This makes the pressure inside our chest less than atmospheric pressure so that air is pushed by the higher pressure into our lungs.
- Air is breathed out (**expiration**) when we contract our chests. This makes the pressure inside our chests greater than atmospheric pressure so that air is pushed by the higher pressure from our lungs.

Two main ways are used to expand and contract our chest:

- diaphragm muscles are used to move the diaphragm up or down (Figure 5.5)
- intercostal muscles are used to move the ribs up and down (Figure 5.6).

NB: The diaphragm muscles and intercostal muscles are used together but, for ease of explanation, have been treated separately in Figure 5.5 and Figure 5.6. In both cases, when positions **a** are retained, volume *decreases* and pressure *increases*. Air is forced out of the lungs, helped also by the natural elasticity of the lung tissue.

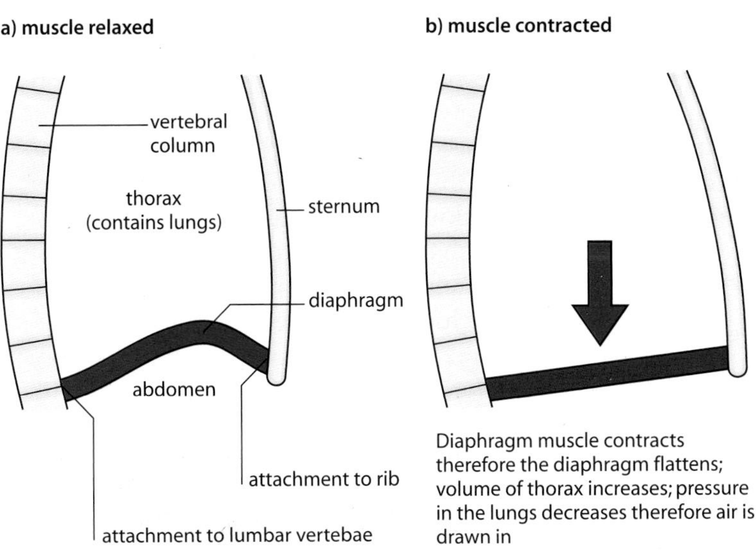

Figure 5.5 Breathing mechanisms (diaphragm).

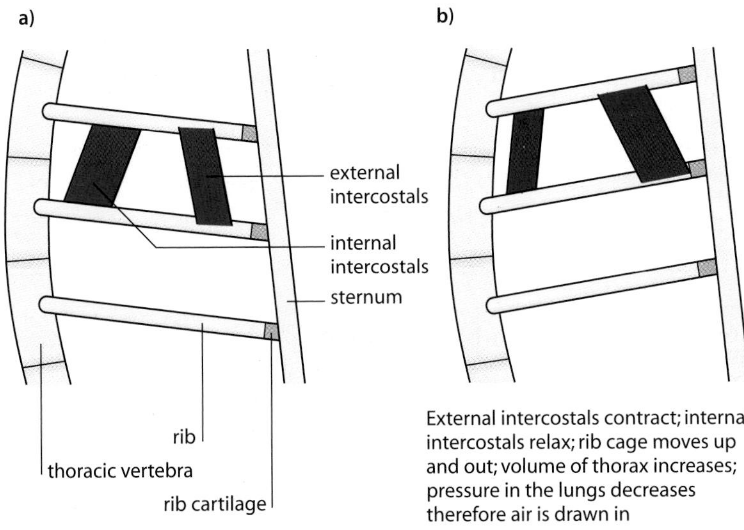

Figure 5.6 Breathing mechanisms (intercostal muscles and rib cage).

Q6: The diaphragm and intercostal muscles are used for gentle breathing. During forced expiration, the abdominal muscles also contract pushing the abdominal organs up against the diaphragm. As a result, what will happen to: (a) the volume of the thorax? (b) the pressure in the lungs?

Effects of exercise on breathing

The short term effects of exercise are:

- an increase in breathing rate
- an increase in the depth of breathing
- an increase in the amount of carbon dioxide in expired air.

The long-term effects of regular exercise include:

- an increase in the number of capillaries in the lungs
- an expansion of the alveoli
- the intercostal muscles and diaphragm muscles become larger and stronger.

Control of breathing rate

Figure 5.7 illustrates control of breathing by the nervous system. Within the medulla of the brain is a respiratory centre. You are never aware of this centre but it controls the rate of breathing by sending impulses to the intercostal muscles and diaphragm muscles. The respiratory centre in the medulla responds to:

- conscious thought
- a reflex
- carbon dioxide levels in the blood (Figure 5.8).

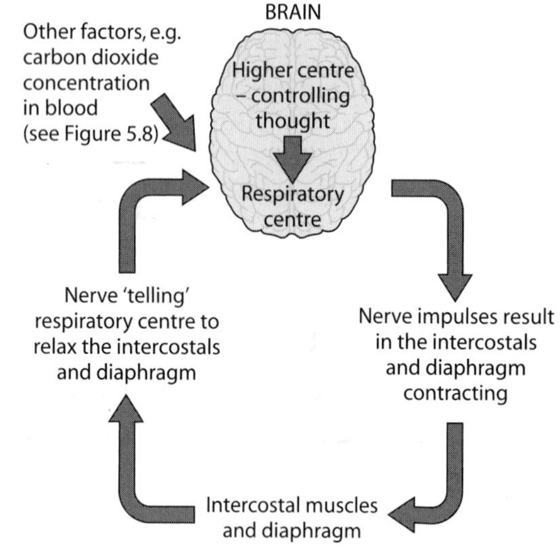

Figure 5.7 Control of breathing by the respiratory centre in the medulla.

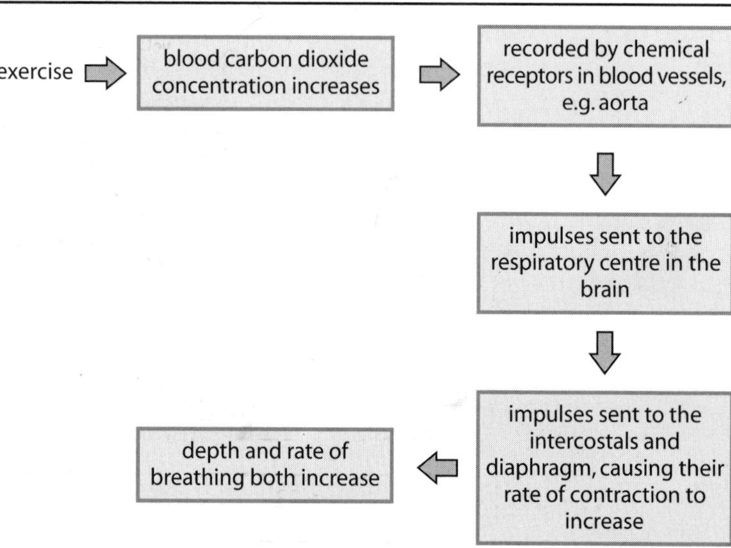

Figure 5.8 The effect on the breathing rate of carbon dioxide concentration in the blood.

Artificial resuscitation (respiration)

Sometimes a person who has had an accident stops breathing. This slows gas exchange in the lungs. To prevent damage to organs, especially the brain which is very sensitive to lack of oxygen for its own respiration, efficient gaseous exchange must begin within a few minutes.

During artificial resuscitation air is moved into, and out of, the lungs of the injured person, substituting for their own breathing movements. It should be continued until the person begins to breathe for themselves again or until aid from a breathing machine is available. The most commonly used method is **mouth-to-mouth resuscitation** (also called 'the kiss of life'). To perform mouth-to-mouth resuscitation successfully you should:

- place the injured person in the position shown in Figure 5.9
- place one hand under the neck and one on the forehead and gently tilt the head backwards to open the air passageway
- push the chin up to lift the tongue and search for and remove any debris (including false teeth) in the mouth
- pinch the nostrils of the injured person, take a deep breath, seal the mouth with your lips and breathe out deeply
- repeat four times
- check that the chest of the injured person is rising and falling indicating that normal breathing has begun again
- if not, continue until the injured person resumes normal breathing or until qualified medical help arrives.

NB: It is essential that an ambulance and medical help are requested.

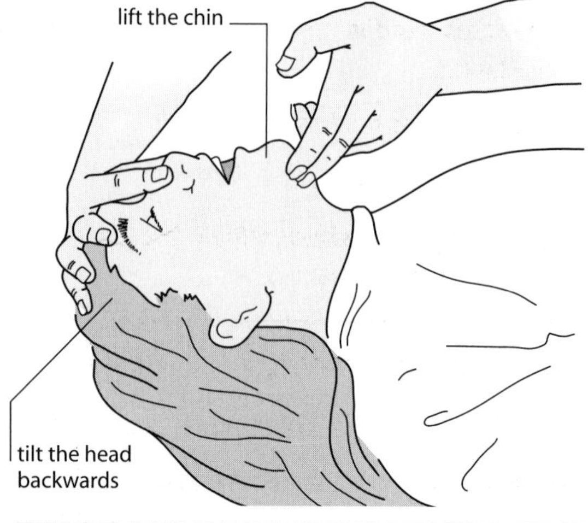

Figure 5.9 Artificial resuscitation.

Practical 5.1 To determine whether expired air contains more carbon dioxide than inspired air

Requirements
- Glass tubing through two bungs
- Two conical flasks
- Lime water
- Dilute solution of disinfectant

1 Set up the apparatus as shown in Figure 5.10.

2 Close tap 2 and open tap 1. With the mouth over tube X (which has been sterilised with disinfectant solution), breathe in several times.

3 Close tap 1 and open tap 2. With the mouth over tube X, breathe out several times.

4 Observe flasks A and B as you breathe.

5 Lime water turns milky when carbon dioxide is passed into it.

6 In which flask, A or B, does the lime water turn milky?

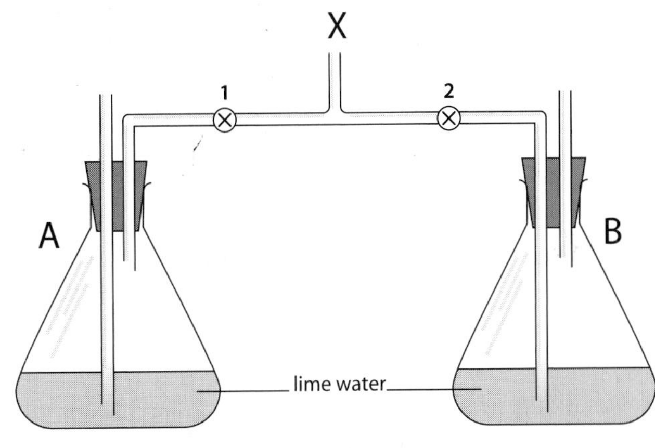

Figure 5.10 Apparatus for Practical 5.1.

Practical 5.2 To determine whether expired air contains more water than inspired air

Requirements
- Two pieces of blue cobalt chloride paper

1 Take two pieces of blue cobalt chloride paper.

2 Leave one in the air untouched.

3 Breathe onto the other.

4 The paper should turn pink more quickly with expired air.

Practical 5.3 To measure tidal volume and vital capacity

Requirements
- Bell jar marked in dm^3
- Trough
- Three wedges
- Tubing
- Dilute solution of disinfectant

1 Set up the apparatus as seen in Figure 5.11, ensuring that the bell jar is full of water.

2 Record the initial volume.

3 Take a deep breath in then breathe out fully down the sterilised mouthpiece.

4 Measure the drop in volume in the bell jar.

5 This is the vital capacity in dm^3.

6 By repeating the experiment, only this time exhaling normally, the tidal volume can be measured.

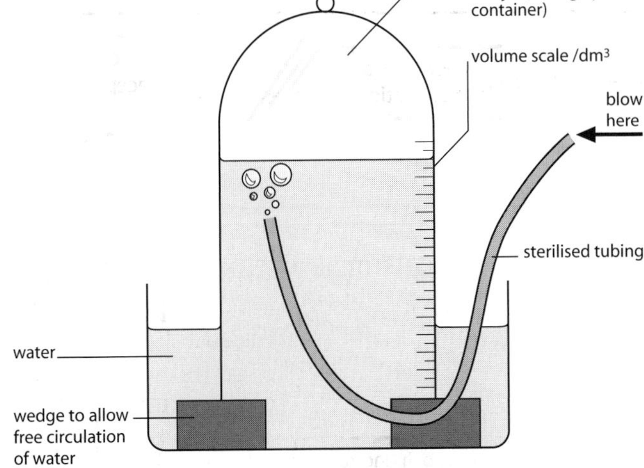

Figure 5.11 Apparatus for Practical 5.3

Practical 5.4 To measure lung volumes using a spirometer

SAFETY: This should only be demonstrated by a competent person.

Requirements
- Spirometer
- Instruction manual
- Fresh soda lime
- Dilute solution of disinfectant
- Chart recorder

1 Set up the apparatus using the instruction manual which will come with the apparatus. Figure 5.12 illustrates a conventional spirometer.

2 Following instructions in the manual, use the apparatus to answer the following questions.

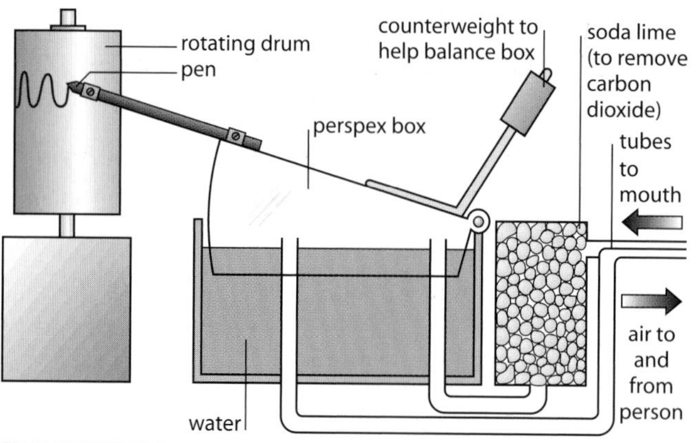

Figure 5.12 Plan of spirometer.

3 What will happen to the volume of air in the box when you: (a) breathe in? (b) breathe out?

4 (a) What will happen to the total volume of air in the box as you breathe in and out five times? (b) Explain your answer.

Using a chart recorder, the movements of the bell can be recorded to give a spirometer trace (Figure 5.13).

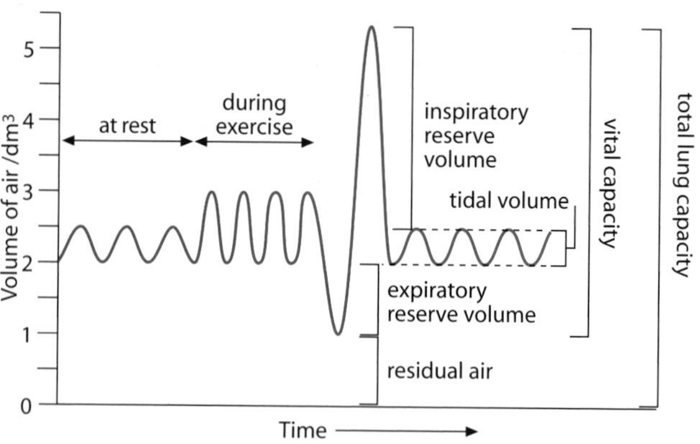

Figure 5.13 Spirometer trace.

5 Using Figure 5.13 and Table 5.4, work out volumes for the following: (a) tidal volume (at rest); (b) inspiratory reserve volume; (c) expiratory reserve volume; (d) vital capacity; (e) total lung capacity; (f) residual (reserve) volume.

6 What will happen to the inspiratory reserve volume during exercise?

7 Why will there always be a residual volume?

Table 5.4 Terms used to describe lung volume

Lung volume	Definition
Tidal volume	Volume breathed in or out in one cycle
Total lung capacity	Maximum volume of air in the lungs
Residual (reserve) volume	Volume of air in the lungs after forced expiration
Vital capacity	Maximum volume of air forced out after the deepest inspiration
Inspiratory reserve volume	Extra volume of air that can be inspired above the tidal volume
Expiratory reserve volume	Extra volume of air that can be expired above the tidal volume
Dead space	Volume of air in the trachea or bronchi that is expelled without reaching the alveoli

Practical 5.5 To determine whether there is more oxygen in inspired than expired air

Requirements
- Two gas jars
- Tubing
- Two covers
- Dilute solution of disinfectant
- Two candles
- Matches

1 Collect a sample of expired air in a gas jar using Figure 5.14.

2 Place a cover over the end of the gas jar and remove it from the water.

3 Remove the cover and quickly invert the gas jar over a lighted candle.

4 Time how long the candle takes to go out.

5 Repeat with a gas jar of atmospheric air.

6 In which air, atmospheric or expired, did the candle burn for the shorter time? What does this indicate?

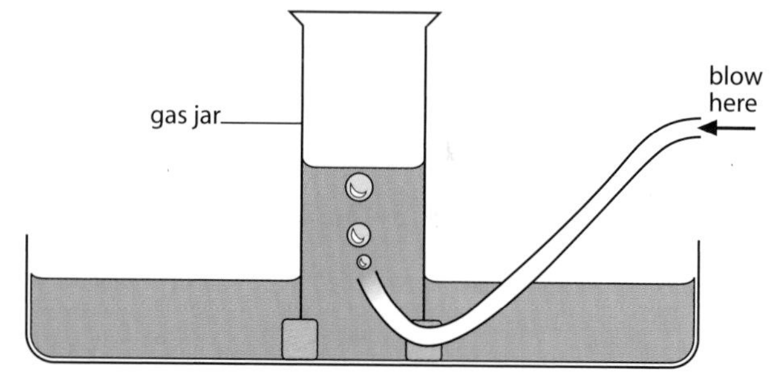

Figure 5.14 Apparatus for Practical 5.5.

Summary

- Respiration is the release of energy when food (especially glucose and lipid) is broken down, and the use of this energy to make adenosine triphosphate (ATP).
- In aerobic respiration oxygen is used. The waste-products are carbon dioxide and water.
- In anaerobic respiration oxygen is not used. In bacteria and in animals, lactate is produced as the sole waste-product. In fungi and in plants, the waste-products are ethanol and carbon dioxide.
- The oxygen debt is the amount of oxygen needed to get rid of the lactate produced during vigorous exercise in humans. When the lactate has been removed, the oxygen debt has been repaid.
- Respiration in yeast cells is exploited commercially in brewing and in bread-making.
- Breathing draws fresh air into the lungs and expels stale air from the lungs.
- The breathing system consists of the nose, larynx, trachea, bronchi, bronchioles and alveoli.
- C-shaped rings of cartilage support the trachea yet allow expansion of the oesophagus when swallowing.
- Gas exchange is the transfer of gases between the alveoli and the blood.
- Characteristics of the respiratory surface are: thin-walled; good blood system; large surface area.
- Breathing mechanisms involve the intercostal muscles, the rib cage and the diaphragm muscles.
- Inspired air differs from expired air in oxygen content, carbon dioxide content, amount of water vapour, temperature and purity.
- During exercise the breathing rate increases, the depth of breathing increases and the amount of carbon dioxide in expired air increases.
- Artificial resuscitation is used to restore a person's breathing.
- Control of the breathing rate is by conscious thought, by a reflex and due to the carbon dioxide levels in the blood.
- A spirometer is a piece of apparatus used to measure lung volumes, e.g. tidal volume, vital capacity, by the production of a spirometer trace.

Self check

See page 231

CHAPTER 6

Excretion and osmoregulation

In this chapter you will learn how the kidneys help to keep the chemical composition of our blood constant. You will also learn how the kidneys work and how they can be regulated by hormone action.

Major sources of metabolic waste

Before looking at the work of the kidneys, you need to be familiar with two important definitions.

- **Metabolism**: Thousands of chemical reactions going on in our cells keep us alive. Together, these reactions make up our **metabolism**. They are also sometimes called metabolic reactions.
- **Excretion**: Many metabolic reactions produce waste products that are not useful to us. In fact, they can be toxic if allowed to become concentrated in the body. The removal of these waste-products from our bodies is called **excretion**.

Table 6.1 summarises the major sources of metabolic waste and shows how each is excreted.

Table 6.1 Summary of human excretory processes

Metabolic waste	Source of waste	How waste is excreted
Carbon dioxide	Aerobic respiration	Removed from the blood in the alveoli and breathed out of the lungs during expiration
Mineral salts	Absorbed from food in excess of needs	Removed from the blood in sweat glands and deposited on the surface of the skin. Removed from the blood by the kidneys and incorporated in urine
Water	Absorbed from food in excess of needs; produced by some metabolic reactions	Breathed out of lungs during expiration. Removed from the blood in sweat glands and evaporated in sweat. Removed from the blood by the kidneys and incorporated in urine
Urea	Breakdown of surplus amino acids in the liver (deamination)	Small amount removed from the blood in sweat glands and deposited on the surface of skin. Most removed from the blood by the kidneys and incorporated in urine
Blood pigments	Breakdown of haemoglobin from old red blood cells in the liver	Released into the gut as part of bile

Q1: Is the removal of faeces from our gut an example of excretion? Explain your answer.

Many of the methods of excretion described in Table 6.1 are described elsewhere in this book. The removal of carbon dioxide from the body is described in Chapter 5, the release of bile is described in Chapter 3 and sweat formation is described in Chapter 7. In the remainder of this chapter we will concentrate on the production of urine by the kidneys.

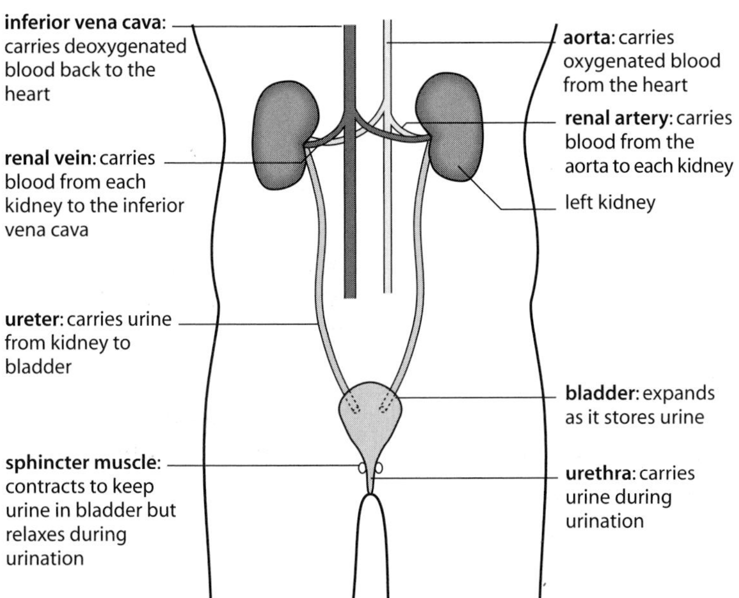

Figure 6.1 The human urinary system.

The urinary system

The kidneys are paired organs which form part of the urinary system.

Figure 6.1 shows the other structures in the urinary system and their relation to the kidneys.

In the kidneys, all small molecules are removed from the blood. Most are then returned to the blood before it leaves the kidneys. However, any that are not needed or are surplus to the body's needs become part of a fluid called **urine**. The urine passes from the kidneys to the bladder where it is stored. When the bladder is full, the urine is passed out of the body during **urination**.

Kidney functions

The functions of the kidneys are summarised in Table 6.2 below. Note that the kidneys have functions other than excretion. You only need to be familiar with the first two functions described.

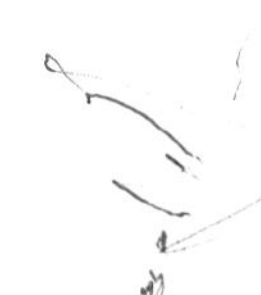

Kidney structure

If you buy a lamb's kidney from a supermarket and slice it in two at home, you will see that it looks like Figure 6.2 on page 48. The outside layer is called the **cortex**. It has a dark red colour because it is full of blood vessels. The inner **medulla** is pink because it has fewer blood vessels than the cortex. Urine flows down small tubes in the pyramids into a region at the top of the ureter called the **pelvis**.

Table 6.2 Summary of kidney functions

Function	How achieved
Excretion	Urea (and certain other waste substances) are removed from the blood and incorporated into urine
Controls the osmotic potential (concentration of dissolved substances) of the blood (osmoregulation)	Surplus water is removed from the blood and incorporated into urine
Controls the pH of blood	Surplus hydrogen ions are neutralised or removed from the blood and incorporated into urine
Endocrine organ	Releases hormones that increase blood pressure to the kidney. Also affects production of red blood cells

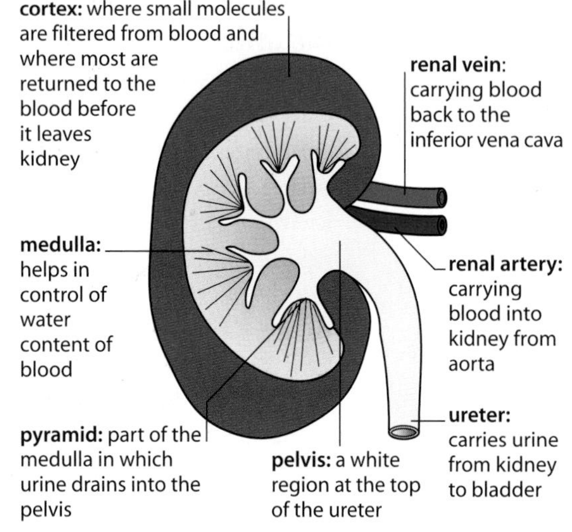

Figure 6.2 Vertical section through a kidney.

afferent blood vessel
efferent blood vessel
glomerulus
Bowman's capsule
first coiled tubule
second coiled tubule
second coiled tubule from another nephron
collecting duct
loop of Henlé
pyramid
pelvis

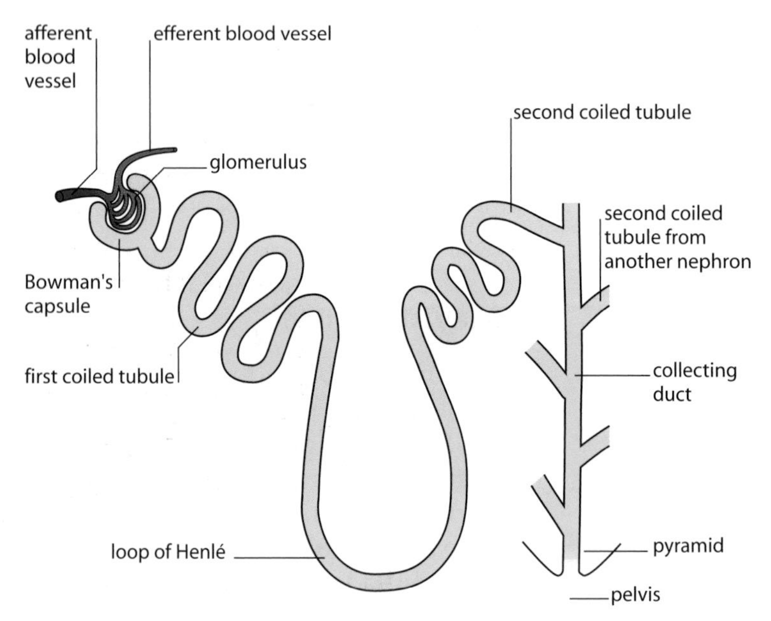

Figure 6.3 A single kidney tubule (nephron).

Kidney tubules (nephrons)

Each kidney contains about one million microscopic tubules called nephrons. It is in these nephrons that blood is filtered and urine is formed.

Figure 6.3 shows the structure of an individual nephron. It is composed of a long tube, with two coiled regions. In between the two coiled parts is a long loop, the **loop of Henlé**. One end of the nephron is blind and has a cup-like shape, the **Bowman's capsule**, enclosing a knot of blood capillaries called the **glomerulus**. The other end leads into a larger tube, called the **collecting duct**, which passes down into the **pyramid**.

If you examine a prepared slide of a section through a kidney under a microscope you are unlikely to see the whole of one nephron as clearly as this. Can you explain why?

Q2: Using Figures 6.1 and 6.3 list, in their correct sequence, the parts of the urinary system through which urine passes following its production in the tubule.

Figure 6.4 shows the position of the nephrons inside a kidney. Remember when you look at Figure 6.4 that each kidney has about one million nephrons inside it. Figure 6.5 is a photomicrograph of a section through the cortex. You can clearly see a cross section through a Bowman's capsule.

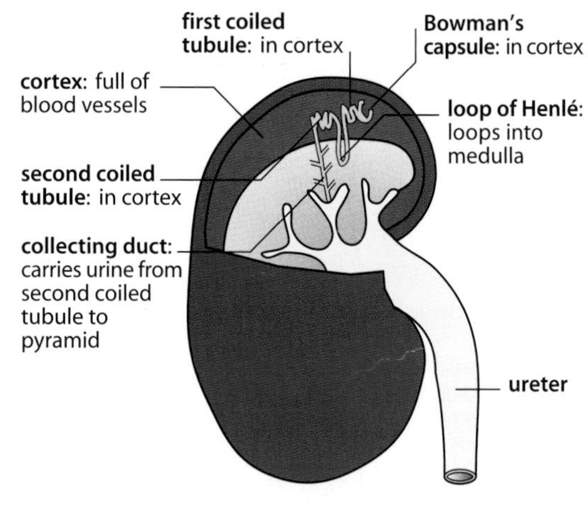

Figure 6.4 Partial vertical section through a kidney showing the position of the nephrons.

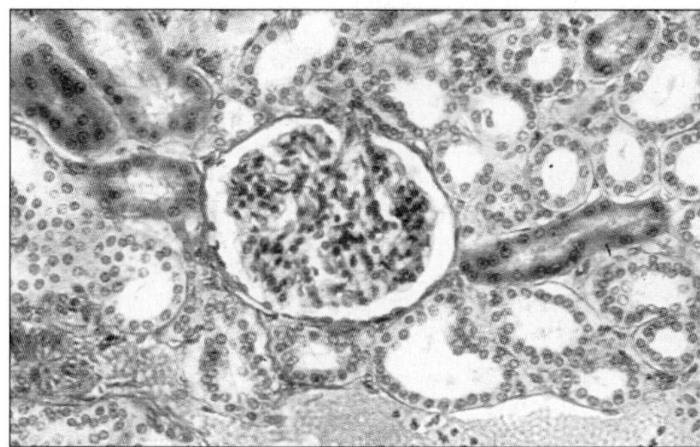

Figure 6.5 Photomicrograph of a Bowman's capsule and glomerulus.

Q3: Using Figure 6.4, explain why the cortex of the kidney is much darker in colour than the medulla.

Two main processes take place in the nephrons:

- **ultrafiltration** of blood plasma from the glomerulus into the Bowman's capsule
- **selective reabsorption** from the nephrons back into the blood capillaries around them.

Ultrafiltration

Filtration is a process which separates particles of different sizes. The term **ultrafiltration** is used when the particles being separated are very small, i.e. molecules or ions.

Figure 6.6 shows how ultrafiltration occurs. Blood in the glomerulus is under high pressure. This comes about because the blood vessel entering the glomerulus has a larger internal diameter than the vessel leaving the glomerulus, creating a build-up of pressure in the glomerular capillaries. Like all capillaries, the walls of those in the glomerulus possess small pores (holes). The membrane lining the inner surface of the Bowman's capsule also has small pores. The pressure inside the glomerular capillaries forces substances that are small enough to get through these pores from the blood into the Bowman's capsule. This movement of molecules is shown by the green arrows in Figure 6.6.

The mixture of small molecules which forms inside the Bowman's capsule is called the **ultrafiltrate**. It normally contains mainly water with dissolved amino acids, glucose, mineral salts and urea. Red blood cells and large molecules, such as proteins, remain in the blood.

Q4: Explain why red blood cells and blood proteins will not normally be part of the ultrafiltrate.

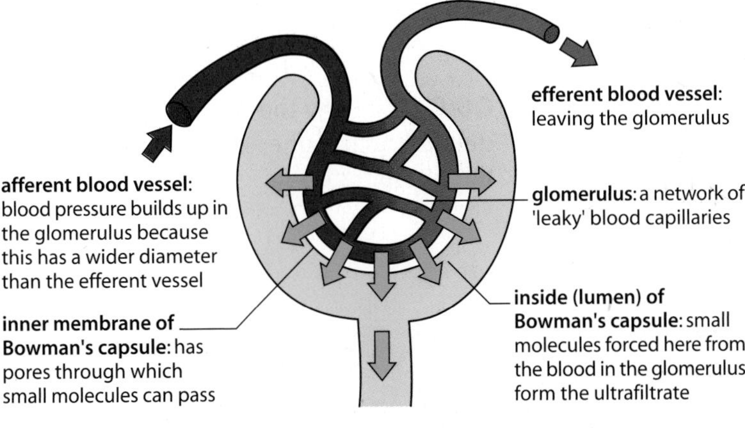

Figure 6.6 Ultrafiltration in the glomerulus and Bowman's capsule.

Selective reabsorption

Look back at Figure 6.3. All substances that are in the ultrafiltrate in the Bowman's capsule could eventually pass right through the nephron and into the collecting ducts leading to the pelvis. This does not happen because most are **reabsorbed** into blood capillaries from various parts of the nephron.

First coiled tubule

Figure 6.7 shows how the efferent blood vessel from the glomerulus forms a second capillary network around the first coiled tubule. The cells lining this part of the tubule absorb substances from the ultrafiltrate and pass them back into the bloodstream. Figure 6.7 also shows the proportion of different molecules that are normally reabsorbed from the ultrafiltrate in this way. Table 6.3 shows how the kidney is adapted to help this reabsorption process.

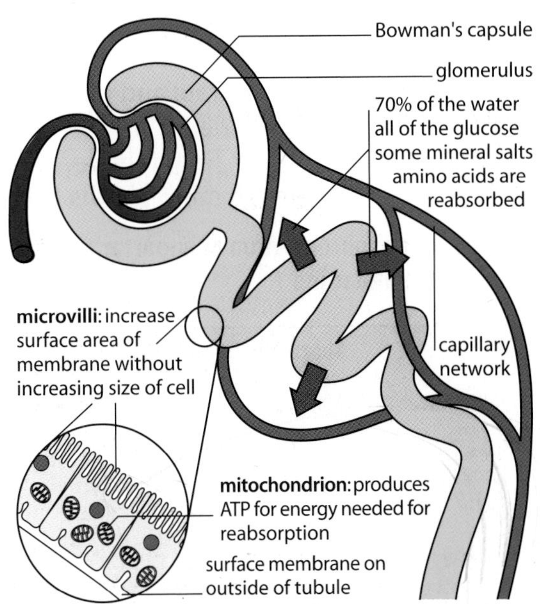

Figure 6.7 The upper part of a single nephron with a high-power view of a cell lining the first coiled tubule.

Table 6.3 How the kidneys are adapted for reabsorbtion

Feature	Explanation of how this helps reabsorption
Tubules are long	Increases surface area for reabsorption
Tubules are coiled	Allows tubules to be long but contained within a small space
Each kidney has over a million tubules	Increases surface area for reabsorption
Cells lining the tubule have microvilli on their inner surface membrane	Increases the surface area of each cell lining the tubule without increasing its overall size
Cells lining the tubule have many mitochondria in their cytoplasm	Mitochondria produce ATP which is a source of energy for the reabsorption process

Q5: Reabsorption does not occur by diffusion alone. Knowing that diffusion is a passive process (page 8), explain why other processes must be involved.

Loop of Henlé

The loop of Henlé works in a complicated way to increase the salt content of the tissues in the medulla. This helps in the reabsorption of water from the ultrafiltrate in the second coiled tubules and collecting ducts. You are not expected to be familiar with the complex processes involved.

Second coiled tubule and collecting duct

The second coiled tubule and collecting duct are also surrounded by a network of capillaries. The cells lining these parts of the tubule can absorb materials from the ultrafiltrate and pass them into the blood capillaries.

Cells lining the second coiled tubule absorb mineral salts from the ultrafiltrate and pass them back into the capillary. However, the major function of the second coiled tubule and collecting duct is to reabsorb water. The amount of water reabsorbed by both depends on the amount of water in the blood. If the blood is very dilute, e.g. after drinking large amounts of fluids, less is reabsorbed from the ultrafiltrate, resulting in a greater quantity of dilute urine. If the blood is too concentrated, e.g. after excessive sweating or eating large amounts of salty food, more water is reabsorbed, resulting in a lesser quantity of more concentrated urine.

Figure 6.8 shows a summary of reabsorption along the whole length of a nephron. Notice that urea has not been reabsorbed from the ultrafiltrate. Table 6.4 illustrates another way of summarising the events that occur in the nephrons. It compares the composition of blood plasma, ultrafiltrate and urine. By studying the table and thinking about what has happened as the ultrafiltrate passes along the nephron, you should be able to explain the different concentrations of each substance in the three fluids.

Table 6.4 The concentration of important substances in plasma, ultrafiltrate and urine

	Approximate concentration in g per dm^3		
Substance	**Plasma**	**Ultrafiltrate**	**Urine**
Urea	0.03	0.03	3.00
Water	91.00	99.00	96.00 (variable)
Glucose	0.10	0.10	0.00
Mineral salts	0.40	0.70	1.20 (variable)
Protein	8.00	0.00	0.00

Q6: Explain why the concentration of urea is much higher in the urine than in the ultrafiltrate.

small molecules, e.g. water, salts, urea, glucose, amino acids **ultrafiltered**

from renal artery

some water, some salts **reabsorbed**

to renal vein

some water **reabsorbed** (under the control of ADH)

70% water, all of the glucose, some salts, some amino acids **reabsorbed**

some water **reabsorbed**

urine: mixture of urea, water and salts. Moves down pelvis, ureter, to bladder, released via urethra

Figure 6.8 Summary of ultrafiltration and selective reabsorption.

Osmoregulation

This process involves the regulation of the concentration of the body fluids through control of the water content and salt content of the blood. We need only concern ourselves here with control of the water content of the blood. If a person loses water from his blood, e.g. by excessive sweating during exercise, the following will occur:

- blood becomes more concentrated
- this is detected by the hypothalamus at the base of the brain
- **antidiuretic hormone** (**ADH**) is produced by the hypothalamus and released from the pituitary body
- ADH travels via the bloodstream to the kidney where it makes the cells lining the second coiled tubules and collecting ducts more permeable to water
- more water is reabsorbed from the ultrafiltrate
- less urine is formed
- blood becomes less concentrated.

Figure 6.9 below summarises these events diagrammatically. It also shows how the reverse happens when a person has drunk a lot of fluids.

Variations in urine composition

You will have realised that the composition of urine changes according to certain factors. Among these factors are:

- **diet** – a high protein diet will increase the concentration of urea in the urine due to deamination of the surplus amino acids. Excessive water intake (including water-based drinks) will result in more dilute urine. Some drugs, such as caffeine in tea, coffee and cola, or alcohol, depress ADH release causing the urine to become more dilute
- **exercise** – the more a person exercises the more concentrated their urine will be due to increased loss of fluid through sweating
- **weather** – in cold weather less sweat is produced, so the urine is more dilute. In hot weather the reverse happens.

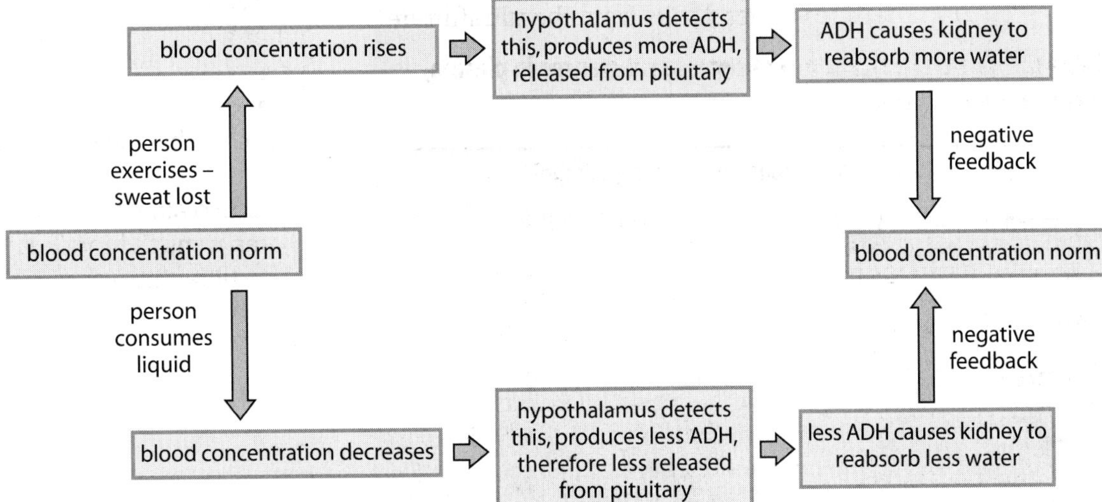

Figure 6.9 Summary of osmoregulation.

Kidneys and health

Kidney failure

If for some reason the nephrons cease to function properly, a person is no longer able to control the volume or composition of the blood. If steps are not taken to correct or compensate for the malfunction, death is the likely outcome. Kidney failure can be treated in one of two ways:

- dialysis using an artificial kidney (kidney machine)
- a kidney transplant.

Dialysis

Figure 6.10 shows a patient on a kidney machine. Notice that tubes run between her forearm and the machine. One tube is attached to a fine tube (**catheter**) inserted into an artery in her arm and the second to a catheter inserted in a vein. In this way, blood flows from her artery through the kidney machine and back into her vein.

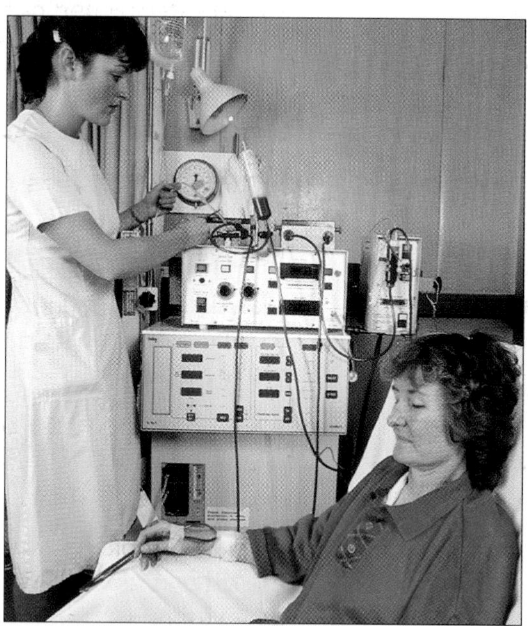

Figure 6.10 A patient undergoing dialysis.

Figure 6.11 represents part of a kidney machine. The blood from a patient is in the centre of the diagram. It is separated from the dialysis fluid by partially permeable membranes. This fluid has the same concentration of blood components as 'normal' blood. Because the blood is surrounded by partially permeable membranes:

- blood proteins and red blood cells will not leave the patient's blood
- there will be no net movement of soluble substances such as glucose because their concentration in the blood is the same as in the dialysis fluid
- any excess soluble substance in the blood, e.g. urea, will pass into the dialysis fluid by diffusion and so be removed from the blood.

Q7: Suggest why a child who depends on dialysis should not be allowed to eat salted crisps or drink cola other than during the first two hours of dialysis treatment.

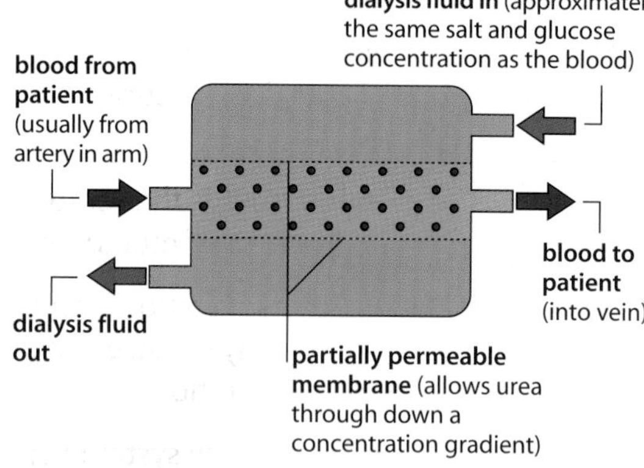

Figure 6.11 A simple representation of the inside of a kidney machine.

Kidney transplants

A transplant involves removing a healthy kidney from one person (the **donor**) and surgically inserting it into the abdomen of a person whose own kidneys do not work (the **recipient**). For skilled surgeons this is a relatively simple operation. A problem arises, however, when some white blood cells in the recipient recognise the new kidney as foreign tissue and attack it. This is called **tissue rejection**. If unchecked, the recipient's white cells will attack the cells of the transplanted kidney and destroy them, resulting in the failure of the transplanted kidney. Tissue rejection can be reduced by:

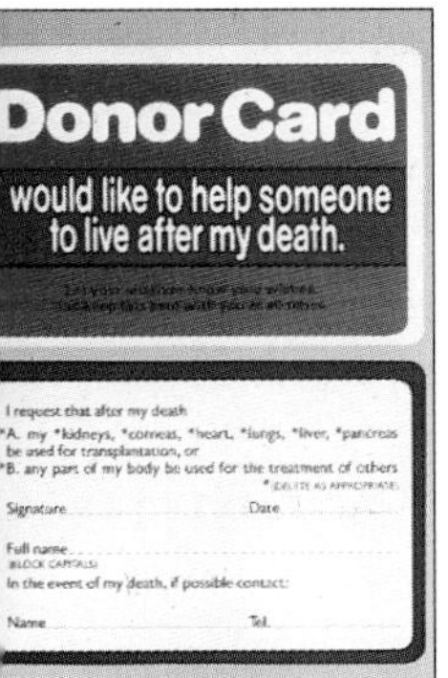

Figure 6.12 A donor card. Many people carry these to indicate that they wish their organs to be used in surgery.

- matching the tissue types of donor and recipient
- injection of immunosuppressant drugs which suppress the action of the white cells of the recipient.

Successful kidney transplants enable people suffering kidney failure to lead normal lives. Many healthy people carry donor cards like the one shown in Figure 6.12. This enables organs such as kidneys to be used fairly quickly in transplants if a card carrier suffers a fatal accident.

Diabetes insipidus

Diabetes insipidus is a disorder caused by a hormonal imbalance involving the production of ADH (antidiuretic hormone) by the hypothalamus. It makes the kidneys overactive or prevents them from reabsorbing water into the bloodstream. People suffering from this type of diabetes produce large volumes of dilute urine. It must not be confused with diabetes mellitis, where the body fails to regulate the concentration of sugar in the blood (see page 55).

Some people secrete much less ADH than is normal. If you look back to Figure 6.9 you will see how this reduces the ability of the second coiled tubules and collecting ducts to reabsorb water. Consequently, more water than normal is lost in the urine.

Q8: Explain why diabetes insipidus could be a life-threatening disorder.

Summary

- Metabolism is the name given to all of the chemical reactions going on inside our cells.
- Excretion is the removal of the waste products of metabolism.
- Osmoregulation is the maintenance of our body fluids, e.g. blood, at a constant concentration.
- The urinary system comprises the kidneys, ureters, bladder and urethra.
- In cross section, a kidney can be seen to be made up of the cortex (dark) and the inner medulla (light).
- The kidney tubule/nephron is the working unit of the kidney. It is made up of the Bowman's capsule, first coiled tubule, loop of Henlé and a second coiled tubule leading into the collecting duct.
- The glomerulus is a knot of blood capillaries surrounded by the Bowman's capsule.
- Ultrafiltration is the filtration of small particles under pressure.
- Selective reabsorption occurs in the kidney. Substances from the ultrafiltrate that are still needed by the body are reabsorbed into the blood.
- ADH (antidiuretic hormone) controls the amount of water in the blood.
- Factors affecting urine composition include diet, exercise and environmental temperature.
- Dialysis, using a kidney machine, is used to treat patients with damaged or diseased kidneys.
- A kidney transplant involves the removal of a healthy kidney from a donor and its insertion into the body of a recipient.
- Diabetes insipidus is a disorder whereby the kidneys produce large amounts of dilute urine.

Self check
See page 232

CHAPTER 7

Homeostasis

In this chapter you will learn about homeostasis and the importance of negative feedback systems. As examples of homeostasis, you will learn about the regulation of the water balance and sugar level of the blood and of the temperature of the body.

Definition of homeostasis

Homeostasis is the maintenance of a constant internal environment within the body. It includes:

- control of the water balance of the blood
- control of blood sugar level
- control of body temperature
- control of blood urea level.

Each of these internal factors is maintained by a separate mechanism that is specific for that factor. However, all the mechanisms for homeostasis share common features:

- a specific sensor is able to detect the value of the factor being monitored
- any deviation from the desired value (norm) is corrected so that the norm is more-or-less maintained
- the corrective mechanism involves negative feedback.

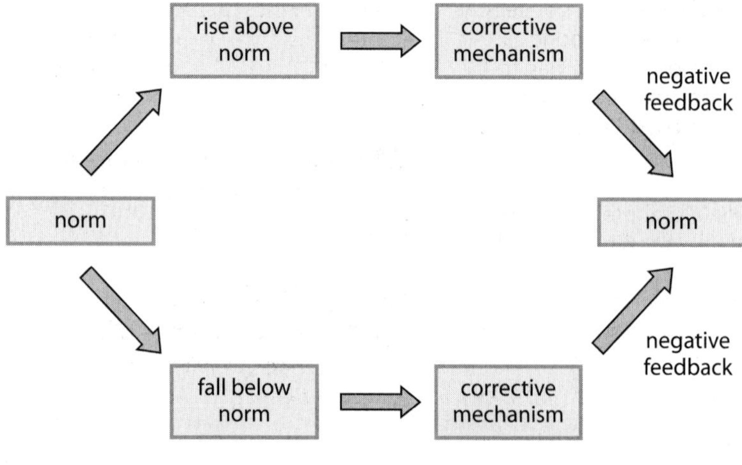

Figure 7.1 Homeostasis.

Negative feedback

This is a control mechanism in which a change from the norm triggers off a response, or responses, which allow the norm to be re-set. Look at Figure 7.1 which represents homeostasis. The top half of the diagram shows what would happen if the internal factor in question rose above its norm value. The corrective action taken by the body would cause the opposite (i.e. negative) effect to what was happening. As a result, the factor would fall back to its norm value. The bottom part of the diagram shows that if the factor fell below its norm the corrective action would again have the opposite (negative) effect, causing it to rise to its norm value.

ADH and water balance is an example of homeostasis that has already been covered in Chapter 6.

Blood sugar regulation

The sugar carried in the blood is glucose. The level of glucose in the blood is closely monitored and has a norm of approximately 80 mg per 100 cm^3 blood.

Q1: What effect would osmosis have on body cells if: (a) blood glucose levels became too high? (b) blood glucose levels became too low? Explain your answers.

Q2: If the blood sugar level dropped too low, what cellular process would be greatly reduced?

The regulation of glucose involves the pancreas and the liver (see Figure 7.2).

- In the pancreas are groups of special cells known as **Islets of Langerhans**. These cells secrete two hormones, **insulin** and **glucagon**.
- If the blood sugar level rises, e.g. after a heavy meal, these cells detect this and release *more* insulin and *less* glucagon.
- The insulin travels to the liver and 'tells' it to do a number of things:
  (i) convert glucose to glycogen (stored in the liver and muscles)
  (ii) convert glucose to fat.
- As a result, the blood sugar level falls.

Q3: (a) Using Figure 7.2 as an example, make your own flow chart to show what would happen if there were a drop in the blood sugar level; (b) Does negative feedback also occur in this case?

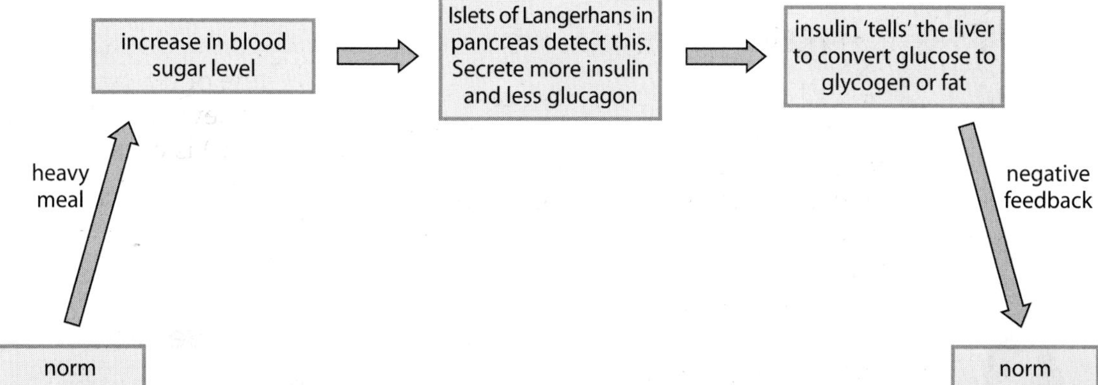

Figure 7.2 The body's response to an increase in blood sugar level.

Diabetes mellitus

Some people have such a high blood sugar level that they cannot reabsorb all of it in the kidneys. A symptom of this condition is the presence of glucose in the urine.

Q4: Describe a test you could use to show the presence of glucose in urine.

There are two forms of diabetes mellitus:

- **Juvenile-onset** (**type**) – usually found in persons under the age of 20; the production of insulin stops and daily injections of insulin are needed.
- **Mature-onset** (**type**) – usually found in persons over the age of 35; the amount of insulin produced by the pancreas is often adequate but cells in the liver no longer respond to it meaning that more insulin has to be produced to get the same effect; can usually be controlled by a low-sugar diet.

Mature-onset diabetes is often associated with obesity. Dieting to reduce weight often improves this condition.

In the past, the insulin used to treat juvenile-onset diabetes has been obtained from pigs or cattle but this can lead to side effects. Advances in genetic engineering have now enabled us to produce synthetic human insulin. For more information on this see Chapter 20.

Another possible way of treating the condition may eventually be by gene therapy in which the human insulin gene is placed inside the patient, so producing the insulin needed constantly as the body requires it.

Q5: Insulin is a protein and so cannot be given orally. Why is this?

Q6: Explain why insulin injections are not normally given to people with mature-onset diabetes.

Temperature regulation

Any significant variation in the internal temperature could have damaging effects on the body's enzymes (page 11). **Endothermic** animals (also called homoiotherms or warm-blooded animals) are able to keep their body temperature fairly constant despite changes in the temperature of the environment or despite internal fluctuations, e.g. when exercising or when a female ovulates (see Chapter 11). Humans are endotherms and maintain a constant internal (core) body temperature of about 37°C. **Ectotherms**, on the other hand, cannot control their body temperature which fluctuates according to environmental temperature variations. Reptiles and fish are examples of ectotherms.

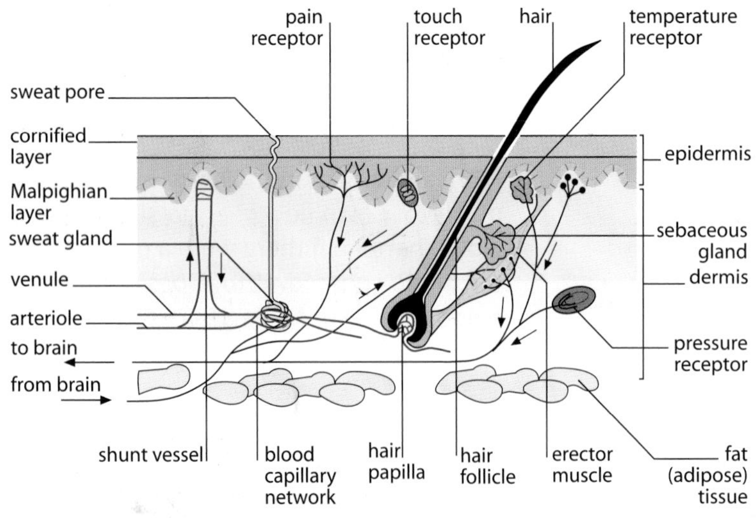

Figure 7.3 Structure of human skin.

Skin structure

The skin is an important organ in helping us to resist infection (page 130) and to avoid dehydration. It also has a major part to play in controlling our body temperatures. Figure 7.3 shows a section through the skin and illustrates its complex nature. Table 7.1 summarises the structure and functions of the skin.

Q7: Using Table 7.1, list six different functions of the skin.

Table 7.1 Structure and functions of the skin

Structure	Functions
1 Epidermis	
Cornified layer	Made up of dead cells containing keratin. It protects the underlying tissues against damage by friction. It also prevents loss of water and entry by pathogens. It is constantly lost and is replaced by new cells from the layer below
Malpighian (germinal) layer	A single layer of cells which actively divide, replacing cells that are lost from the surface of the skin. These cells contain melanin which protects underlying tissues against ultra violet light
2 Dermis	
Sweat glands	Absorb water and inorganic ions from blood in the capillaries around them and secrete this onto the surface of the skin
Arteries and capillaries	Carry blood (containing heat) to the skin and so help in temperature regulation
Hairs and hair erector muscles	Temperature regulation (hairs are raised and lowered by the muscles)
Sebaceous glands	Secrete sebum which prevents the skin from cracking; helps to waterproof the skin and also inhibits the growth of bacteria
Receptors	Detect temperature, pain, touch, pressure
3 Adipose (fat) layer	This is a layer of triglycerides (page 14) under the skin (subcutaneous). It slows down heat loss or heat gain as well as acting as a reserve energy store

Heat can be gained or lost from the body in four ways:

- radiation
- conduction
- convection
- evaporation of water.

These terms are explained in Table 7.2.

Table 7.2 Ways in which heat can be gained and lost

How heat is lost or gained	Explanation
Radiation	Transfer of heat to or from the body to other objects (via the air)
Conduction	Transfer of heat to or from the body by direct contact with another object, e.g. radiator, window
Convection	Transfer of heat to or from the body via moving air
Evaporation	The loss of heat used to change water from a liquid to a vapour, e.g. when water leaves the skin surface or gas exchange system

Figure 7.4 summarises the ways in which heat is gained or lost by the body. The response by humans to heat *gains* are explained in more detail below. The response to heat *losses* is the reverse of these changes.

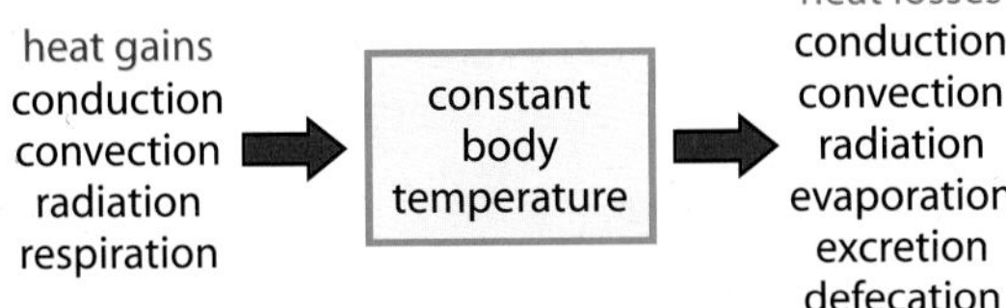

Figure 7.4 Summary of heat losses and gains.

Response to heat gains

- Sweating (Figure 7.5)
- Flattening of hairs on the skin (Figure 7.6). This is of negligible value in humans
- Vasodilation and dilation of shunt vessels (Figure 7.7)
- More blood in the circulation – blood which is stored in the liver and spleen is released into the circulation. More blood therefore reaches the skin surface, therefore more heat is lost.
- Metabolic rate falls. This is a long-term effect under the control of the hormone thyroxine
- Lack of shivering – this spasmodic contraction of voluntary muscle to produce heat does *not* occur.

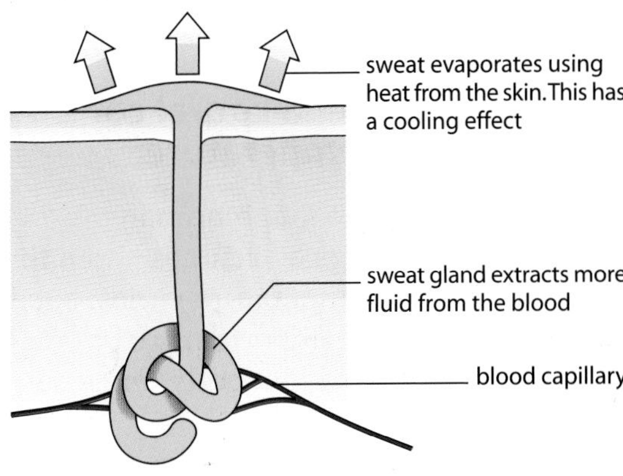

Figure 7.5 Sweating.

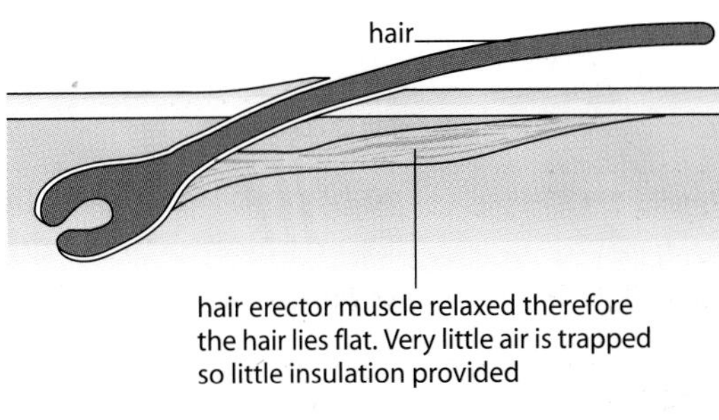

Figure 7.6 Reaction of hairs on the skin.

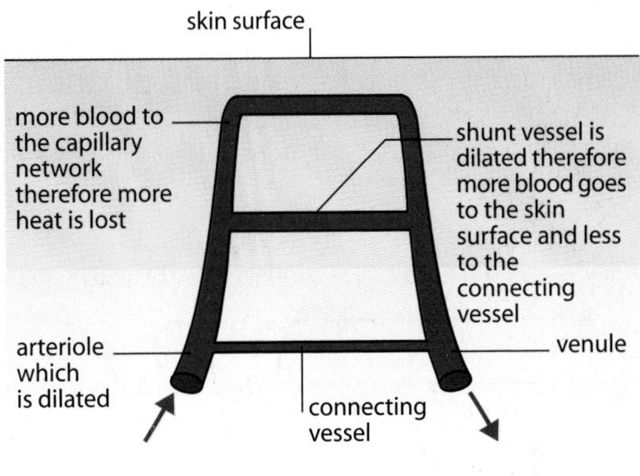

Figure 7.7 Vasodilation and shunt vessels.

Q8: Generally, people living in hot climates have little adipose tissue beneath their skin. Explain the value of this condition.

Q9: How would you expect cold conditions to affect: (a) the rate of sweating? (b) the position of hairs on the skin? (c) arterioles and shunt vessels in the skin? (d) volume of blood in the circulation? (e) metabolic rate? (f) shivering?

Behavioural control of body temperature

Although humans show many physiological changes when the environmental temperature varies, behaviour also plays an important part in maintaining a constant body temperature.

Q10: List three behavioural changes that could occur if the environmental temperature: (a) rises well above the norm; (b) falls well below the norm.

Role of the brain in temperature regulation

The hypothalamus in the brain acts as a thermostat and is sensitive to changes in blood temperature. If the temperature of the blood entering the hypothalamus falls, it sends impulses to organs causing them to reduce heat loss. The reverse happens if the temperature of the blood entering the hypothalamus rises.

An experiment was performed to show the role of the hypothalamus in temperature regulation. In this experiment, a person sat in a special calorimeter which allowed readings of the skin temperature, the hypothalamus temperature and the rate of sweating to be taken. (The temperature of the hypothalamus can be taken by placing a temperature probe down the outer ear so that it touches the eardrum.) Periodically the person drank an quantity of iced water.

The results of such an experiment are shown in Figure 7.8. Initially, with a high external temperature:

- the internal body temperature was high
- the rate of sweating was high
- the skin temperature was low.

On drinking the cold water:

- the internal body temperature dropped. This was caused by the cold water cooling the blood flowing around the stomach
- the rate of sweating decreased. This was caused by the cooled blood reaching the hypothalamus. The hypothalamus 'sensed' this and sent impulses to the sweat glands causing them to reduce the rate of sweat production
- the skin temperature increased. This was caused by the reduction in the rate of sweating.

NB: The temperature receptors in the skin seemed to play little part in this response as skin temperature in the experiment rose.

Figure 7.8 Results of Benzinger's experiment.

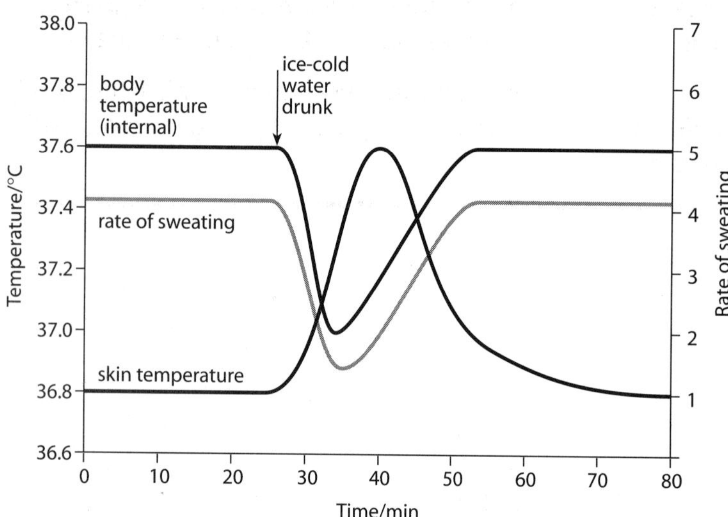

Role of the temperature receptors in the skin

These sense changes in the external temperature and are very useful in:

- informing the brain of these changes so that the brain can alter behaviour, e.g. if the person feels a cold draught he/she may close a window.
- protection, e.g. if a person picks up an object which is very hot then he/she rapidly drops it.

Hypothermia

This is the medical term given to a marked drop in body temperature as a result of prolonged exposure to low temperatures. It is most likely to occur in:

- very young babies – as their temperature regulation mechanisms are not fully developed
- people exposed to severe cold, e.g. on mountain tops or after falling into cold water
- old people – as their temperature regulation mechanisms are less effective.

Also they may lack money for fuel or for heat-saving measures, e.g. proper roof insulation.

Hypothermia results in a reduced metabolic rate which can lead to coma and death.

The principle of hypothermia is used in heart-lung operations. By reducing the blood temperature, the heart and brain need less oxygen and therefore can withstand reduced or interrupted blood flow for short periods. This gives surgeons sufficient time to operate.

Brown fat

This is a special type of fat cell found particularly in the newborn. When the fat is oxidised it gives out a great deal of energy as heat which is a safeguard for the baby. Brown fat cells possess many mitochondria which do not produce ATP but instead release the energy as heat.

Summary

- Homeostasis is the maintenance of a constant internal environment within the body.
- Negative feedback is a control mechanism in which a change from the norm triggers a response which results in a change back to the norm.
- Islets of Langerhans are groups of cells in the pancreas which secrete insulin and glucagon.
- Insulin is a hormone which reduces blood sugar level.
- Glucagon is a hormone which increases blood sugar level.
- The skin performs several important functions, one of which is a role in temperature regulation.
- Endotherms are animals that maintain a virtually constant body temperature.
- Ectotherms are animals whose body temperature is governed by the environmental temperature.
- Heat can be lost by radiation, convection, conduction and evaporation.
- Heat can be gained by radiation, convection and conduction and generated internally by respiration.
- The hypothalamus is part of the brain which is sensitive to changes in the blood temperature.
- Temperature receptors in the skin sense changes in external temperature or if an object is very hot.
- Hypothermia is a medical term given to a marked drop in body temperature.
- Brown fat is used to generate heat quickly instead of using the energy to make ATP.

Self check
See page 234

CHAPTER 8

Skeleton and muscles

In this chapter you will learn about the structure and functions of the skeleton. In addition you will study joints, how muscles work and their use in bending and lifting. Health issues and injuries are also covered in this chapter.

Functions of the skeleton

The skeleton has several functions:

- **protection** – e.g. the cranium of the skull protects the brain and the ribcage protects the lungs and heart
- **support** – the skeleton supports the soft body tissues allowing us to stand
- **movement** – bones provide a solid structure for muscle attachment
- **manufacture of blood cells** – the marrow of some bones produces blood cells
- **store of calcium** – calcium is very important in, e.g., muscle contraction and blood clotting. The bones provide a store of calcium ions.

Major bones of the skeleton

For convenience, the skeleton can be divided into:

- **axial skeleton** – the skull, itself comprising cranium and mandible (Figure 8.1); the vertebral column (Figures 8.2, 8.3 and 8.4); the ribs and sternum (Figure 8.5)
- **appendicular skeleton** – the pectoral girdle (Figures 8.6a and 8.7); the pelvic girdle (Figures 8.6b and 8.7); the limbs (Figure 8.6).

Axial skeleton

Skull

The **cranium** protects the delicate tissues of the brain. It is made from many individual bones that fuse together. The joints between these bones can be seen as **sutures** in Figure 8.1. The flat bones of the skull continue to make red blood cells throughout our lives.

The **mandible** articulates against the cranium and allows us to feed and to speak.

Q1: The bones of the skull are not fused by the time a baby is born. Instead, they are able to move over each other without damaging the baby's brain. Suggest one advantage of this.

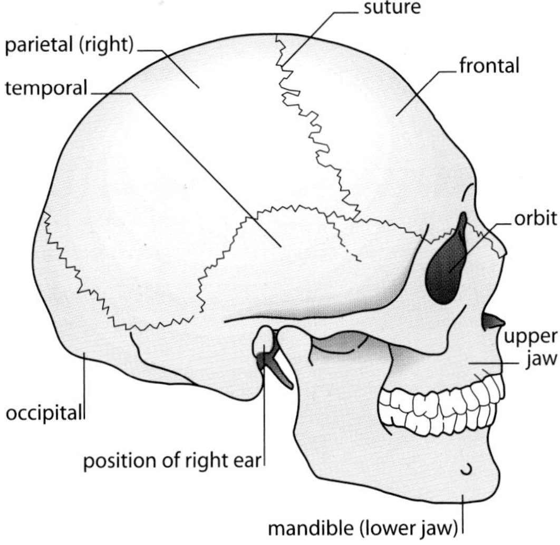

Figure 8.1 Human skull.

Vertebral column

The vertebral column gives support to the body, provides attachment for the back muscles and protects the delicate tissues of the spinal cord. There are 33 vertebrae in a human, although some are fused (Figure 8.3). Each vertebra has the general structure shown in Figure 8.2. However, vertebrae have slightly different functions according to their positions along the spine. These functions are summarised in Table 8.1 and the differences in structure of vertebrae from the neck (cervical), chest (thoracic) and small of the back (lumbar) are shown in Figure 8.4.

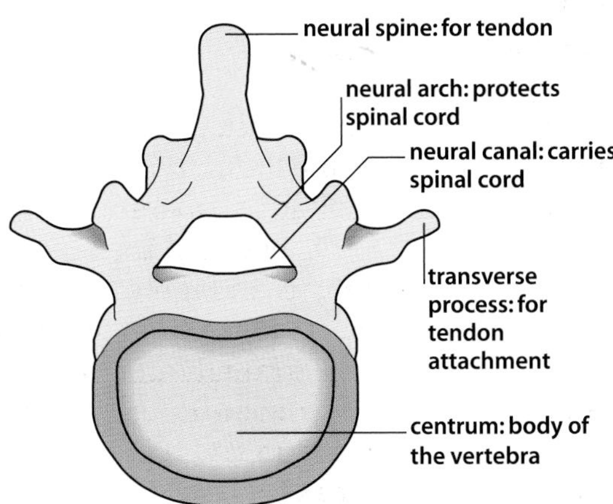

Figure 8.2 Generalised vertebra.

atlas vertebra
axis vertebra
7 cervical (neck) vertebrae
12 thoracic vertebrae (connected to a rib on each side)
5 lumbar vertebrae (largest and strongest)
5 sacral vertebrae (fused together forming the sacrum)
4 caudal vertebrae (fused together forming

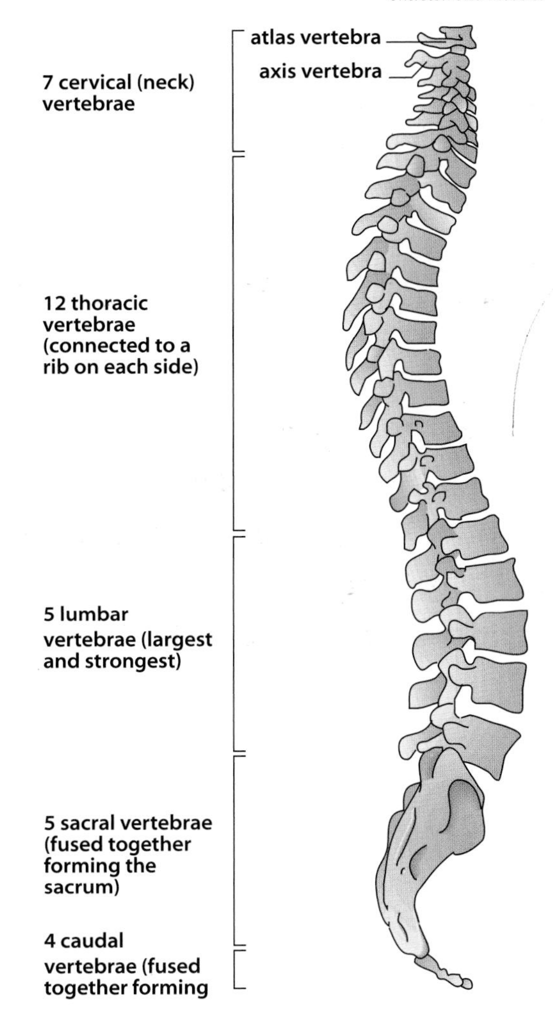

Figure 8.3 Human vertebral column.

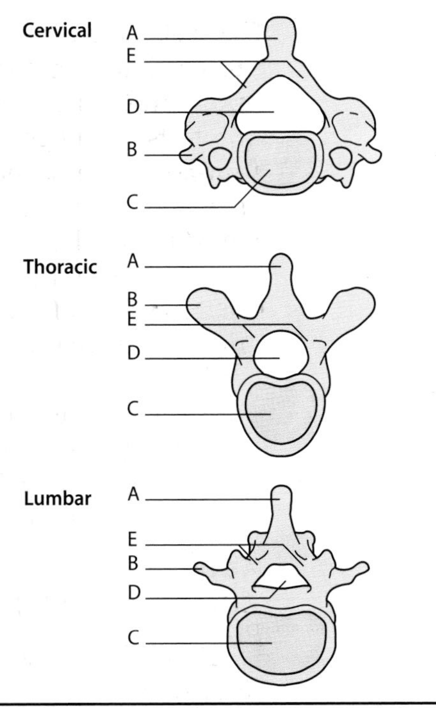

Figure 8.4 Cervical, thoracic and lumbar vertebrae.

Table 8.1 Summary of vertebral functions

Vertebrae	Number	Special features
Cervical	7	First two are the **atlas** and **axis** which allow rotation and nodding of the head
Thoracic	12	Articulate (join) with the ribs
Lumbar	5	Support the upper body – large, to withstand stress
Sacral	5	Fused together to support the pelvic girdle
Caudal (coccyx)	4	Greatly reduced in humans; no special function

Q2: Use the information in Figure 8.2 on page 69 to name the structures labelled A to E in Figure 8.4.

Ribs and sternum

Together with the sternum (or breast bone), twelve pairs of ribs form a protective cage around the heart and lungs. They are also vital in bringing about the breathing movements that draw fresh air into our lungs and force stale air out of our lungs (page 41). The head of each rib articulates with the centrum of a thoracic vertebra (Figure 8.5). The uppermost ten pairs of ribs join to the sternum by cartilage. The lowest two pairs of ribs do not: for this reason they are called 'floating ribs'.

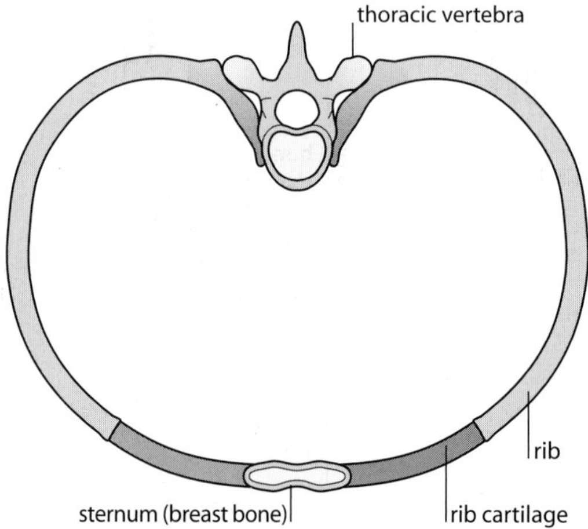

Figure 8.5 Arrangement of ribs, sternum and thoracic vertebrae.

Appendicular skeleton

Pectoral girdle

The pectoral girdle is made from the **scapula** (shoulder blade) and **clavicle** (collar bone) on each side of the body. Figure 8.6a shows that these bones do not fuse, so that the pectoral girdle is flexible. This gives our shoulders great manœuvrability.

Pelvic girdle

The pelvic girdle is formed by the fusion of six bones that grow separately in a fetus. They fuse not only with each other but also with the five sacral vertebrae giving a girdle that is rigid (Figure 8.6b). This is advantageous in ensuring that the thrust developed by our leg muscles is not lost.

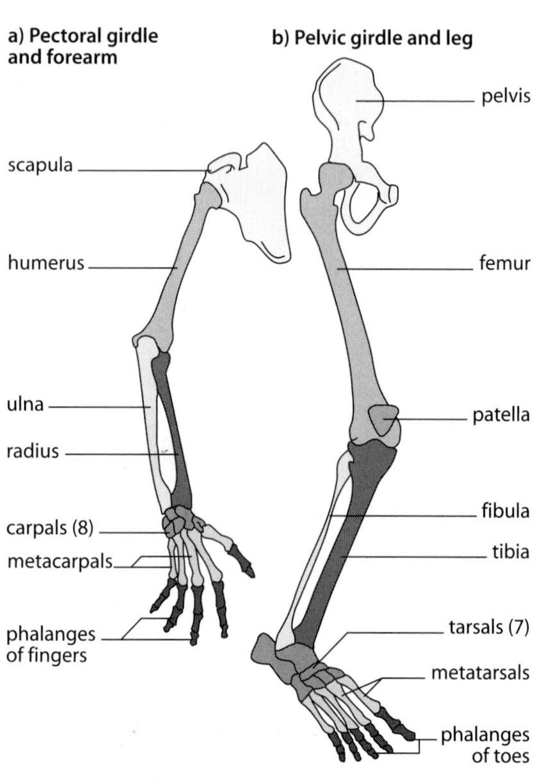

Figure 8.6 Limbs and girdles compared.

Limbs

The arms and legs are built on the same pattern called a **pentadactyl** (five digits) limb. Note how corresponding bones in the two limbs in Figure 8.6 have been given correponding shading.

NB: The radius in the forearm is the one nearest the thumb regardless of whether the palm is turned upwards or downwards.

Figure 8.7
Human skeleton.

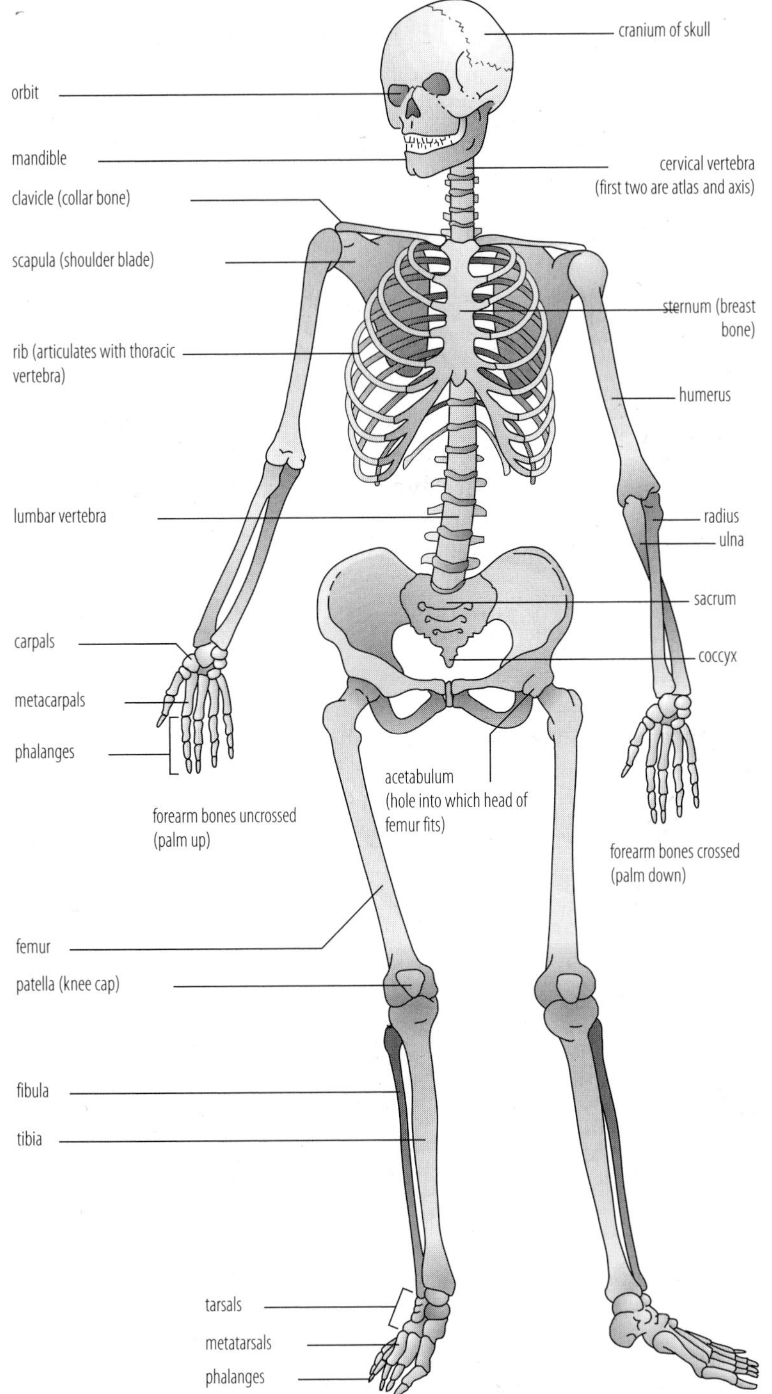

Structure of bone and cartilage

Bone and cartilage are two tissues (see page 5), each made of cells that secrete a non-living **matrix** around themselves. In bone tissue, the bone-secreting cells (**osteocytes**) secrete a rigid matrix of protein and calcium salts. In cartilage tissue, the cartilage-secreting cells (**chondrocytes**) secrete a flexible matrix of protein.

Figure 8.8 shows the microscopic structure of two types of bone tissue and of cartilage tissue: it also shows their distribution in a limb bone. Notice that the limb bone is not solid but contains a marrow-filled cavity. This gives a structure that is strong yet light. In a fetus and young child, the marrow of limb bones produces blood cells. During childhood, these bones stop making red blood cells, but they continue to make some white blood cells throughout life.

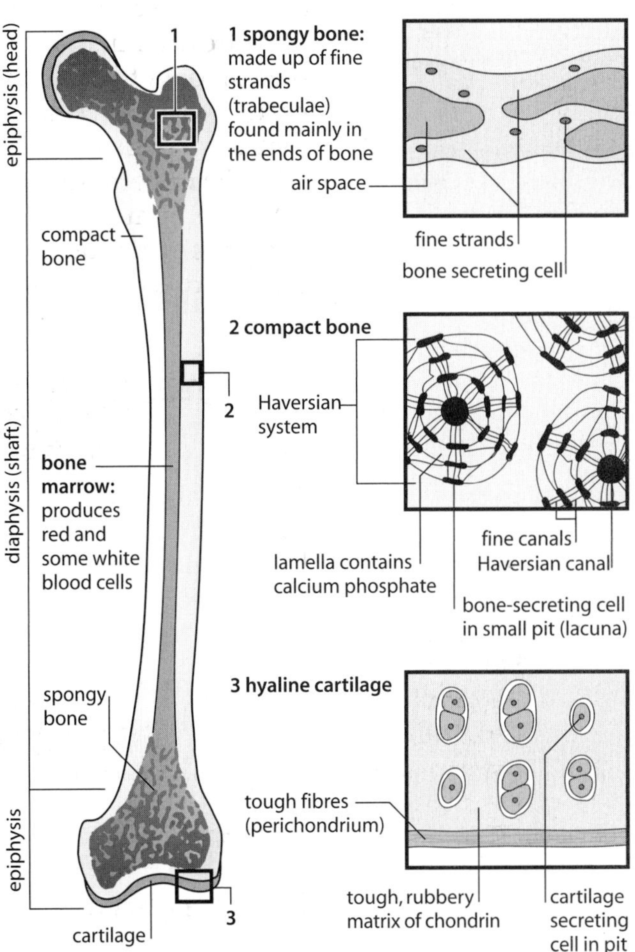

Figure 8.8 LS of a long bone with detail of tissues.

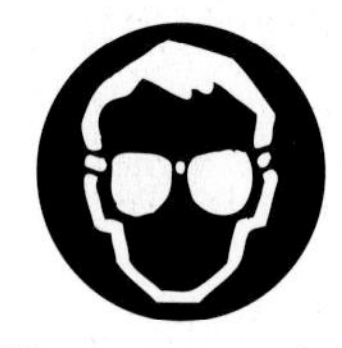

Wear eye protection

CORROSIVE
Hydrochloric acid

Practical 8.1 To demonstrate that bones contain mineral salts

Requirements
Two pieces of rib bone from a chicken
Dilute hydrochloric acid
Two beakers
Forceps
Eye protection

1 Take two small pieces of bone. Place one in dilute hydrochloric acid and the other in water. (Hydrochloric acid dissolves mineral salts from the bone but leaves the protein intact.)

SAFETY: Take care when using hydrochloric acid. Refer to the safety procedures on page viii.

2 What factor(s) should be kept constant in this experiment?

3 Leave the bones in these solutions for 2 to 3 days.

4 Remove the bones using the forceps and wash them carefully in tap water.

5 Feel the two pieces and record your results.

6 What is the difference between the two bones at the end of the experiment?

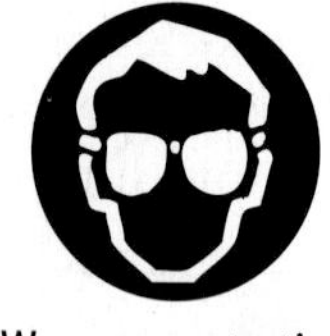

Wear eye protection

Practical 8.2 To demonstrate that bones contain organic material

Requirements
One piece of rib bone from a chicken
Crucible
Forceps
Bunsen burner and tripod
Either gauze or clay triangle (to hold crucible on tripod)
Red litmus paper
Matches
Eye protection

1 Place a small piece of bone in a crucible.

2 Place the crucible on a tripod; heat the crucible strongly using a Bunsen burner.

3 As the bone burns, test the fumes given off with a piece of moist red litmus paper.

4 Allow the bone to cool then test the pliability of the bone.

5 Explain your results.

Joints and ligaments

Joints occur wherever two bones meet. They can be divided into three groups:

- **immoveable** (fixed joints), e.g. bones of the cranium of the skull
- **slightly moveable** e.g. joints between adjacent centra of the vertebral column
- **freely moveable** (synovial joints), e.g. hip, knee, joint between centrum of thoracic vertebra and head of rib.

Q3: Where would you find other: (a) immoveable joints? (b) slightly moveable joints? (c) synovial joints?

Synovial joints are adapted to allow friction-free movement, otherwise the bones might rub against each other causing pain and damage. These adaptations are summarised in Table 8.2. Synovial joints can be further classified according to the range of movement they allow. Figure 8.9 shows a number of synovial joints and the range of movement possible.

Ligaments are another type of connective tissue. Like bone and cartilage, ligaments are made from cells that secrete a non-living matrix around themselves. In this case, the matrix contains fibres of an elastic protein. This gives ligaments strength but elasticity, making them ideal for holding bones together at a joint.

Immovable joint: bones of the skull fused together

parietal bone
frontal bone
temporal bone
suture

Pivot joint: The odontoid peg of the axis fits into the atlas. This gives rotation of head and atlas; nodding of the head is due to the skull moving on the atlas – a hinge joint.

articulating process for skull
canal for spinal cord
atlas
axis
odontoid peg
articular process

Ball and socket joint: This allows freedom of movement in any plane. Also seen in the hip joint

ligament: holds bone to bone
scapula
humerus
cartilage: prevents bones rubbing together
synovial fluid: lubricates the joint
synovial membrane: produces synovial fluid

Hinge joint: This allows freedom of movement in one plane. Also seen in the knee

humerus
ligament
synovial membrane
ulna
cartilage
synovial fluid

Gliding joint: The two articulating surfaces are flat therefore slide over one another easily. This gives flexibility but limited strength. Also seen in the ankle. Having limited strength means that those parts are easily sprained

ulna
radius
ligament
carpals
metacarpals

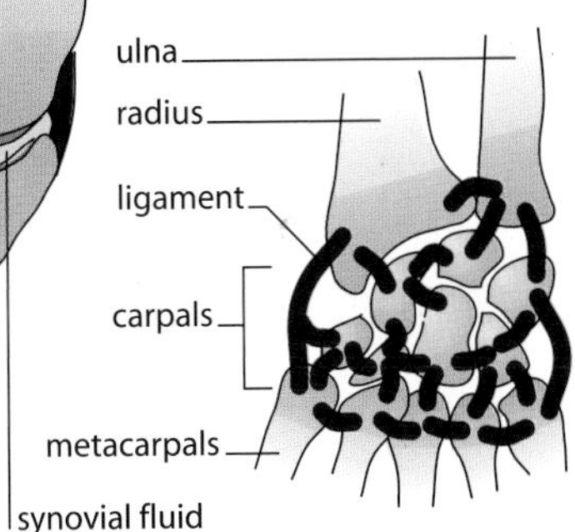

Figure 8.9 A range of joints in the human skeleton.

Q4: Figure 8.10 shows an X-ray of a knee. Name the parts labelled 1, 2 and 3 and state one function of each.

Figure 8.10 X-ray of the knee joint.

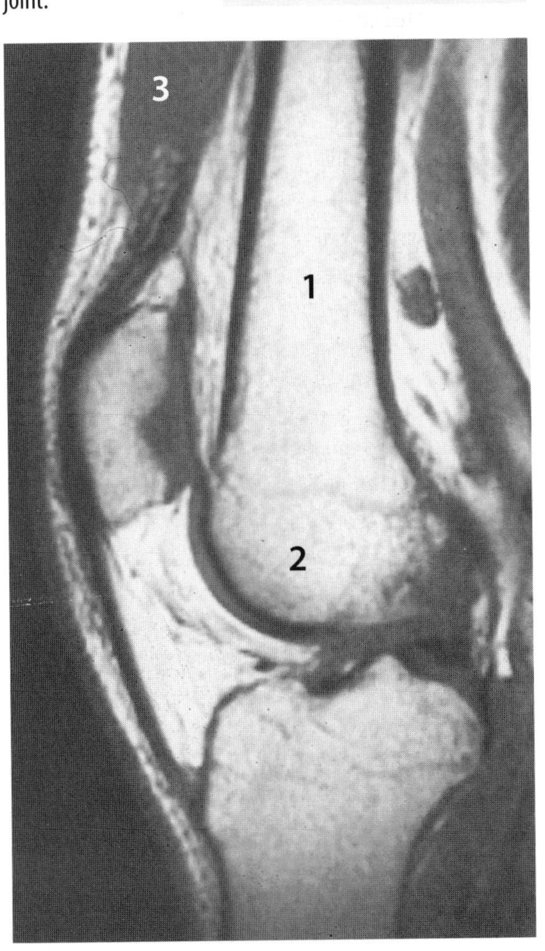

Table 8.2 Summary of parts and functions of a synovial joint

Part	Function
Cartilage	Prevents bone from rubbing on bone
Ligament	Holds bone to bone
Synovial membrane	Produces synovial fluid
Synovial fluid	Lubricates the joint/nourishes the cartilage

Disorders of the skeleton

Osteoporosis is the most common of all bone diseases, especially in old age. It results chiefly from a reduction in the amount of organic material in bone tissue. There are several causes:

- lack of stress on the bone, generally through inactivity in older people
- deficiency of protein in the diet
- deficiency of vitamin D in the diet (vitamin D is needed for absorbing and using the calcium and phosphorus needed for the bone matrix)
- reduced secretion of oestrogen in post-menopausal women. For this reason, many women choose to follow a course of treatment involving synthetic oestrogen (hormone replacement therapy or HRT).

Arthritis is the name given to a number of diseases that affect the joints. Wearing away of the cartilage at the joints is known as **osteoarthritis** and is very common in older people. **Rheumatoid arthritis** is a much more complex disorder and is thought to result from the sufferer's immune system attacking their own cartilage.

Slipped disc: Pieces of tough cartilage (known as fibrocartilage) are found between the centra of adjacent vertebrae and are known as discs. Occasionally, the centre (nucleus) of a disc may be displaced, so pressing on the nearest spinal nerve (see Chapter 9). This causes a great deal of pain.

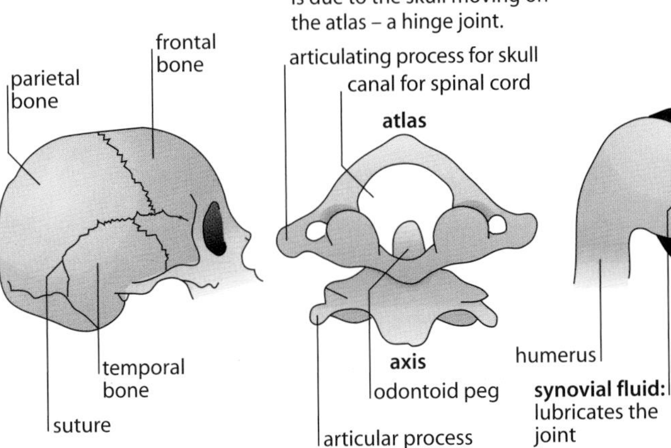

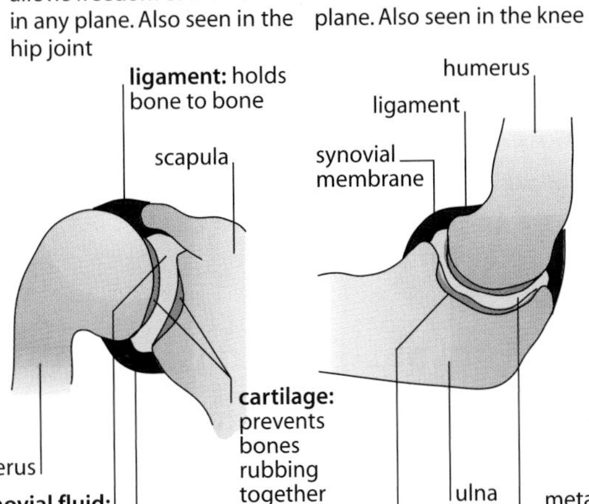

Muscles and tendons

There are three types of muscle tissue:

- **cardiac** – found only in the heart (see page 31)
- **smooth** (also called involuntary muscle)
- **striped** (also called voluntary muscle and skeletal muscle).

Smooth (involuntary) muscle

The appearance of this muscle tissue is shown in Figure 8.11.

- Smooth muscle tissue is made up of tapered cells whose cytoplasm lacks stripes.
- The cells are arranged in sheets.
- These sheets of cells may be arranged in a circular or longitudinal pattern.
- These muscles carry out many automatic contractions (i.e. you do not think about them as they are not under conscious control).

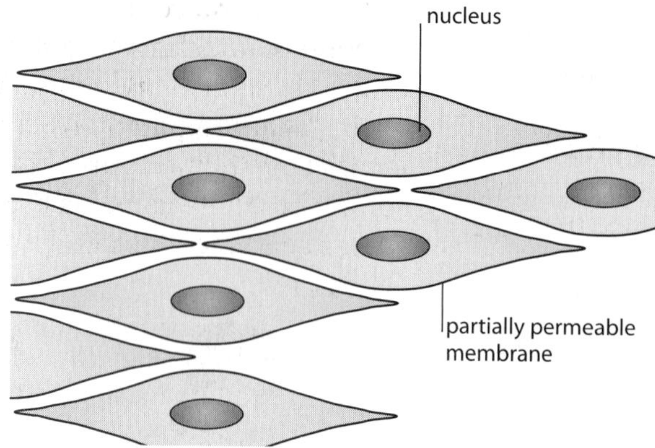

Figure 8.11 Smooth muscle tissue.

Q5: Suggest parts of the body where you might find smooth muscle.

Striped (voluntary) muscle

The appearance of this muscle tissue is shown in Figure 8.12.

- Striped muscle tissue is made up of a large number of cylindrical muscle cells (fibres) separated by connective tissue.
- The cytoplasm of these cells has characteristic stripes (Figure 8.12c).
- The stripes are caused by protein fibres that enable the muscle cells to contract.
- Each muscle is attached to bone by tendons (apart from the tongue).
- Whole muscles work **antagonistically** (in opposition) in pairs to move bones.
- Contraction of striped muscles can be controlled by conscious decision.

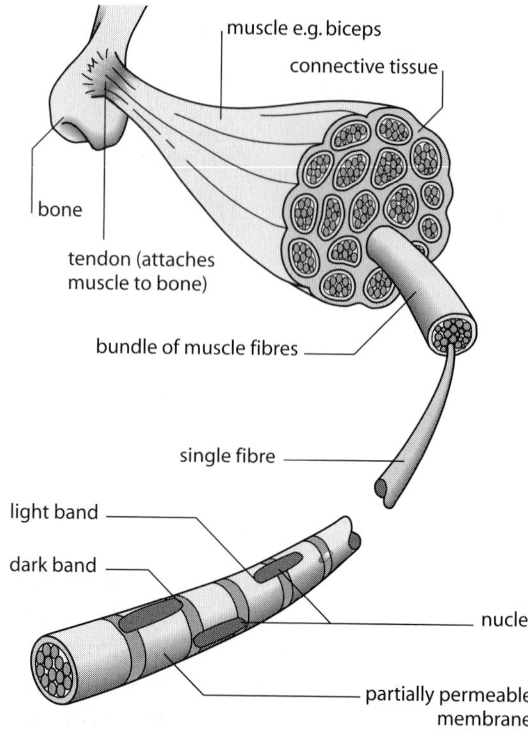

Figure 8.12 Composition of skeletal muscle.

How striped muscles work

Striped muscles can be classified according to the movement they bring about, e.g:

- **rotators** – bring about rotation of the limb
- **extensors** – cause a straightening of the limb (increase angle between bones)
- **flexors** – cause a bending of the limb (decrease angle between bones).

Q6: Figure 8.13 represents the bones and muscles of a human arm. The biceps and triceps muscles work antagonistically, i.e. when one contracts the other relaxes and vice versa. (a) What will happen to the arm when the triceps contracts? (b) What will happen to the arm when the biceps contracts? (c) What sort of muscle is the triceps? (d) What sort of muscle is the biceps?

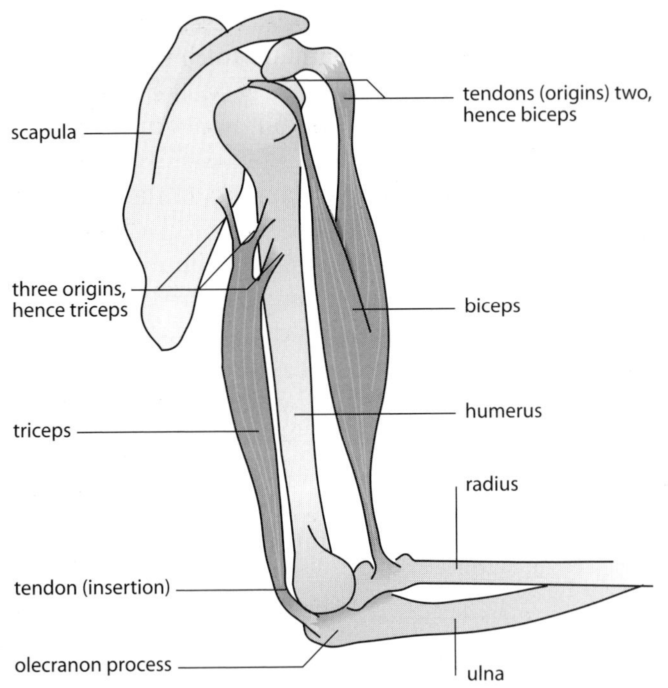

Figure 8.13 Antagonistic muscles of the arm.

Muscle fatigue

When the muscles are contracted for long periods, they tire (e.g. see how long you can hold your arms above your head). Another way of saying this is that muscles become **fatigued**. Muscles can stop contracting because nerve cells run out of the chemical messenger with which they stimulate muscles (see page 74). Alternatively, the muscles themselves may run out of energy and so be unable to respond to nervous stimulation.

Q7: (a) What type of respiration begins to be used during strenuous exercise? (b) Consequently, what waste product will accumulate in muscles during strenuous exercise? (c) Suggest why pain (cramps) is associated with muscle fatigue.

Muscle tone, posture, bending and lifting

Muscle tone

No muscle is ever totally relaxed. Some fibres are always contracted and this gives the muscle its tone. The advantages of this are:

- muscles are maintained in a permanently active state and so are capable of rapid contraction when required
- the body is kept upright and the internal organs in position.

Twitchy fibres

Recent research has shown that there are at least two types of voluntary muscle fibre.

- **Slow twitch** – mainly use fatty acids as their source of energy and, since they have a store of lipid, fatigue slowly.
- **Fast twitch** – mainly use glucose as their source of energy and, because they lack an energy store, fatigue quickly.

It has been found that slow twitch muscle fibres develop more extensively in athletes who do distance running, whilst the fast twitch type develop more in sprint training.

Posture

We have a *good* standing posture if :

- the head is balanced on the top of the vertebral column
- the vertebral column is balanced on its point of attachment to the pelvic girdle
- the knee joints are straightened
- the feet are squarely on the ground.

In this position (Figure 8.14) the muscles of the body are using as little energy as possible to maintain the position of the body.

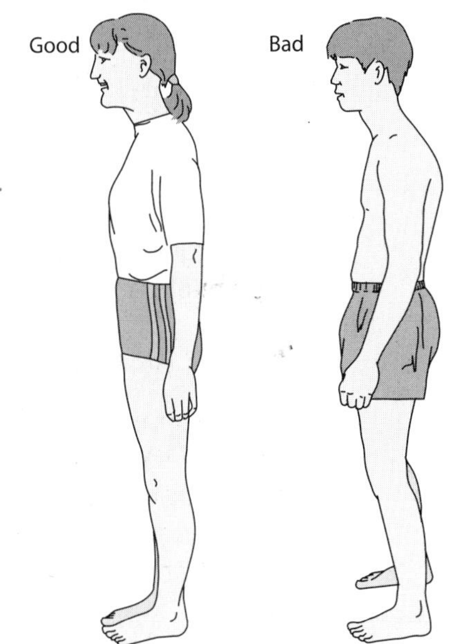

Figure 8.14 Posture.

Bad posture leads to:

- more energy being needed by the muscles to keep the body upright, leading to fatigue and backache
- digestive system being compressed therefore working less efficiently
- breathing system being compressed therefore working less efficiently
- main blood vessels becoming compressed therefore carrying less blood.

Prolonged bad posture may lead to a deformed vertebral column and flat feet.

Bending and lifting

Poor posture during lifting (poor lifting technique) can damage the back. The intervertebral discs are particularly at risk from damage since they are designed to withstand being squashed (compression) but not being stretched (tension).

To prevent damage, the following good lifting technique should be followed:

- keep the vertebral column as straight as you can to prevent stretching the discs
- keep the lifted object as close to you as possible so as to reduce the leverage exerted by the object
- use your legs and hips to help support the lifted weight
- always bend from the knees as this allows the legs to support the lifted weight.

Foot care

The many bones of the feet are linked with cartilage to form a flexible arch which supports the weight of the body. Many problems associated with feet are due to ill-fitting footware, both in childhood and adulthood.

Young children

As children's bones contain a lot of flexible cartilage, tightly-fitting shoes can permanently damage their feet. The rules to be followed are:

- babies should go barefoot to allow rapid, unrestrained foot growth
- shoes for young children should allow plenty of room for the child's foot to grow
- feet should be measured when the child is standing so that its weight will spread the feet out.

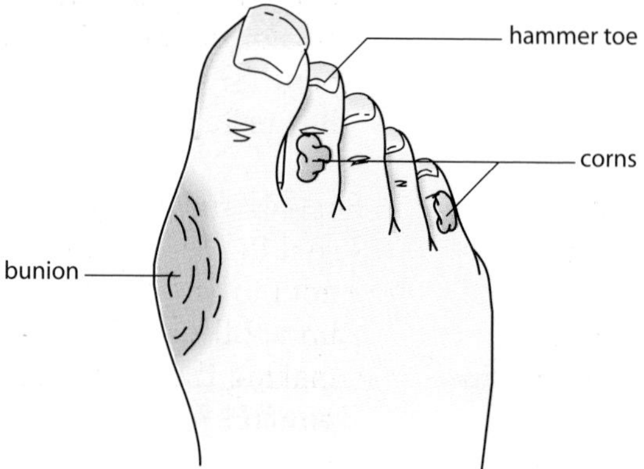

Figure 8.15
Problems caused by ill-fitting shoes.

Teenagers and adults

A number of problems can be caused by ill-fitting shoes:

- **backache** – caused by poor posture due to high heels which throw the foot forwards in the shoe
- **corns** – hard, painful patches of skin caused when toes rub against the inside of the shoes
- **bunions** – painful, swollen joints at the base of the big toe caused by wearing narrow, pointed shoes or high-heeled shoes. These can cause the bones to become deformed
- **hammer toe** – the big toe is pushed inwards and crushes the adjacent toe, causing it to bend so that the end points downwards (Figure 8.15).

Sports injuries

People involved in sports inevitably run the risk of injuries, most of which are likely to involve bones, muscles, tendons or cartilage.

- **Pulled or torn muscles**: the muscle fibres come apart. This is most likely in the hamstring or calf muscles. To treat this as a first aider follow the RICE treatment:

Rest → **I**ce → **C**ompression → **E**levation

Then seek medical help. The time the torn muscle takes to heal will vary depending on the extent of the tear and the treatment given.

- **Tendon rupture:** this most commonly happens to the Achilles tendon in the heel. If a complete rupture has occurred, surgery will be needed to rejoin the two ends. This is followed by having the tendon immobilised in plaster of Paris for about six weeks.
- **Torn cartilage:** this will require an operation using keyhole surgery (see Health issues).
- **Tendonitis:** if muscles are constantly used, strain is put on the tendons with the result that they become inflamed and hurt even at rest. This often happens to tennis players and javelin throwers. Rest is needed to cure this.
- **Sprain:** this occurs when the ligaments around a joint are torn as a result of a sudden wrench. Movement becomes difficult and the area becomes swollen as blood and tissue fluid accumulate. Treatment usually involves immobilisation of the joint.
- **Dislocation:** this occurs when one or more of the bones at a joint becomes forced out of position. The person must immediately see a doctor who will put the bone back in place. Dislocations tend to recur as ligaments become weaker once they have been stretched. In serious cases, surgery may be performed to shorten the ligaments and stop further recurrence.

Health issues

Keyhole surgery (arthroscopy): This involves the introduction of an illuminated instrument into the synovial cavity, usually of the knee joint, via a small cut. This procedure enables the surgeon to see ligaments and cartilage directly and therefore to make a better-informed decision about treatment.

Hip replacement: With the longevity of the population increasing, hip replacement is becoming more and more common. In this operation, a false socket (usually made of plastic) is cemented into the pelvic girdle. An artificial ball (usually stainless steel) is then embedded into the femur and held in place by metal pins. The leg is re-set by fitting the new ball into the new socket (Figure 8.16).

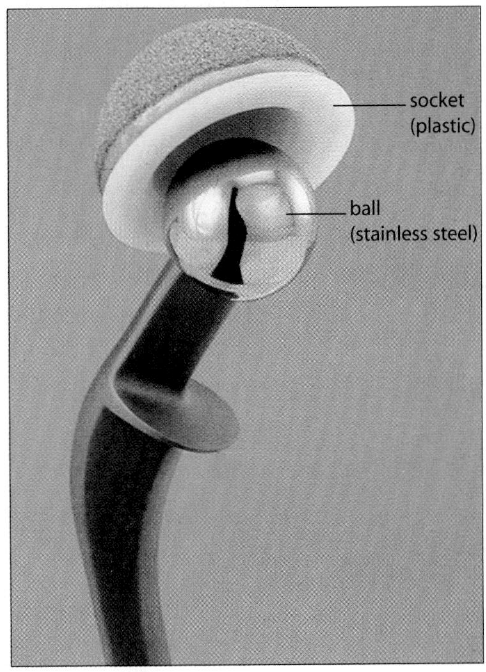

Figure 8.16 An artificial replacement hip joint.

Bone injuries

A cracked or broken bone is called a **fracture**. Fractures are most likely to occur in the limb bones, particularly those of the lower limbs (radius and ulna; tibia and fibula). Fractures are named according to certain features:

- **closed fracture** – bone broken but the overlying skin surface is intact
- **open fracture** – broken ends of the bone come through the overlying skin surface
- **compound fracture** – fractured bone has also caused other injuries, e.g. rib may have penetrated a lung
- **stress fracture** – is a slight crack in the bone. This will usually heal by itself if it is rested.

First-aid for fractures involves:

- sending for an ambulance immediately
- not moving the person and immobilising the broken limb
- making the person as comfortable as possible while they wait for the ambulance.

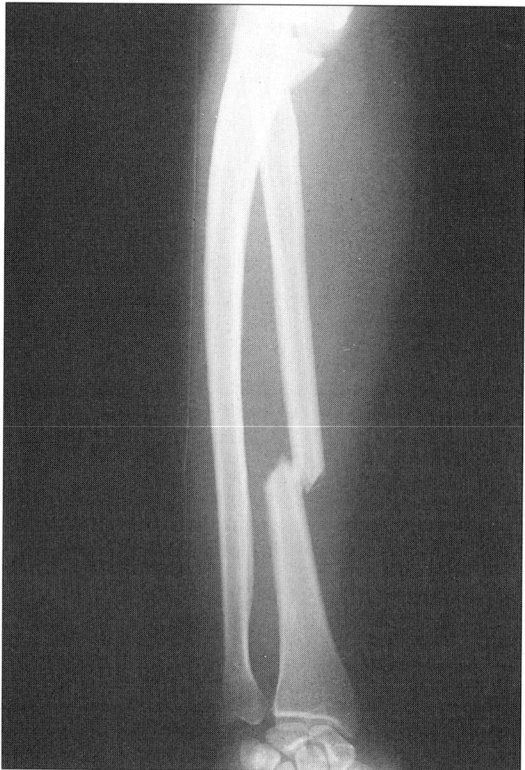

Q8: Figure 8.17 is an X-ray of a damaged radius. Name the type of damage shown.

Figure 8.17 X-ray of a damaged radius.

Summary

- The functions of the skeleton include protection, support, movement, manufacture of blood cells and a store of calcium.
- The axial skeleton is made up of the skull, vertebral column, ribs and sternum.
- The appendicular skeleton is made up of pectoral girdle, pelvic girdle and limbs.
- The vertebral column is made up of 33 vertebrae. Those in the cervical, thoracic, lumbar and sacral region are adapted for particular functions associated with their position.
- There are twelve pairs of ribs, ten of which are attached to the sternum by cartilage. The head of each rib articulates with the centrum of a thoracic vertebra during breathing movements.
- The arm and leg are built on the same pentadactyl limb pattern.
- There are two types of bone tissue – compact bone is found as a tube around the outside of bones; spongy bone is found in their interior.
- Joints can be immovable (fixed), slightly moveable or freely moveable (synovial) joints.
- Cartilage prevents bone rubbing on bone.
- Ligaments hold bone to bone.
- The synovial fluid lubricates the joint and nourishes the cartilage.
- Osteoporosis is a condition where bones become very weak.
- Arthritis is a collective name for diseases of the joints.
- Displacement of the disc between the vertebrae is called a slipped disc.
- There are three types of muscle – smooth (involuntary), cardiac and striped (voluntary or skeletal).
- Skeletal muscles can be classified according to the movement they bring about, e.g. rotators, extensors and flexors.
- Muscles work antagonistically, i.e. when one contracts the other relaxes.

Self check
See page 235

CHAPTER 9

Coordination

In this chapter you will learn how the nervous system and endocrine system work in coordinating the body's activities. You will learn the general arrangement of nerves within the nervous system. You will also study the different types of nerve cells (neurones), the way that they carry impulses along their length and the way in which they communicate with one another in a simple reflex arc.

General features of coordination systems

Look at the gymnast in Figure 9.1. To perform like this, the muscular movements of his body must be finely coordinated. Although his endocrine system will be active (e.g., he will have felt nervous before his event), most of this coordination is done by the nervous system. To work, both the endocrine and nervous systems involve the following:

- **stimulus** – any detectable change in the external or internal environment
- **receptor** – an organ that detects a specific stimulus
- **effector** – an organ (muscle or a gland) that produces a response as a result of stimulus detection.

Q1: Use the flow chart in Figure 9.2 on page 72 to design a flow chart for the response resulting from the stimulus of a telephone call for which you have been waiting.

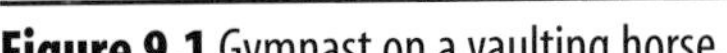

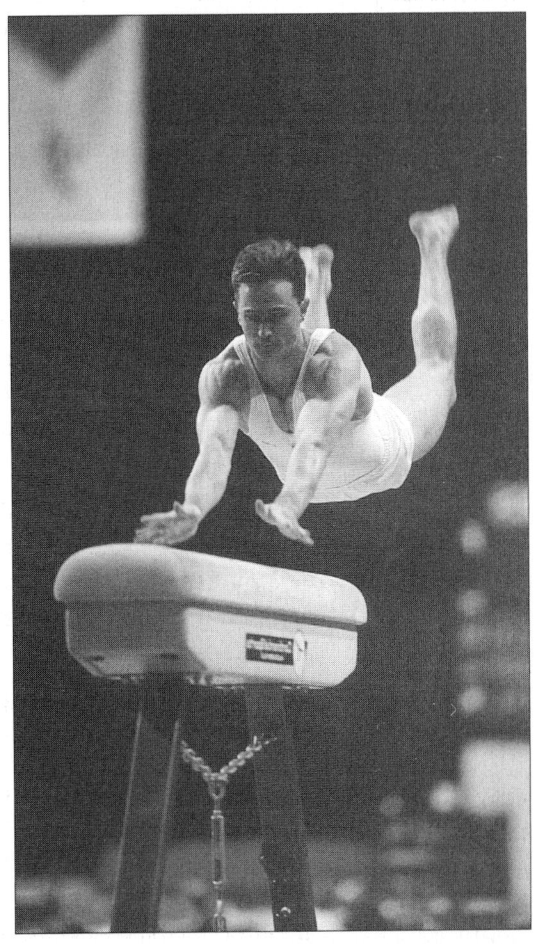

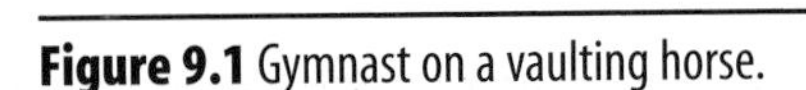

Figure 9.1 Gymnast on a vaulting horse.

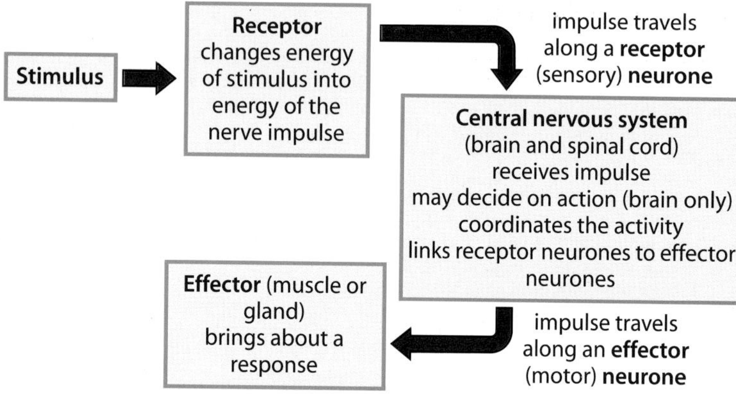

Figure 9.2 Flow chart showing coordination of the body's activities.

Structure of nerves and nerve cells (neurones)

These two terms are often confused. A **neurone** is an individual cell that transmits impulses along its length. A **nerve** is made up of hundreds of neurones (Figure 9.3). To understand this, think of a telephone cable. This is the equivalent of the nerve. The individual wires inside the cable are the equivalent of the neurones. Just like the wires inside the cable, each of the neurones can transmit an impulse.

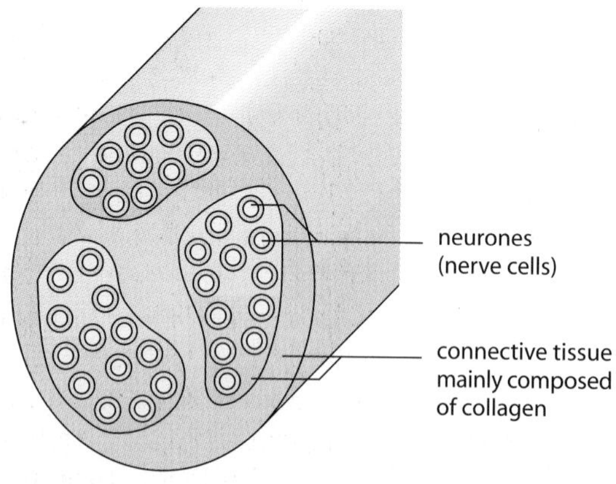

Figure 9.3 T.S. of a nerve shown diagrammatically.

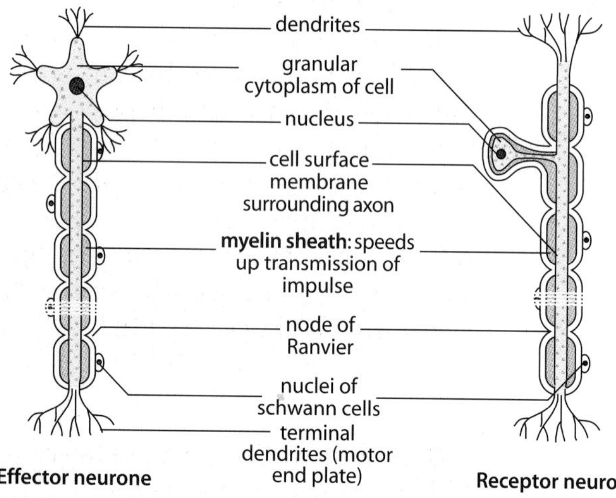

Figure 9.4 Neurone structure.

Nerves

Nerves may be:

- **sensory** (sometimes referred to as receptor nerves or afferent nerves). These nerves contain only neurones that carry impulses *from* receptors *to* the central nervous system (page 75). An example of a sensory nerve is the optic nerve which transmits impulses from the retina of the eye to the brain
- **effector** (sometimes referred to as motor nerves or efferent nerves). These contain only neurones that carry nerve impulses *from* the central nervous system to effectors. Examples of effector nerves are some cranial nerves (leading from the brain)
- **mixed** – contain both sensory and effector neurones. The spinal nerves are examples of mixed nerves.

Neurones (nerve cells)

There are three types of neurone:

- **receptor (sensory) neurones** – carry impulses from receptors to the central nervous system
- **effector (motor) neurones** – carry impulses from the central nervous system to effectors
- **relay neurones** – carry impulses from receptor neurones to effector neurones or from one relay cell to another (e.g. in the brain).

Although they have different functions, these neurones have a similar structure. Figure 9.4 shows the appearance of an effector neurone and a receptor neurone. Note that both neurones have long cytoplasmic extensions from their main cell body. One of these, the **axon**, carries impulses to the target organ. The other receives impulses and is long in a receptor neurone (**dendron**) but short in an effector neurone (**dendrites**). The functions of the other structures labelled in Figure 9.4 are shown in Table 9.1.

Table 9.1 Structure and functions of the parts of the neurones

Structure	Function
Cell body	The main part of the cell containing cytoplasm and the nucleus
Dendron	Part of the neurone that transmits impulses towards the cell body
Axon	Part of the neurone that transmits impulses away from the cell body to the target cell
Myelin sheath	Made of individual cells (called Schwann cells) with abundant fatty material in their surface membranes. They wrap themselves around the axis of the axon and dendron, resulting in faster impulse conduction
Dendrite	Finely branched endings that receive impulses
Node of Ranvier	The gap between adjacent Schwann cells where the myelin sheath is absent

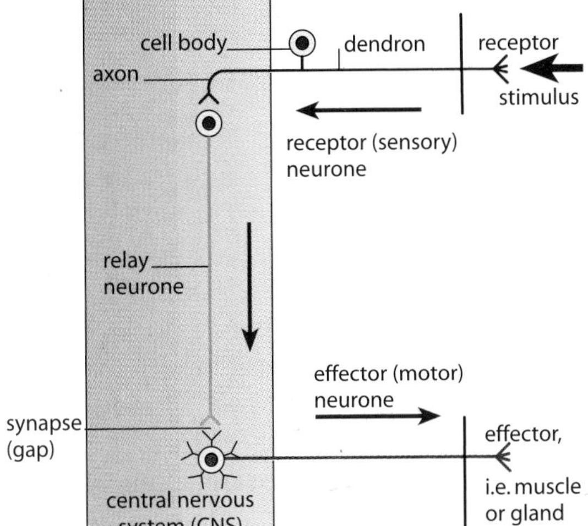

Figure 9.5 Diagrammatic interpretation of a simple reflex arc.

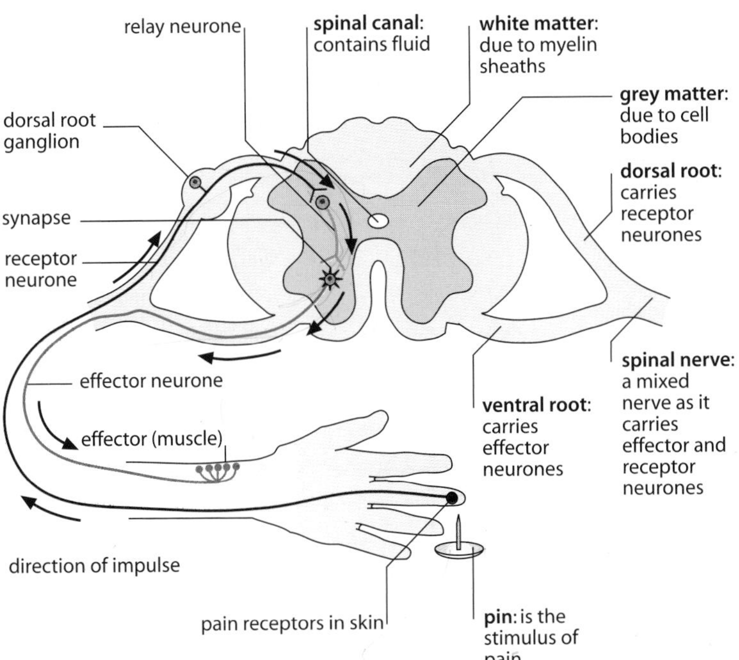

Figure 9.6 A simple reflex arc.

Simple reflexes

Neurones link together to form nervous pathways between individual receptor cells and individual effector cells. Some of these pathways are unlearned, i.e. we have them at birth, and are fixed, i.e. a particular impulse always results in the same response. Such an action is called a **simple reflex** and often involves protective behaviour, e.g. blinking the eye when a foreign object approaches the face. The nervous pathway that controls a simple reflex is called a **simple reflex arc** and is shown diagrammatically in Figure 9.5. The reflex arc that controls withdrawal of the hand from a hot object is shown in Figure 9.6. Although this diagram shows a pathway involving only a single receptor, relay and effector neurone, you should realise that several hundreds of these pathways actually cause withdrawal of the hand.

In contrast to a simple reflex, learned behaviour is governed by nervous pathways that are established well after birth. They usually involve the cerebrum of the brain, so that conscious thought occurs. Unlike the fixed nature of simple reflexes, learned behaviour is complex since a great variety of responses can result from a single stimulus.

Q2: List three differences between a simple reflex and a voluntary act.

Q3: Copy the table below and fill in the blanks. The first example has been done to help you. (You might need to use other chapters of this book to gain the information you need.)

Reflex	Stimulus	Receptor	Response	Purpose
1 Withdrawal of hand	Pin prick	Pain receptors in skin	Arm muscles contract	Protection against further damage
2 Production of saliva				
3 Blinking of eye				
4 Narrowing (constriction) of pupils				
5 Knee jerk				

How a neurone works

A neurone produces an impulse which is like an electrical current passing along its length. This current involves changes in electrical charges on the inside and outside of the neurone. The electrical charges are produced by ions, of which the most important are sodium (Na^+) and potassium (K^+).

The key processes shown in Figure 9.7 occur in the surface membrane of a neurone before, during and after an impulse passes along a neurone:

- at rest, the surface membrane of a neurone is **polarised** (more positive charges on the outside and more negative charges in the cytoplasm)
- an impulse starts when this balance of charges is reversed (**depolarisation**)
- this depolarisation continues down the neurone
- **repolarisation** occurs soon after.

Synapses

As can be seen from Figure 9.5 and 9.6, impulses must be able to get across gaps (**synapses**) between adjacent nerve cells. Figure 9.8 shows how this is achieved. When an impulse arrives at the end of a neurone it causes the release of chemical transmitters (**neurotransmitters**) on to its target cell. These transmitters cause the depolarisation of the surface membrane of the target cell.

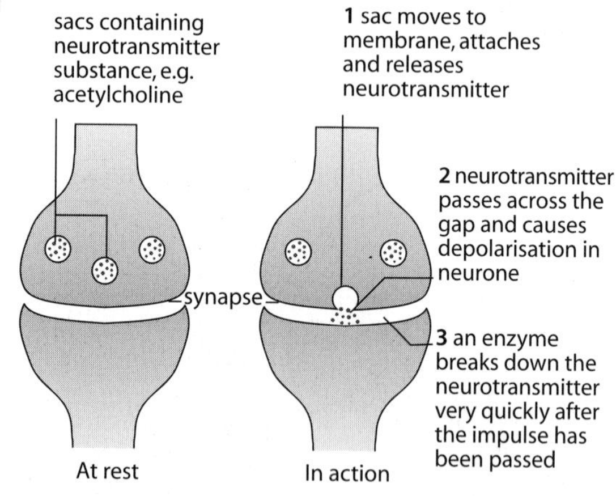

Figure 9.8 Conduction across a synapse.

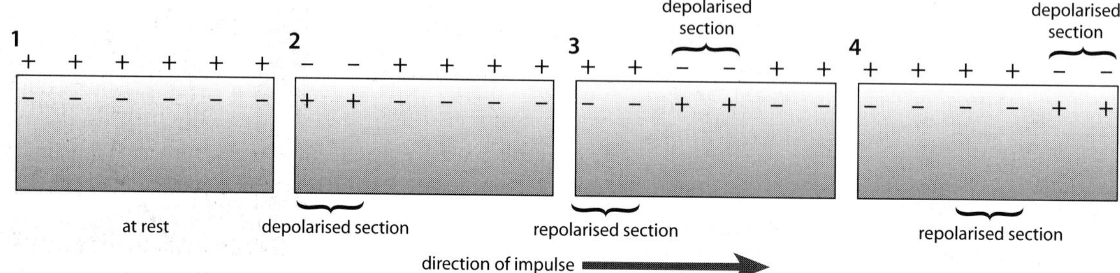

Figure 9.7 Conduction of nerve impulses.

Drugs and the nervous system

Many drugs affect the neurotransmitters at synapses or, indeed, mimic their actions. You will read more about drug actions in Chapter 14.

Alcohol blocks the release of neurotransmitters across synapses, particularly in the brain.

Amphetamines are commonly called 'speed'. The reason for this is that they mimic the action of a neurotransmitter that speeds up the heartbeat.

Q4: What will happen to a person's reflexes if he/she has been drinking alcohol?

The nervous system can be considered as consisting of two parts: the central nervous system (CNS) and the peripheral nervous system (PNS).

NERVOUS SYSTEM	
Central Nervous System (CNS) (brain and spinal cord)	Peripheral Nervous System (PNS) (nerves linking the CNS to all parts of the body)

Central nervous system (CNS)

The CNS consists of the brain and spinal cord. Each of these has:

- **white matter** – mainly the axons and dendrons of neurones. It appears white in colour because these parts of the neurones are surrounded by Schwann cells with their fatty myelin
- **grey matter** – mainly the cell bodies of neurones. It appears grey in comparison with the white matter because these parts of the neurone are not surrounded by myelin
- **cerebrospinal fluid** – circulates within membranes (**meninges**) around the outside of the CNS and also inside a canal within the CNS.

Q5: Suggest a role for the meninges and fluid in the CNS.

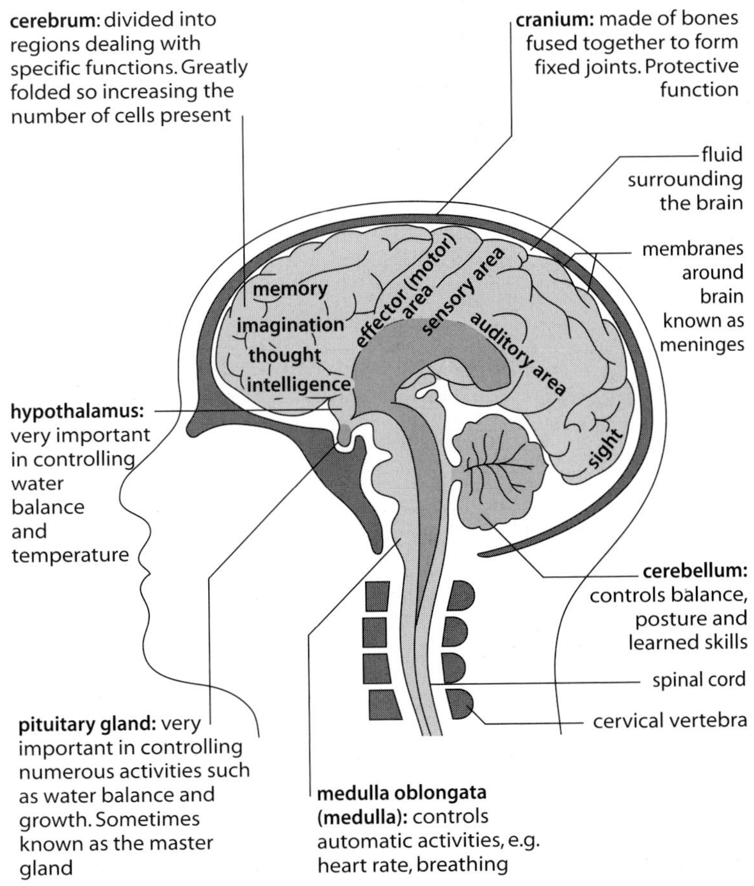

Figure 9.9 VS human head.

The brain

The brain is responsible for the control of many actions, some of which we are conscious of but many of which we are not. Figure 9.9 shows the main regions of the human brain and summarises their function. Figure 9.10 shows a photograph of a brain scan that can be used when diagnosing illnesses of the brain.

NB: the right side of the brain coordinates the left side of the body and vice versa.

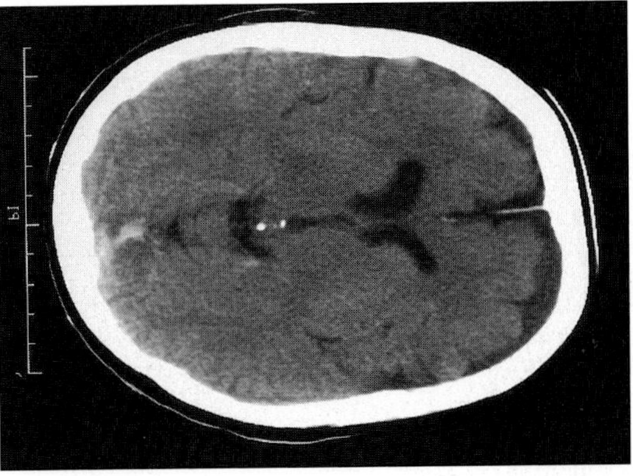

Figure 9.10 Brain scan (CT scan).

Spinal cord

The spinal cord runs from the brain to the lumbar region of the back and is protected by the vertebrae (page 61). Along its length, its structure is similar to the cross-section shown in Figure 9.6.

Peripheral nervous system

This consists of nerves running to, and from, the central nervous system. It can be represented in two parts:

- the nerves which control the **voluntary** activities of the body
- the nerves which control the **involuntary** (**autonomic**) activities of the body, e.g. heart beat.

Q6: Suggest another involuntary activity controlled by the autonomic nervous system.

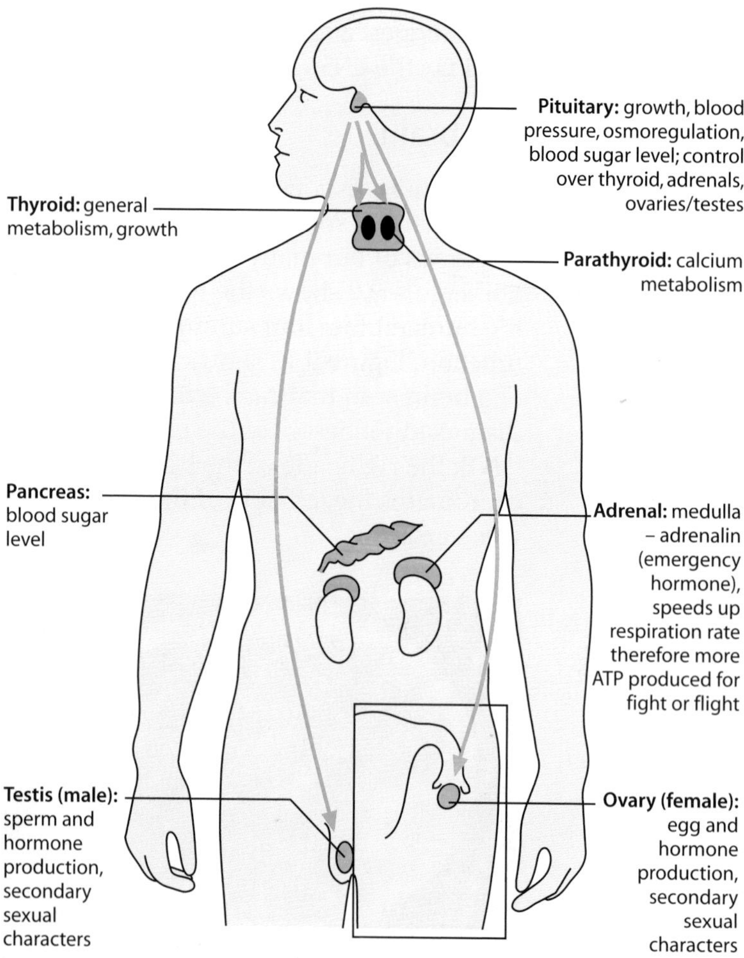

Figure 9.11 Position of the main endocrine glands.

Endocrine system

Endocrine glands secrete chemicals directly into the bloodstream. This is in contrast with **exocrine** glands, e.g. salivary glands, that secrete substances into ducts. The chemicals released by endocrine glands act as chemical messengers and are known as **hormones**.

The location of some of the major endocrine glands, together with the function of some of the hormones they secrete, is summarised in Figure 9.11. Many of these activities are covered elsewhere in this book:

- ADH and water balance – Chapter 6
- insulin/glucagon and blood sugar levels – Chapter 7
- thyroxine and body temperature – Chapter 7
- sex hormones – Chapter 11.

NB: one of the glands in Figure 9.11 acts as both endocrine and exocrine gland. This is the pancreas and its two functions are:

- **endocrine** – islets of Langerhans secrete hormones (insulin and glucagon) into the bloodstream
- **exocrine** – pancreatic cells secrete digestive enzymes into the duodenum via the pancreatic duct.

Generally, responses coordinated by hormones tend to be much slower than responses coordinated by nerves; they also tend to affect more regions of the body.

Q7: Suggest two other differences between nervous coordination and hormonal coordination.

Summary

- The nervous system and the endocrine system coordinate the body's activities.
- A receptor is a structure that detects a stimulus.
- An effector is an organ that carries out a response to a stimulus.
- A reflex action is a rapid, automatic response to a specific stimulus.
- The nervous system is made up of the central nervous system (brain and spinal cord) and the peripheral nervous system.
- A nerve is made up of large numbers of nerve cells known as neurones.
- Sensory (receptor, afferent) nerves contain neurones that carry nerve impulses from receptors to the CNS. Effector (motor, efferent) nerves contain neurones that carry nerve impulses from the CNS to effectors. Mixed nerves contain both receptor and effector neurones.
- Voluntary actions are governed by conscious thought. In-born, fixed actions are called simple reflexes and are controlled by simple reflex arcs.
- The nerve impulse passes down a neurone as a result of changes in the balance of electrical charges on the inside and outside of a neurone.
- Release of chemicals (neurotransmitters) enables nerve impulses to bridge the small gap (synapse) between adjacent neurones.
- Specific areas of the brain coordinate particular activities. The right side of the brain governs the activities of the left side of the body and vice versa.
- Endocrine organs secrete chemicals (hormones) directly into the bloodstream, whereas exocrine organs secrete chemicals into ducts.

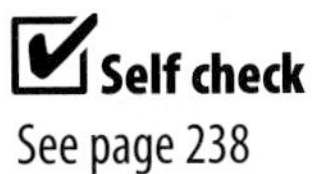

See page 238

CHAPTER 10

Sensory perception

In this chapter you will learn about a number of receptors in the body but will concentrate on the eye and ear.

Function of a receptor

Receptors contain cells that detect stimuli. To do this, they convert the energy of the stimulus into the energy of a nerve impulse. A single receptor can only respond to one specific stimulus.

Exteroceptors are sensitive to external stimuli; **interoceptors** are sensitive to internal stimuli. Table 10.1 summarises the main exteroceptors and interoceptors and shows the stimuli to which each is sensitive.

Table 10.1 Stimuli detected by body receptors

Stimulus	Receptor	Location
External	*Exteroceptors*	
Sound	Sound-sensitive cells	Cochlea of the inner ear
Light	Rod and cone cells	Retina of the eye
Smell	Chemoreceptors	Nose
Taste	Chemoreceptors	Nose and tongue
Temperature	Heat-sensitive cells	Dermis of the skin
Pressure	Pressure-sensitive cells	Dermis of the skin
Touch	Touch-sensitive cells	Dermis of the skin
Pain	Pain-sensitive cells	Dermis of the skin
Gravity	Gravity-sensitive cells	Utriculus of the inner ear
Internal	*Interoceptors*	
Blood concentration	Osmoreceptors	Hypothalamus of the brain
Blood temperature	Temperature receptors	Hypothalamus of the brain
Tension in muscles	Proprioceptors	Tendons

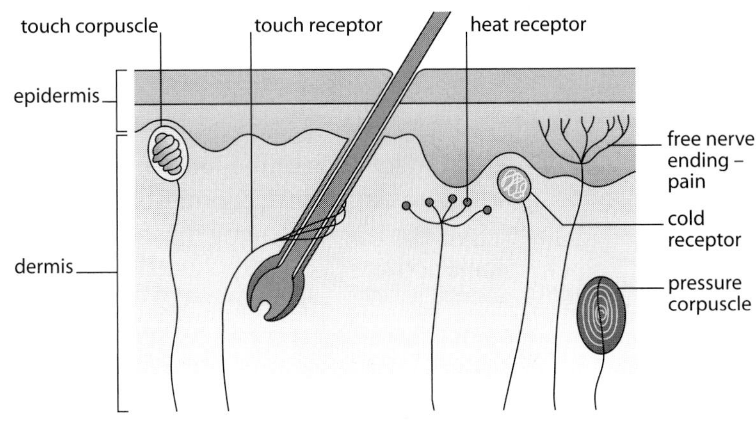

Figure 10.1 Receptors in the skin.

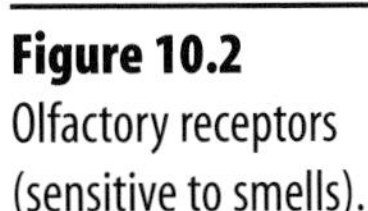

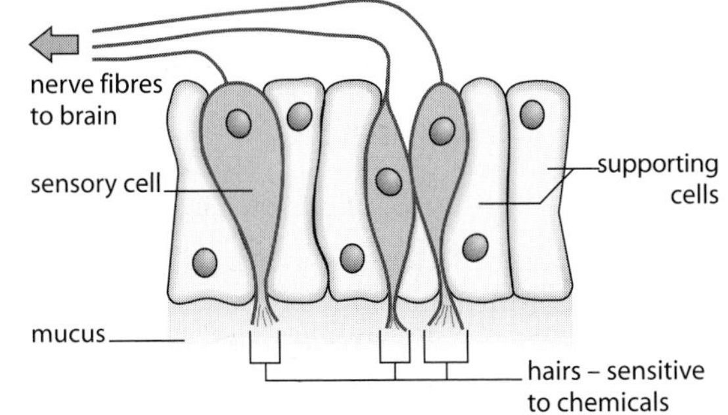

Figure 10.2 Olfactory receptors (sensitive to smells).

Receptors in the skin

In Figure 10.1 you can see receptors in the skin that are sensitive to touch, pain, pressure and temperature.

Olfactory Receptors

These are found in the nasal cavity (Figure 10.2). They contain cells that detect chemicals which have dissolved in the mucus lining this cavity. These give us our sense of smell and help with our ability to taste.

Q1: Using Figure 10.1 to help you, state precisely where you would find receptors for touch, pain, pressure, temperature.

Q2: Where in the body would you expect to find the highest concentration of touch receptors?

Practical 10.1 To investigate the density of touch receptors in various parts of the skin

DANGER
Sharp object

Requirements

Compasses, pair with blunt points
Ruler, graduated in mm

1 Obtain a pair of blunt compasses and adjust the points so that they are about 2 cm apart.

SAFETY: take care when using the compasses.

2 Blindfold a volunteer.

3 Touch the volunteer's skin gently on the back of the hand with the two points simultaneously.

4 Record how many points the volunteer feels.

5 Repeat with the points 1 cm and 3 cm apart.

6 Repeat on different parts of the body, e.g. back of neck, finger tips, sole of foot, forearm.

Taste Receptors

Taste receptor cells are found in groups, called **taste buds**, in the epidermis of the tongue (Figure 10.3). Like olfactory receptors, they detect dissolved chemicals - in this case those that are dissolved in the mucus lining our mouths. Individual taste receptor cells respond to only one of the following stimuli:

sweet sour salt bitter

Figure 10.4 shows that receptors specific for these stimuli are located together in different regions of the tongue.

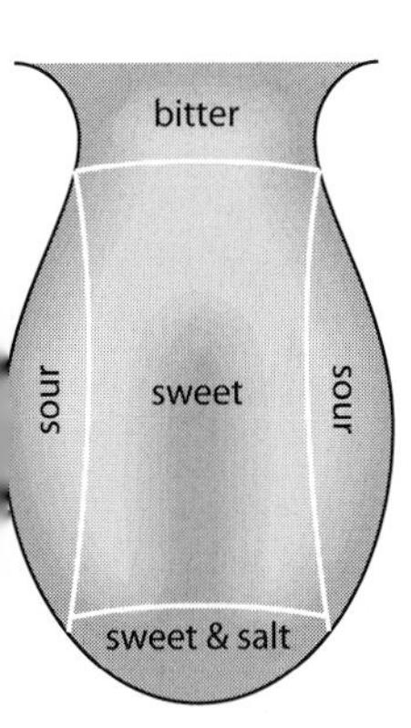

gure 10.4 Taste regions the tongue.

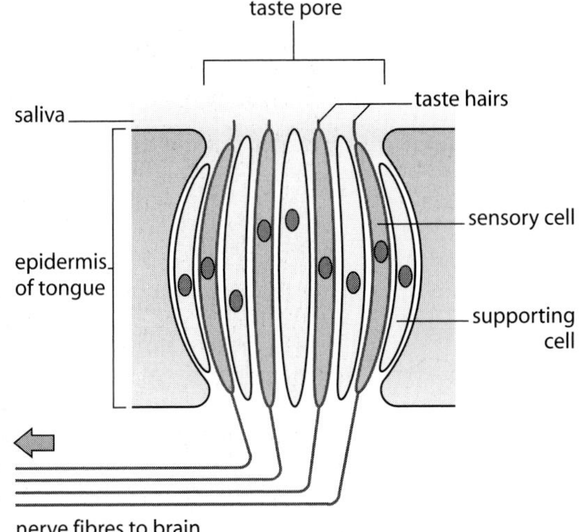

Figure 10.3 A taste bud.

Q3: Impulses from olfactory receptors and taste receptors are carried to the brain. (a) How do you know that this is true? (b) Use information from Chapter 9 to name the type of neurone that will carry nerve impulses from these receptors to the brain.

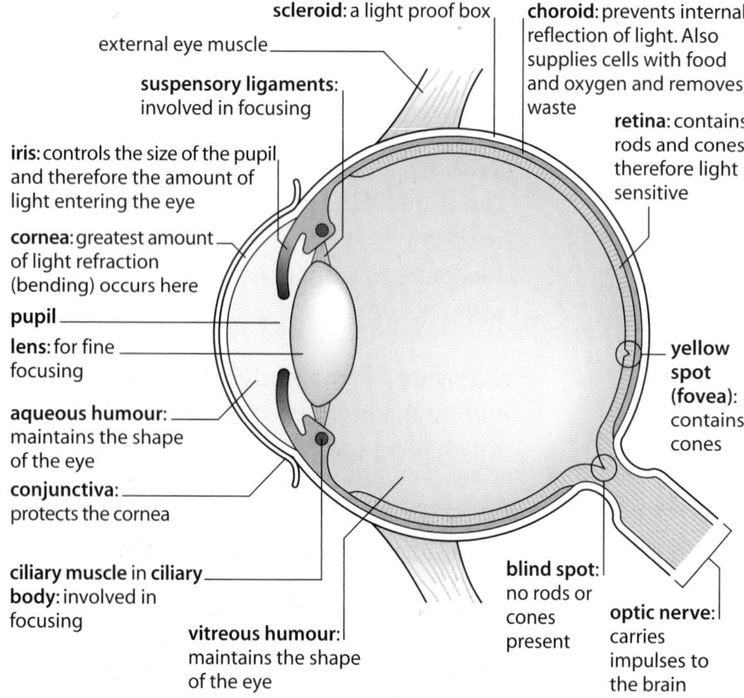

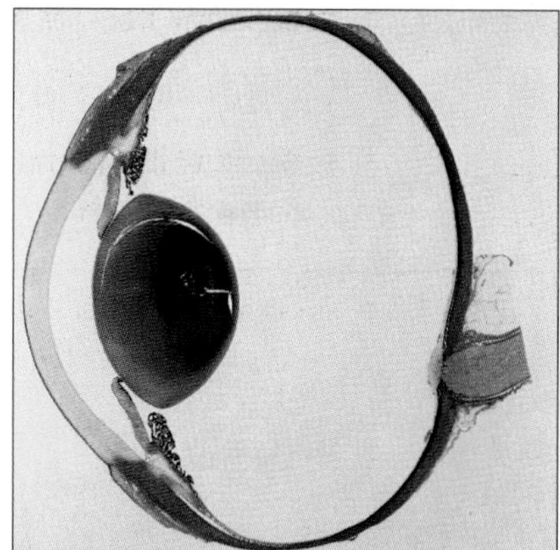

Figure 10.5 VS human eye (diagram and photograph).

The eyes

Each eye is situated in a bony socket of the skull, called an **orbit**, and has a number of muscles attached to it so that it can be moved. The **eyelids**, **eyelashes** and **tears** (from tear glands) help to protect the eye from damage. Figure 10.5 shows a vertical section through the eye and summarises the functions of the various parts. It also shows a photograph of a section through an eye.

Q4: Use Figure 10.5 to name one function for each of the following structures: iris; retina; choroid; optic nerve; cornea; lens; ciliary muscle; conjunctiva; scleroid.

Response of the eye to dim and bright light

The **iris** gives us our 'eye colour'. It contains involuntary muscle arranged in two layers: **radial** and **circular**. Like skeletal muscles, these muscles act as an antagonistic pair in each iris. They control the size of the pupil in response to the amount of light falling on the eye (Figure 10.6).

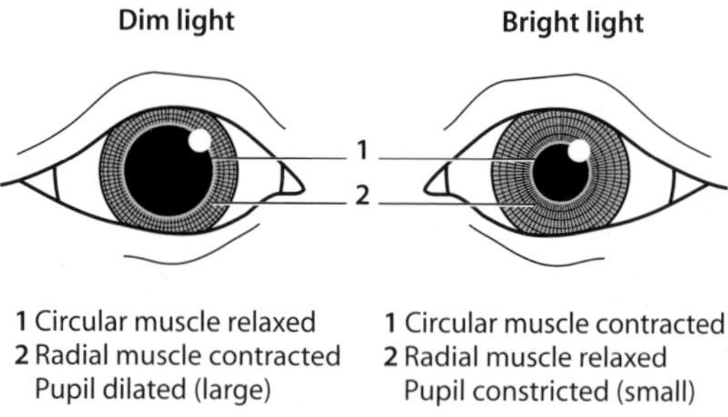

Figure 10.6 Response of the eye to dim and bright light.

Image formation

Light is made of small particles (photons) that travel in straight lines called **rays**. We are able to see objects if light rays strike them, rebound off them and enter our eyes. When light rays from an object enter the eye they are bent (**refracted**) mainly by the cornea and the lens. This leads to the rays being focused to form an image on the retina. As a result, impulses are sent to the cerebrum of the brain. In fact, the images that form on the retina are imperfect. The focusing process turns them upside down and back-to-front and the structure of the retina leaves 'holes' in them. The cerebrum interprets the images, turning them the right way up and the right way around and filling in the 'holes'.

Accommodation

Although most of the bending of light is done by the cornea, it is the lens that can change its shape, allowing us to focus near and distant objects. The ciliary muscle shown in Figure 10.5 can contract and relax, pulling on the suspensory ligaments that hold the lens or releasing the tension on them. This causes the lens to change shape.

Figure 10.7 shows an unaccommodated eye: in this condition distant objects are focused on the retina but near objects are out of focus. Figure 10.8 shows an accommodated eye in which near objects are focused on the retina but distant objects are out of focus.

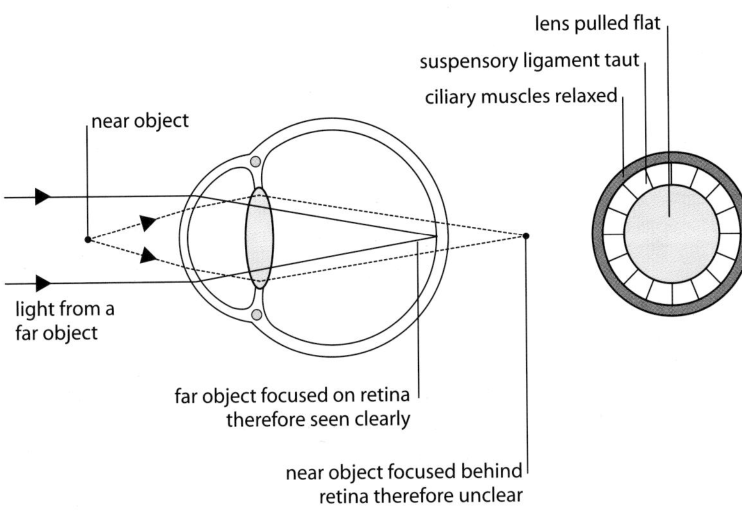

Figure 10.7 Unaccommodated eye (distance vision).

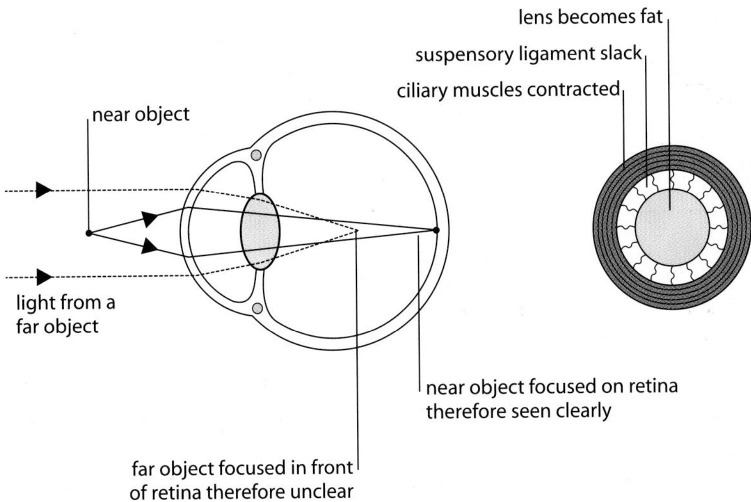

Figure 10.8 Accommodated eye (close vision).

Q5: Draw a table like the one shown below. Use Figures 10.7 and 10.8 to help you to complete the table.

	Unaccommodated eye	Accommodated eye
Ciliary muscle		
Suspensory ligaments		
Lens shape		
Focal length		
Distance of focused object		

Defects of the eye

The ability of the lens to focus images on the retina is affected by the size of the eyeball, the shape of the lens and the ability of the lens to change shape. If any of these factors changes adversely, the eye will not focus images clearly.

Long sight (hypermetropia)

This condition results in images from distant objects being focused on the retina while those from near objects are focused behind the retina, so they are seen as out-of-focus. Figure 10.9 shows how this defect can be corrected by using a converging (convex) lens in spectacles or contact lenses.

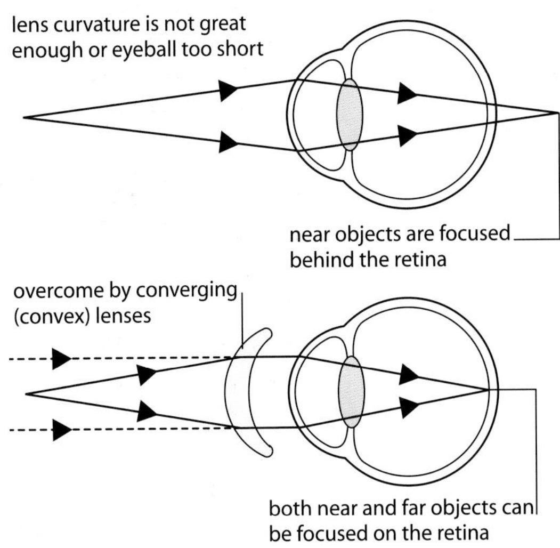

Figure 10.9 Long sight and its correction.

Short sight (myopia)

Short-sighted people are able to focus images from near objects on the retina but those from distant objects are focused in front of the retina, so they are seen as out-of-focus. Figure 10.10 shows how this defect can be corrected by using a diverging (concave) lens in spectacles or contact lenses.

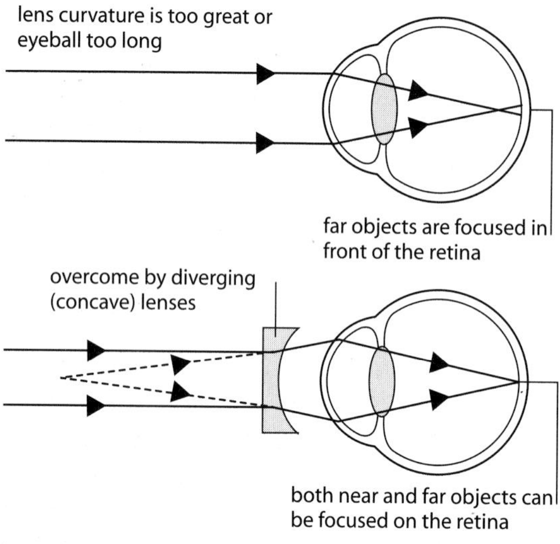

Figure 10.10 Short sight and its correction.

Old sight (presbyopia)

Over the age of 40, the elasticity of the lens is gradually lost, eventually leaving it in a more-or-less fixed shape suitable only for distance vision. Sufferers of 'old sight' generally use spectacles for reading that have a single converging lens or bifocal lenses.

Astigmatism

Astigmatism occurs if the cornea or lens has an uneven curvature. If so, one part focuses the light too much but another part does not focus the light enough. Usually most of the image seen is out of focus. Special lenses must, therefore, be fitted that counteract this uneven curvature. Soft contact lenses cannot be used, glass or hard plastic must be used instead.

Retina

This is the light-sensitive part of the eye and contains the light-sensitive cells shown in Figure 10.12.

- **Rods:** work in dim light. Their light-sensitive pigment (**rhodopsin**) is broken down (bleached) by light even of low intensity, resulting in an impulse passing to the brain. When a person goes from light to dark conditions it takes some time before they can see clearly. During this time (called **dark adaptation**), rhodopsin that was fully bleached by the bright light is re-synthesised.
- **Cones:** work only in bright light as their pigment (**iodopsin**) is not broken down by dim light. They are found mainly in the **fovea** and allow us to see colour. It is thought that there are three types of cone, each being sensitive only to blue, red or green light. Depending on what type and what ratio of cones are stimulated, the brain interprets impulses from the cones as a colour.

Cataracts and glaucoma

Cataracts occur when the lens becomes opaque or milky with age (Figure 10.11). Nowadays, the opaque lens can be removed surgically and replaced with an artificial one or with a transplant. Sight is therefore restored.

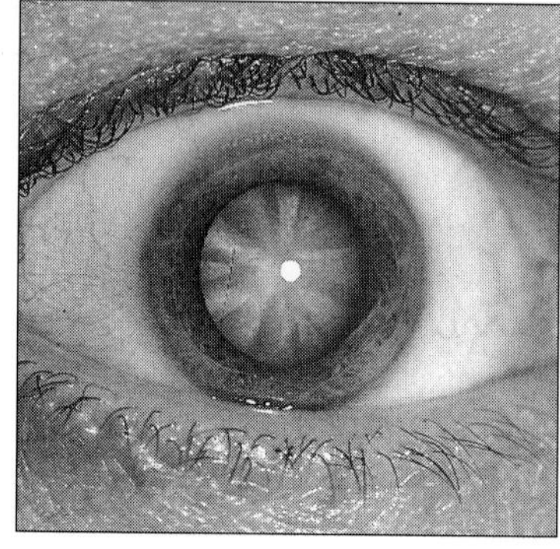

Figure 10.11 Photograph showing cataract.

Glaucoma: If aqueous humour is formed at a greater rate than it is reabsorbed, the pressure inside the eyeball will increase. This requires immediate treatment either by the use of drugs or by an operation to drain the excess fluid. If this does not occur, the pressure can build up and the person may lose the sight in the affected eye.

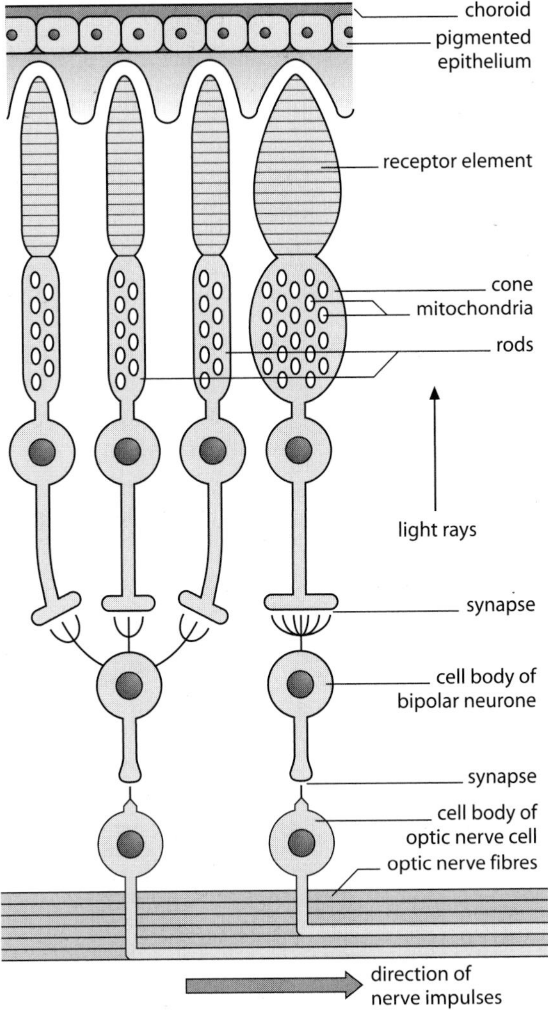

Figure 10.12 Section through the retina.

Q6: What type of neurone will carry impulses from the rods and cones to the brain?

Figure 10.12 shows a number of interesting features of the retina. Firstly, note that light must pass through the neurones before it stimulates the rods and cones.

Also note the way in which rods and cones form synapses with receptor neurones. Several rods synapse with a single receptor neurone. This makes the retina more sensitive to dim light but reduces the detail that can be distinguished in dim light. In contrast, each cone synapses with a single receptor neurone. This enables the retina to distinguish detail more clearly as impulses are sent down different receptor neurones from the different parts of the image.

Binocular vision

Because we have two eyes, our field of vision is greater than if we had a single eye. More importantly, because the fields of vision of the two eyes overlap, much of what we see is seen at a slightly different angle by both eyes (Figure 10.13). This is known as **stereoscopic vision** and enables our brains to judge depth of field (3-D effect).

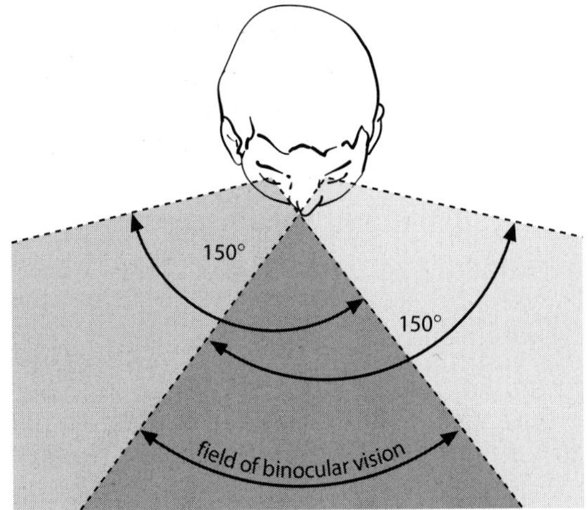

Figure 10.13 Human field of binocular vision.

The ears

Figure 10.14 shows the structures within an ear that enable us to:

- detect sound, i.e. to hear
- detect movements of the head, therefore helping our balance
- detect gravity, therefore helping our balance.

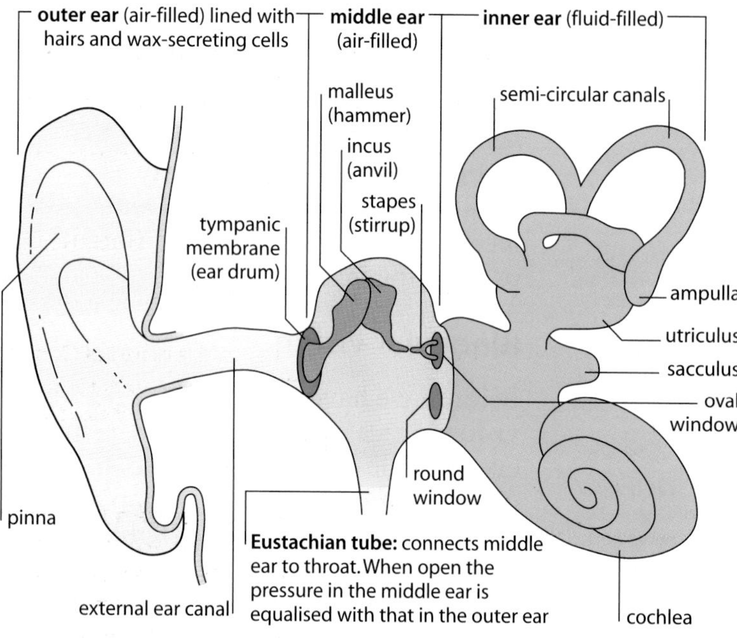

Figure 10.14 VS human ear.

Q7: Using Figure 10.14, name the three ossicles in the correct order from the ear drum to the oval window.

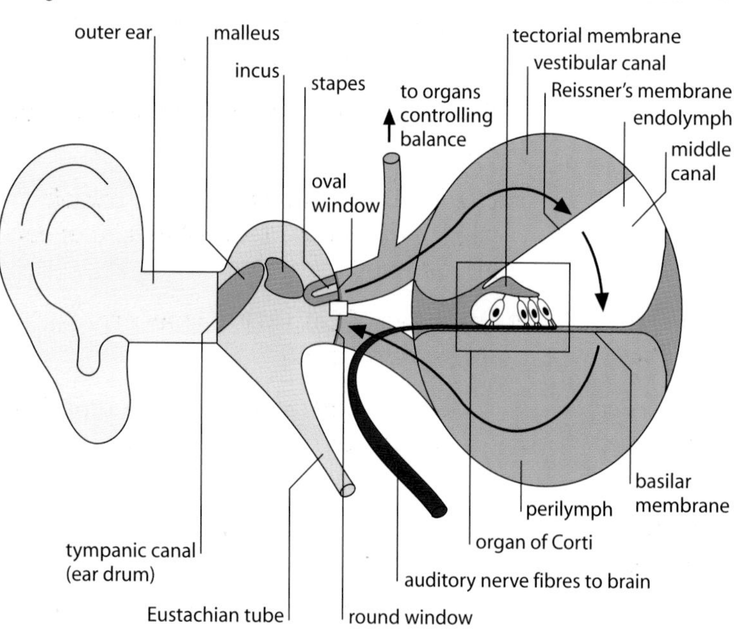

Figure 10.15 Detailed section through the ear.

Hearing

Sound travels through air (or water) as **pressure waves**. When these waves enter the outer ear, they strike the ear drum causing it to vibrate. These vibrations cause the three small bones (**ossicles**) in the middle ear to vibrate.

Vibrations of the ossicles are now passed on to the **oval window**, which vibrates causing vibrations in the **perilymph** (fluid) in the vestibular canal. Eventually these vibrations stimulate a mound of sensory cells in the cochlea called the **organ of Corti**. Figures 10.15 and 10.16 show how this is achieved.

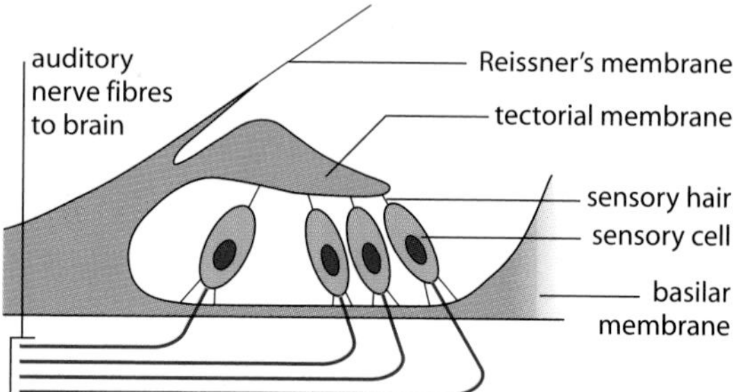

Vibrations cause the basilar membrane to move up and down. This in turn causes the sensory hairs to be alternately crushed and stretched. These movements stimulate the sensory cells which send impulses to the brain along the auditory nerve. The brain interprets these impulses as different types of sound.

Figure 10.16 Section through cochlea showing organ of Corti.

Q8: Suggest how deafness might result if a person were constantly subjected to a loud noise.

Balance

Mounds of sensory cells in the **ampulla** of each semi-circular canal (Figure 10.17) give us our sense of movement. When the head is moved the fluid within the semicircular canals (**endolymph**) moves. This in turn, moves the **cupula** (Figure 10.18), so stimulating neurones that send impulses to the brain. The brain interprets these impulses as movement of the head.

Further mounds of sensory cells in the utriculus give us our sense of gravity. Together these organs stimulate the brain, giving us a sense of balance.

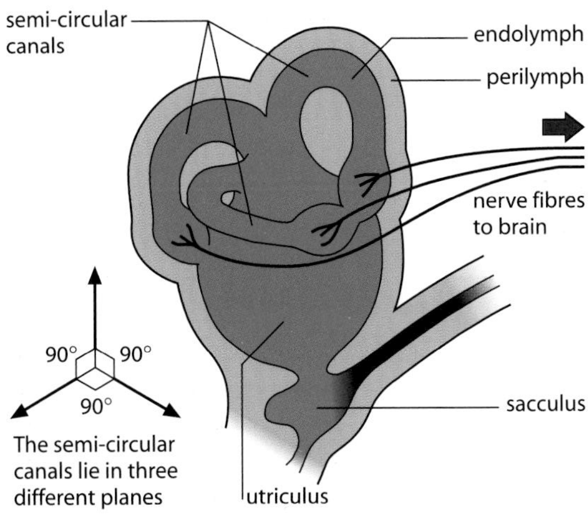

Figure 10.17 Apparatus controlling balance.

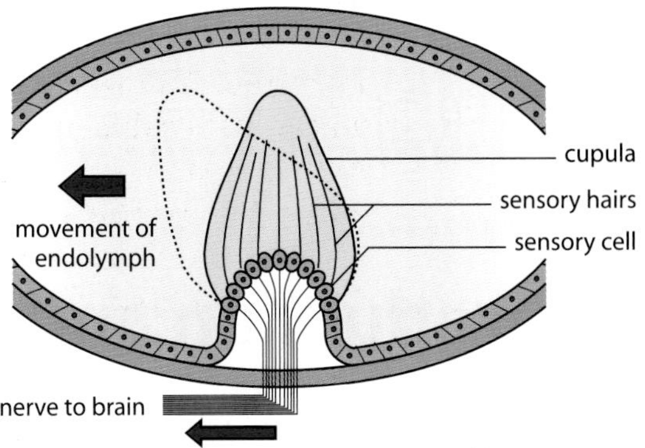

Cupula displaced by movement of endolymph. This pulls on the sensory hairs, stimulating the sensory cells to send impulses along nerve fibres to the brain. The brain interprets these in terms of position.

Figure 10.18 Section through an ampulla.

Loss of hearing

Temporary deafness can be caused by various factors:

- an ear infection may cause fluid to fill the middle ear so that the ear bones do not vibrate properly
- overproduction of wax can block the ear canal, causing hearing to be 'muffled'
- a small child may push a foreign object into the ear canal
- colds may result in the Eustachian tube becoming blocked with mucus. This leads to painful pressure build-up in the middle ear.

Permanent deafness happens as a result of damage to parts of the middle or inner ear:

- in older people the ear bones may become fixed (otosclerosis), so failing to transmit the vibrations. They may be replaced by plastic ones
- damage to the organ of Corti in the cochlea prevents the passage of nerve impulses to the brain.

In some deaf people a hearing aid can be used which either amplifies the sounds, or transmits the vibrations through the skull bones to the cochlea.

Summary

- Many different stimuli are detected by specific receptors in the body.
- Receptors in different parts of the tongue are sensitive to solutions that are sweet, sour, salt or bitter.
- The radial and circular muscles of the iris control the size of the pupil and, therefore, the amount of light entering the eye.
- The cornea and lens refract (bend) light that enters the eye and focus it on the retina.
- Accommodation is the focusing of a near object.
- Defects of the eye include long sight, short sight, old sight and astigmatism.
- The retina is the light-sensitive part of the eye. It contains rods (which work in dim light) and cones (which work in bright light and give us colour vision).
- The ear allows us to hear and gives us our sense of balance.
- The ear is made up of the outer ear (air-filled), middle ear (air-filled) and inner ear (fluid-filled).
- The organ of Corti in the inner ear responds to sound.
- The semi-circular canals and the utriculus help to give us our sense of balance.

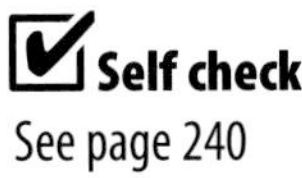
Self check

See page 240

CHAPTER 11

Reproduction and family planning

In this chapter you will learn about the female and male reproductive systems, how women become pregnant, and how couples may choose when to start a family and how many children to have.

The female reproductive system

Once a girl reaches puberty, she starts to release **ova** (eggs) from the **ovaries** in her reproductive system. The structure of the female reproductive system is shown in Figure 11.1. This figure also gives information about the roles played by each of the following structures:

- **vagina**
- **clitoris**
- **cervix**
- **ovaries**
- **oviducts (Fallopian tubes)**
- **uterus (womb)**.

Q1: Why do the vagina and cervix contain muscles?

1 Oviduct (Fallopian tube): narrow tube that carries eggs from the ovary to the uterus

2 Ovary: organ that produces eggs and also female sex hormones

3 Uterus (womb): pear-shaped organ in which a fetus develops during pregnancy

4 Cervix: a ring of muscle at the end of the uterus nearer to the vagina. Allows blood to pass out during periods and sperm to pass through after intercourse

5 Vagina: muscular tube. Very elastic – it can accommodate a penis and, at childbirth, stretches to let the baby out

6 Clitoris: the female equivalent of the penis. When stimulated, for example during sexual intercourse, it can become sexually aroused and stiffen

7 Front of pelvic girdle

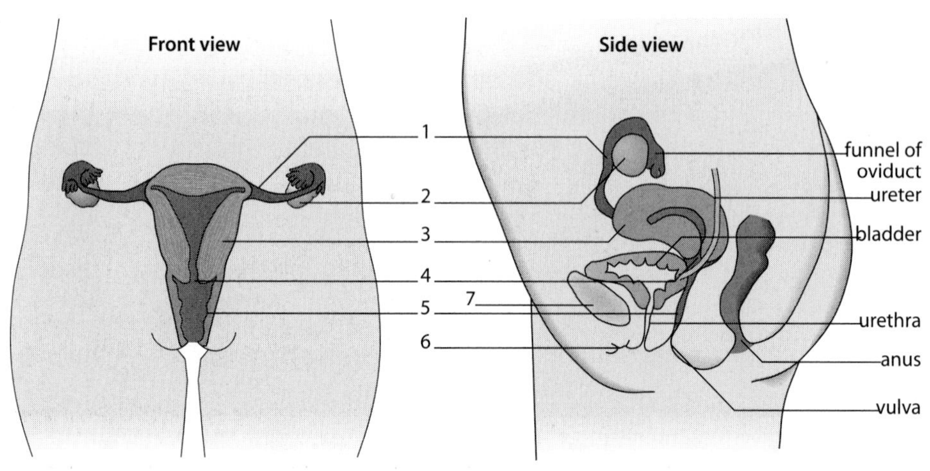

Figure 11.1 The female reproductive system as viewed from the front and side. The side view also shows the urinary system.

1 **Sperm duct:** tube that carries sperm to the penis

2 **Seminal vesicle:** structure that adds secretions to sperm. Sugar is added to provide a source of energy for the sperm

3 **Prostate gland:** another structure that produces secretions such as proteins and salts that are added to the sperm

4 **Urethra:** tube running down the penis. At different times it carries urine or semen

5 **Penis:** the male equivalent of the clitoris. When stimulated, for example during sexual intercourse, it can become sexually aroused and erect

6 **Scrotum:** sac containing the testes. Keeps the temperature of the testes slighly lower than body temperature – essential as sperm cannot survive long at 37°C

7 **Epididymis:** coiled tube in which the sperm mature

8 **Foreskin:** thin skin that covers the end of the penis. Some men have had their foreskin removed. They are said to be circumcised

9 **Testis:** organ that produces sperm and also male sex hormones

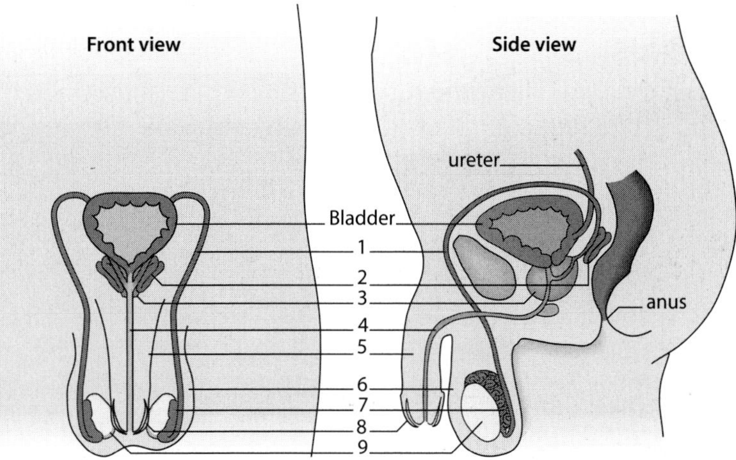

Figure 11.2 The male reproductive system and associated structures as viewed from the front and side. The side view also shows the urinary system.

The male reproductive system

Once a boy reaches puberty, he starts to produce **sperm** from his **testes**. The structure of the male reproductive system is shown in Figure 11.2. This figure also gives information about each of the following structures:

- **scrotum** (also known as the **scrotal sac**)
- **testes** (plural of **testis**)
- **epididymes** (plural of **epididymis**)
- **sperm ducts**
- **seminal vesicles**
- **prostate gland**
- **urethra**
- **penis**
- **foreskin**.

Q2: Distinguish between the functions of the sperm duct, the epididymis and the urethra.

Production of eggs

All the eggs a woman ever has are present in her ovaries at her birth. From the age of puberty an egg is released every four weeks or so, often from one ovary one month and the other the next. Figure 11.3 shows diagrammatically how eggs are produced by the ovaries. Figure 11.4 shows a photograph of a section through a mammalian ovary.

Q3: How many corpora lutea (singular: corpus luteum) are produced for each egg that is released?

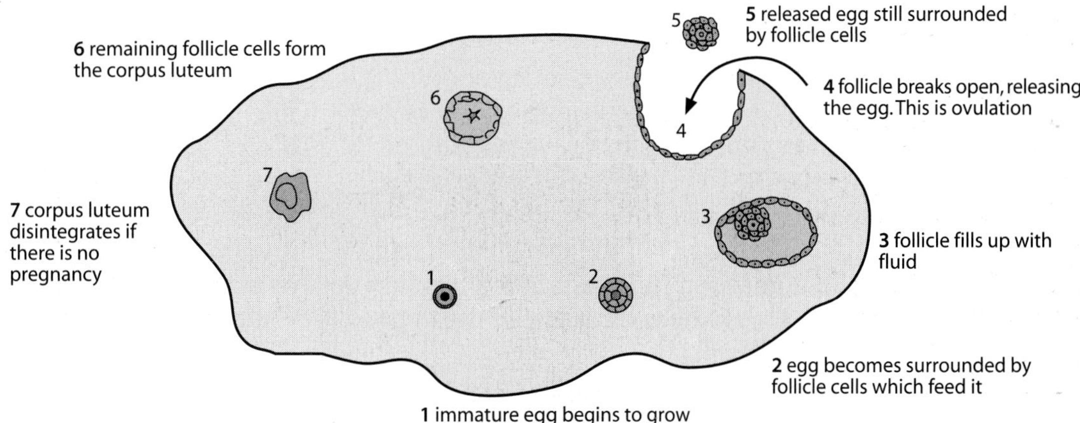

Figure 11.3 The production of eggs in the ovary of a mammal. The various stages have been arranged in order anticlockwise to help you see what is going on. In real life this is not the case.

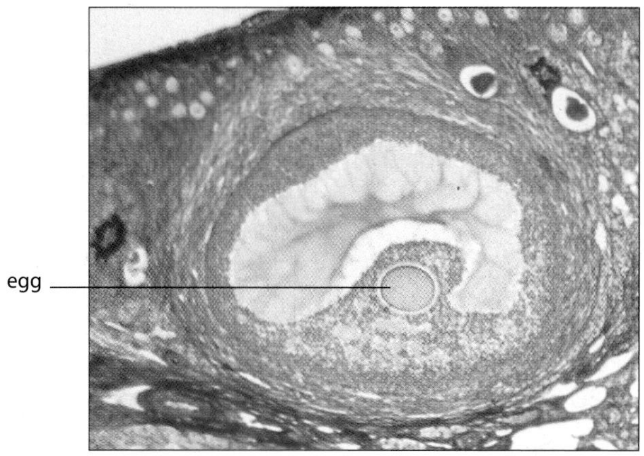

Figure 11.4
A photomicrograph showing a section through a follicle in an ovary. Notice the large egg. Magnification x 50.

Eggs are produced as a result of the type of cell division called meiosis (see page 154). Meiosis results in the formation of **gametes**. In a woman these gametes are eggs. As a result of meiosis each egg contains only 23 chromosomes – the haploid number in humans. This is half the number of chromosomes found in all the human cells that are not gametes.

When an egg is released from the ovary, the woman is said to ovulate. **Ovulation** happens roughly halfway between a woman's periods. The egg enters one of the oviducts. Here it is slowly moved towards the uterus by the action of tiny hair-like cilia, whose regular beating carries the egg along, and by contractions of the muscles in the oviduct. The regular pattern of events in a woman's body from the start of one period to the next is called the **menstrual cycle**.

Practical 11.1 The structure of a mammalian ovary

Requirements
Light microscope
Prepared slide of a mammalian ovary, TS

1 Examine a prepared slide of a mammalian ovary under the low power of a light microscope.

2 Try to identify what you see by consulting Figures 11.3 and 11.4.

3 If possible, find a slide which clearly shows a large egg in a large follicle. This means that the egg was soon due to be released from the ovary. If you can't find such an egg, use Figure 11.4.

4 Work out approximately how large an egg is at around the time it is released from the ovary. (There are a thousand micrometres in one millimetre, so 1000 μm = 1 mm.)

5 Are eggs larger or smaller than other mammalian cells?

Note to students
There are several ways you can work out the size of an object under a light microscope. Consult your teacher/lecturer. You can use an eyepiece graticule and a stage micrometer, or an ordinary ruler marked in millimetres and held on the stage within the field of view. Always make a record of the magnification at which you are working and put a scale on any drawings.

The menstrual cycle

The menstrual cycle is a series of changes that take place in the body of a woman to prepare for the possibility of pregnancy. The cycle itself lasts about a month (typically between 25 and 32 days). The events of the menstrual cycle are summarised in Figure 11.5 which shows the changes throughout the cycle in the following:

- lining of the uterus
- development and release of the egg
- levels of two ovarian hormones **oestrogen** and **progesterone**.

Both oestrogen and progesterone cause the lining of the uterus to develop more blood vessels and thicken. Progesterone also stops ovulation from occurring. If a woman becomes pregnant, her corpus luteum goes on secreting progesterone, so preventing the release of another egg. If the woman does not become pregnant, her progesterone levels decline and the end of one menstrual cycle is followed by the start of another.

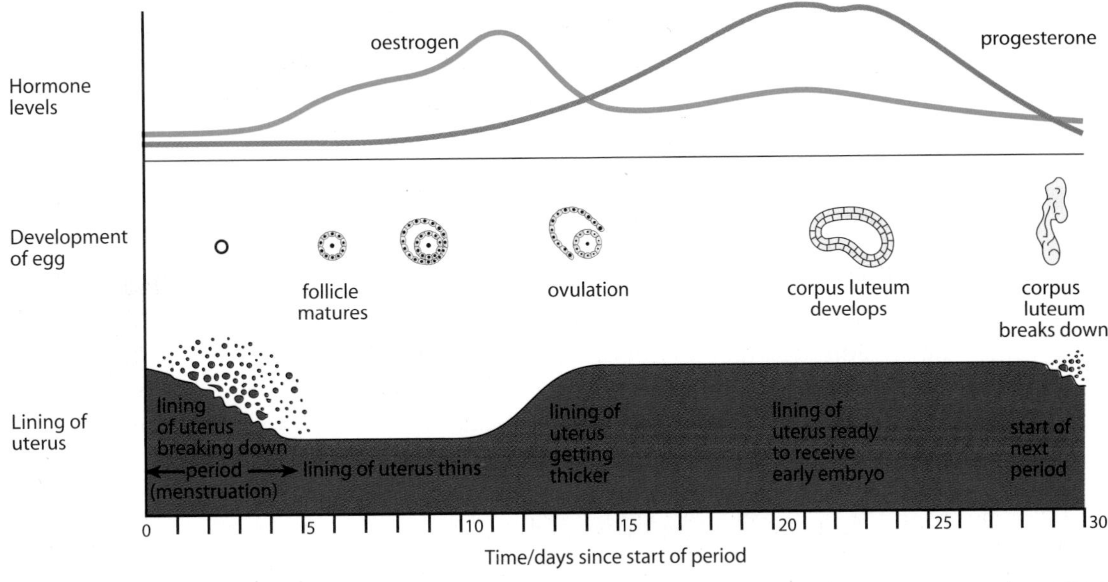

Figure 11.5 The changes that occur during the menstrual cycle. Production of oestrogen and progesterone by the ovaries is due to their stimulation by the hormone FSH which is produced by the pituitary gland. Ovulation itself is triggered by a sudden surge in luteinising hormone (LH), also produced by the pituitary gland.

Q4: What is happening to the levels of oestrogen and progesterone when the lining of the uterus gets thicker during the menstrual cycle?

Q5: What can you say about the levels of oestrogen and progesterone when the lining of the uterus breaks down during the menstrual cycle?

Production of sperm

In males, meiosis results in the production of gametes called **sperm**. Each sperm has 23 chromosomes, just like each egg. From the time of puberty, a man typically produces two or three hundred million sperm each day. Figure 11.6 shows diagrammatically how sperm are produced in the testes and Figure 11.7 shows a photograph of a section through a mammalian testis. Mature sperm are found in the middle of the tubules that are coiled within each testis.

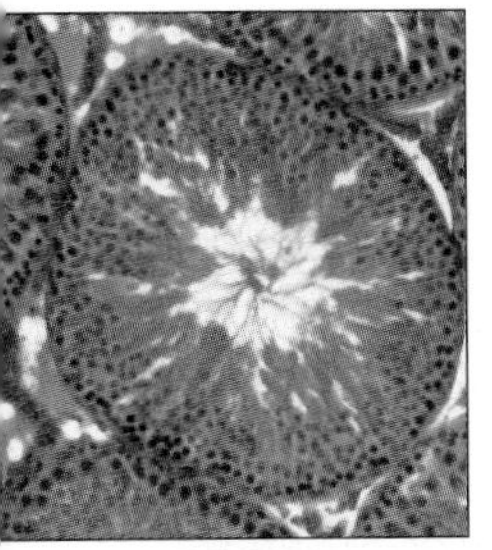

Figure 11.7
A photomicrograph showing a section through part of a mammalian testis.

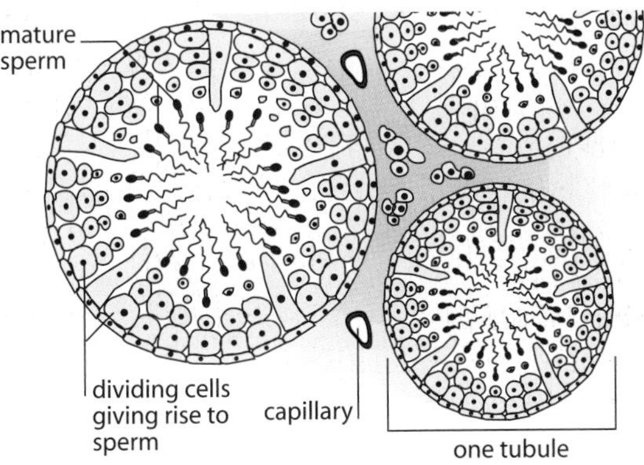

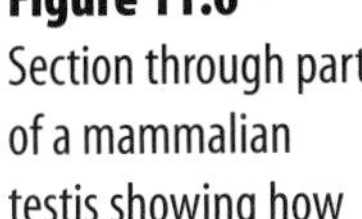

Figure 11.6
Section through part of a mammalian testis showing how sperm are produced.

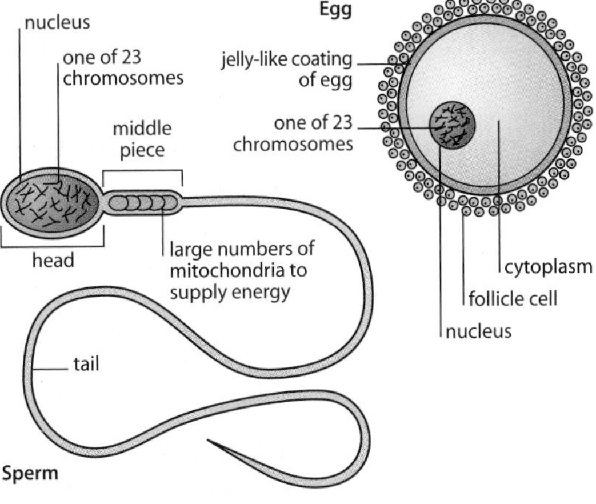

Figure 11.8
Human egg and sperm. These drawings are not to scale; an egg is much larger than a sperm.

Q6: In Figures 11.6 and 11.7, are the sperm that are found in the centres of the tubules mature or immature sperm?

Eggs and sperm differ greatly in size and shape from one another (see Figures 11.8 and 11.11).

Sexual intercourse

For many couples, sexual intercourse is the most intimate way they have of expressing their feelings to one another. However, sexual activity doesn't have to include sexual intercourse. Particularly in the earlier stages of a relationship, it may simply mean hugging or kissing.

Sexual intercourse involves contact between the genitals of two people. So for heterosexuals this means the woman letting the man insert his penis into her vagina. Usually this happens after a period of foreplay in which the couple become sexually aroused through caressing and kissing each other. When a man is sexually aroused, his penis becomes filled with blood and stiffens. When a woman is sexually aroused, her vagina secretes a lubricating fluid and the muscles relax. As a result, the man's erect penis quite easily slides in (see Figure 11.9).

Sexual intercourse generally ends with one or both partners having an orgasm. When a man has an orgasm, semen spurts out of his penis in a process called **ejaculation**. Having an orgasm, whether you are a woman or a man, is usually very satisfying. It is also known as climaxing and you might feel quite sleepy afterwards.

Some people, perhaps around one in twenty, are homosexual. Homosexual women may call themselves lesbians. Homosexual men may call themselves gays. Some lesbians and gays are open about their sexual preferences (see Figure 11.10). Many, though, try and hide the fact for fear of people ridiculing them, discriminating against them or even physically assaulting them.

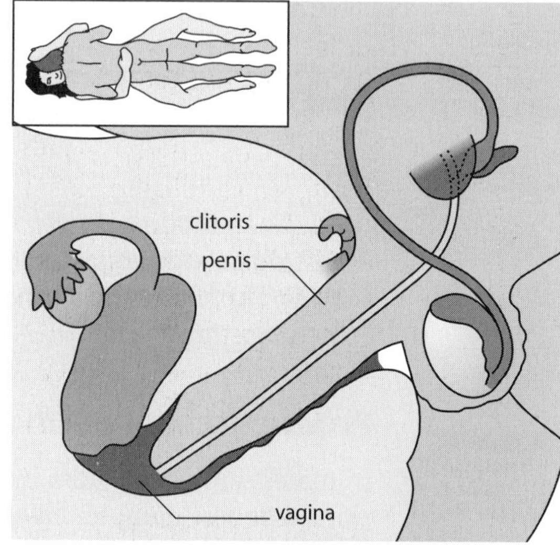

Figure 11.9 There are many positions for sexual intercourse – not all with the male on top!

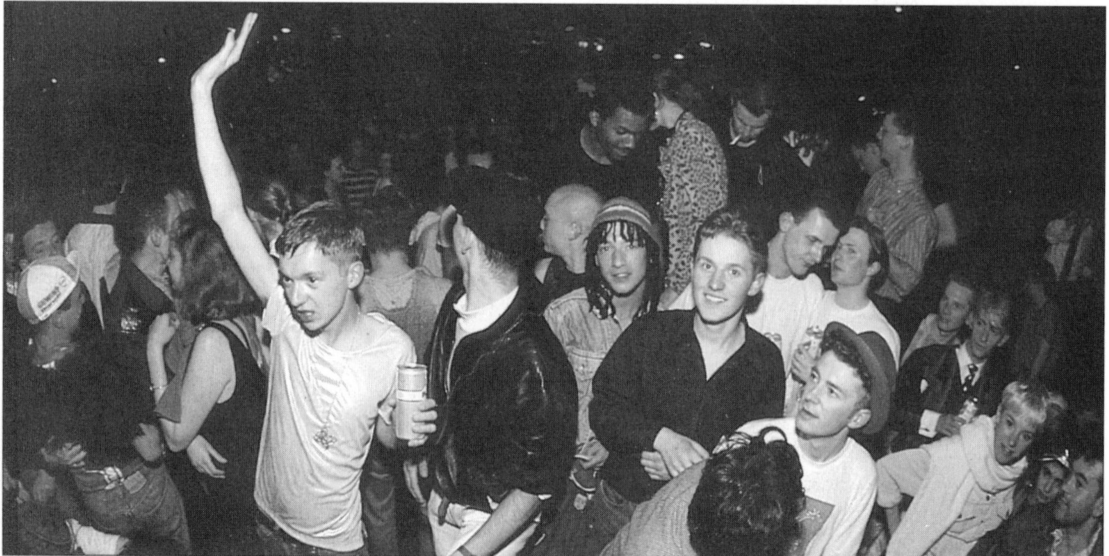

Figure 11.10 Some lesbians and gays are happy for everyone to know about their sexual preferences. Others haven't 'come out', often because they are afraid of what people might say or do to them.

Fertilisation

When a man ejaculates, he only produces about 3 cm^3 of semen. However, this contains some 300 million sperm. **Fertilisation** occurs if one of these sperm gets through the outer layer of the egg (see Figure 11.11). When this happens, the 23 chromosomes of the sperm and the 23 chromosomes of the egg mean that the fertilised egg has 46 chromosomes in all, the usual diploid number. The fertilised cell is called a **zygote**.

Fertilisation takes place in one of the oviducts. There are only two or three days each month when a newly released egg is in its oviduct. These are the days when fertilisation is possible. Another name for fertilisation is **conception**.

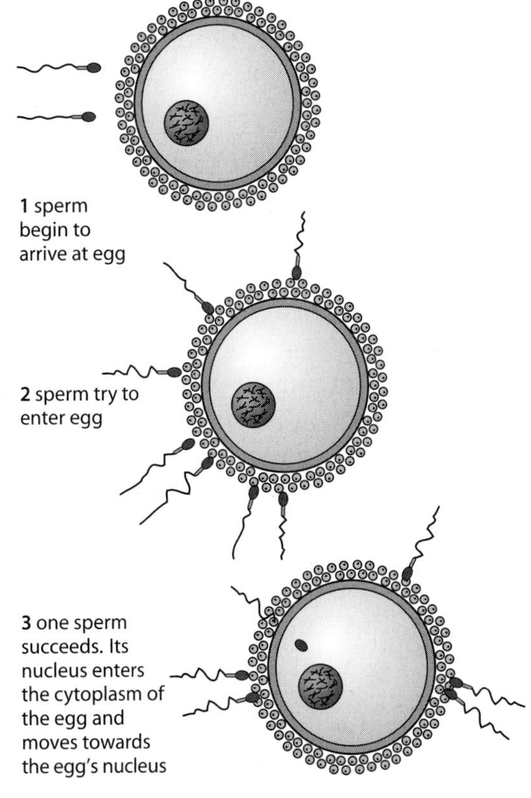

Figure 11.11 Only one sperm manages to get its nucleus past the follicle cells and jelly-like layer of the egg.

Q7: Suppose a particular sperm fertilises an egg. List, in the correct order, the structures through which the sperm passes from where it is produced to where it meets the egg.

Family planning

When a couple take deliberate steps to control the number of children they intend to have, they are practising **family planning**. **Contraception** means the prevention of pregnancy. Exactly when pregnancy starts is a matter of opinion. Some people think it starts as soon as fertilisation occurs. Most people think it starts about a week later when the developing zygote implants into the uterine wall (see page 95).

The following are the various methods of contraception commonly used in the UK.

- **Abstention** – not having sexual intercourse.
- **Withdrawal** – man withdraws his penis from the woman's vagina before he ejaculates.
- **Rhythm method** – woman works out when her fertile period is each month by taking her body temperature and noticing changes in the mucus in her cervix (see Figure 11.12). Couple only has intercourse during the five days after the woman's period has ended or once five days have elapsed from the estimated day of ovulation.
- **Condom** – a thin rubber covering is rolled over the penis of the man before intercourse.
- The **pill** (**combined pill**) – contains the hormones oestrogen and progestogen (an artificial form of progesterone). Prevents ovulation (see Figure 11.13).
- The **pill** (**progestogen-only pill**) – contains progestogen but no oestrogen. Works partly by making the woman's mucus in the cervix thicker, so that the man's sperm can't get through. Also works by preventing a fertilised egg from implanting.

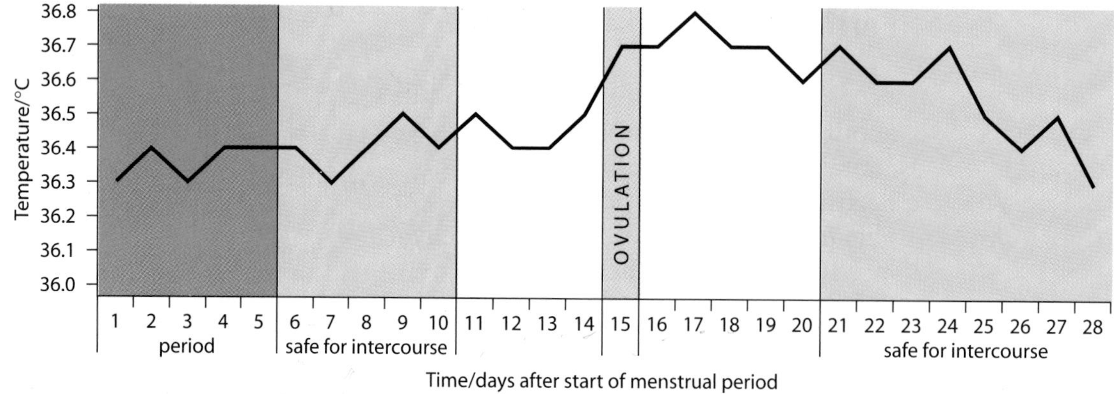

Figure 11.12 The rhythm (or natural) method relies on the woman being able to detect slight changes in her body temperature and cervical mucus. At ovulation the body temperature rises and the mucus becomes thinner (resembling the white of a raw hen's egg). There are also changes in the woman's hormone levels which can be detected by ovulation prediction kits.

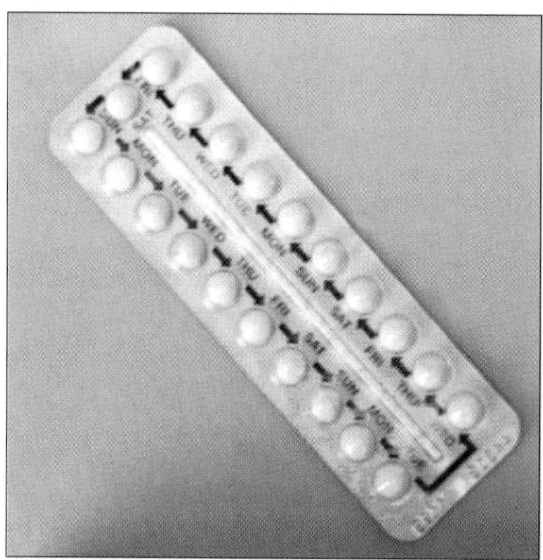

Figure 11.13 The pill has revolutionised the lives of hundreds of millions of women since the 1960s.

- The **intra-uterine device (IUD coil)** – a small piece of plastic that fits in the uterus and prevents a fertilised egg from implanting (see Figure 11.14).

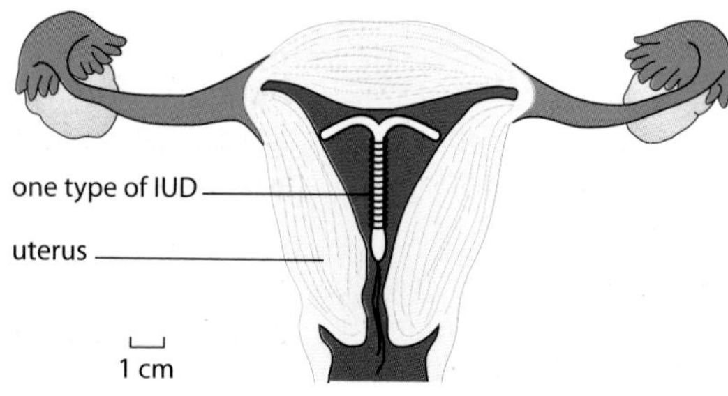

Figure 11.14 An example of an intra-uterine device, showing its position in the uterus once inserted by a doctor.

- The **diaphragm (cap)** – a dome-shaped piece of rubber which covers the entrance to the cervix and prevents sperm from reaching the egg. Used with a spermicidal cream to kill the sperm.
- **Male sterilisation (vasectomy)** – a simple surgical procedure in which the two sperm ducts are cut and tied.
- **Female sterilisation** – a surgical procedure in which the two oviducts are cut and tied.

Q8: Which of the methods of contraception listed operate(s) after conception but before implantation?

The main advantages and disadvantages of these various methods of contraception are listed in Table 11.1 (overleaf). Emergency contraception is also available from a doctor if action is taken quickly. One option is the morning-after (or emergency) pill. This must be taken within three days of unprotected intercourse. The second option is to have an IUD fitted within five days of unprotected intercourse.

Q9: Abortion isn't usually described as a method of contraception, even though it is a form of birth control. Why is this?

Table 11.1 Advantages and disadvantages of the main methods of contraception

Method	Advantages and disadvantages
Abstention	Completely effective but you may miss out on a lot of life
Withdrawal	Very ineffective and somewhat frustrating
Rhythm method	Quite effective but requires a lot of practice; approved by the Roman Catholic Church unlike the other methods below
Condom	Very effective if used carefully; need to have condoms to hand; some couples like them because they can make it take longer before the man ejaculates; other couples find they take away some of the spontaneity of love-making
Combined pill	Very effective provided the woman doesn't forget to take it each day; often reduces period pains; can cause high blood pressure or other medical conditions in some women
Progestogen-only pill	Very effective provided woman doesn't forget to take it each day at the same time
Intra-uterine device	Very effective; needs to be fitted by a doctor
Diaphragm	Very effective; needs to be inserted before sexual intercourse and removed about six hours later; needs to be obtained from a doctor or family planning clinic
Male sterilisation (vasectomy)	Very effective; only needs to be done once but usually irreversible
Female sterilisation	Very effective; only needs to be done once but usually irreversible

In vitro fertilisation

In vitro **fertilisation** occurs when an egg is fertilised by a sperm outside a woman's body. The technique was developed in the late 1970s to help certain infertile couples. For example, even though a woman produces eggs normally and has a healthy uterus, she may be unable to conceive. This could happen if her oviducts have become damaged so that they are unable to carry the fertilised egg into the uterus.

The procedure is as follows.

- A sample of semen is obtained from the father-to-be.
- The woman is given hormone-based drugs to increase the number of eggs she will produce at ovulation.
- Two or three eggs are removed from the woman under anaesthetic just a few hours before they would normally be ovulated.
- The eggs and semen are mixed in a small Petri dish.
- The fertilised eggs are left to develop into young embryos in an incubator at 37°C for two to three days (see Figure 11.15).
- One or more of the embryos are transferred to the uterus in the hope that they implant.
- Hopefully, nine months later one or more healthy babies is born.

If a couple are unable to have children because of problems with the man's sperm, the woman may benefit from **artificial insemination**. Sperm from a donor male is collected and then inserted into her uterus at ovulation.

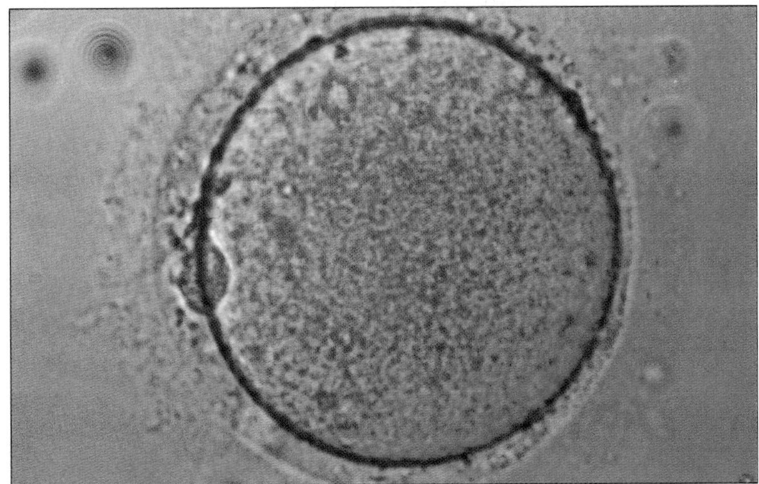

Figure 11.15 In *in vitro* fertilisation a woman's eggs are fertilised outside her body in the laboratory and then transferred to her uterus. The success rate of the technique is improving steadily, but in 1995 was still only about 25% per treatment.

Sex and the law

There are a number of laws in the UK relating to sexual behaviour. The most important are as follows.

- The age of consent (the age at which you may legally have sexual intercourse) is 16 in the case of heterosexual intercourse and 18 in the case of homosexual intercourse between two men. (Lesbianism is not covered by the law.) If you have sexual intercourse with someone under the age of consent you are breaking the law, even if the other person gives their consent.
- Child sexual abuse, sexual harassment, indecent assault, obscene telephone calls and rape (whether out of marriage or within marriage) are all against the law. Any such offence should be reported to the police. Nowadays the police have trained counsellors and you can chose whether to speak to a male or a female about what has happened.
- An abortion is legal up to the 26th week of pregnancy provided there is some risk to the mental or physical health of the mother or offspring.

Useful addresses:

- British Pregnancy Advisory Service (BPAS), Austy Manor, Wootton Wawen, Solihull, B95 6BX. Tel: 0121 643 1461
- Family Planning Association (FPA), 27–35 Mortimer Street, London W1N 7RJ. Tel: 0171 636 7866
- Brook Advisory Centres, 233 Tottenham Court Road, London W1P 9AE. Tel: 0171 580 2991
- Rape Crisis Centre, PO Box 69, London WC1X 9NJ. Tel: 0171 837 1600
- The Gay and Lesbian Switchboard. Tel: 0171 837 7324.

Summary

- The ovaries in a woman's reproductive system produce eggs (ova), each containing 23 chromosomes. Between puberty and the menopause a woman, unless she is pregnant, breast-feeding or very unwell, typically releases one egg every 28 days or so.
- The menstrual cycle is a series of changes that take place in the body of a woman to prepare for the possibility of pregnancy. If a fertilised egg fails to implant, levels of oestrogen and progesterone are low and a period results.
- The testes in a man's reproductive system produce sperm with 23 chromosomes.
- Sexual intercourse involves contact between the genitals of two people. Usually this happens after a time of foreplay. Sexual intercourse generally ends with one or both partners having an orgasm.
- Most people are sexually attracted to members of the other sex (heterosexual attraction). Around one in twenty people are only attracted sexually to members of their own sex (homosexual attraction).
- Fertilisation occurs if a sperm succeeds in penetrating an egg. The fertilised cell is called a zygote.
- Contraception means the prevention of pregnancy. Contraception may be achieved by a number of different methods including the rhythm method, condom, pill, IUD, diaphragm, vasectomy and female sterilisation. Each method has advantages and disadvantages.
- *In vitro* fertilisation occurs when an egg is fertilised by a sperm outside a woman's body. The technique can help some infertile couples to have children.
- Sexual behaviour is regulated by a number of laws designed to protect people from exploitation and harm.

Self check

See page 241

CHAPTER 12

Pregnancy and birth

In this chapter you will learn how a fertilised human egg can develop into a newborn baby. We will examine how a woman's body is able to support the developing child within her, and look at the events surrounding childbirth.

Implantation

Fertilisation takes place in one of the two oviducts. When an egg is fertilised, the cell that results has 46 chromosomes – 23 from the egg and 23 from the sperm. During the next six days or so the fertilised egg is slowly moved down the oviduct, dividing first into two cells (Figure 12.1), then into four cells and then into a ball of cells. Once it reaches the uterus it settles into the lining of the uterus, a process called **implantation** (see Figure 12.2).

Q1: Are the cell divisions that give rise to the ball of cells mitosis or meiosis?

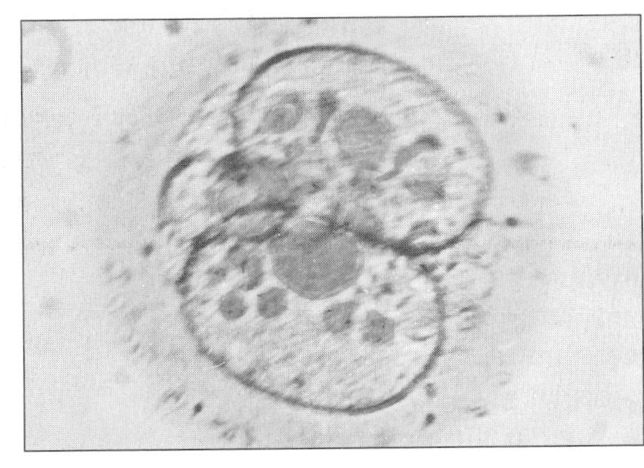

Figure 12.1 Thirty six hours after conception the fertilised egg divides for the first time. Two genetically identical cells result.

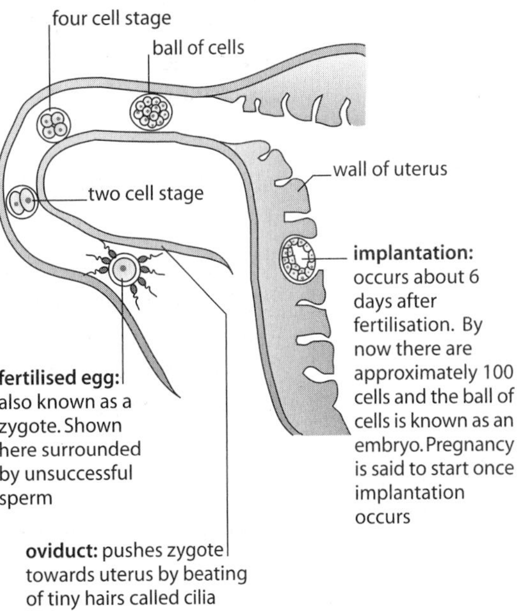

Figure 12.2 The events between fertilisation and implantation.

Pregnancy

Once implantation has happened the woman is said to be **pregnant**. The ball of cells implanted in the lining of her uterus is called an **embryo**. During pregnancy, the embryo greatly increases in size and complexity.

The main stages in the development into a baby ready to be born at the end of pregnancy are summarised as follows.

- One month after fertilisation a human embryo looks a bit like a fish embryo or tadpole (Figure 12.3). The embryo doesn't yet have arms or legs but it is clear where these will develop.

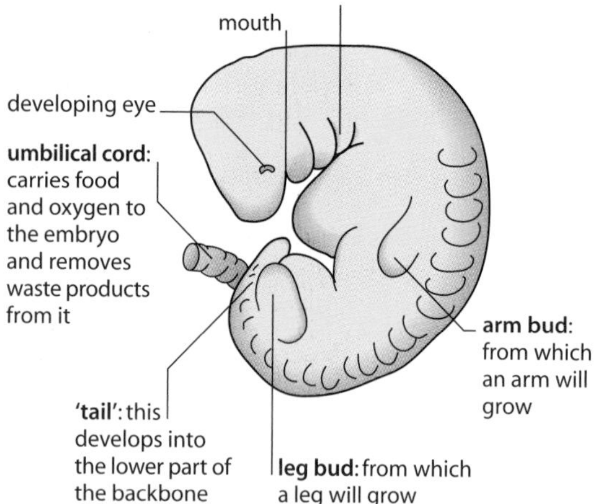

Figure 12.3 Embryo one month after fertilisation.

Q2: One month after fertilisation the embryo is about 4 mm in length. What is the magnification of Figure 12.3?

- Two months after fertilisation the embryo looks much more human. It is now called a **fetus.** It is about 45 mm in length. Most of the organs are formed and the heart is beating.
- Three months after fertilisation the nerves and muscles of the fetus are developing rapidly (Figure 12.4). The fetus is about 90 mm in length.
- Five months after fertilisation the fetus, though only about 180 mm in length, has perfectly formed eyebrows, fingernails, fingerprints and body hair. Its movements may have been felt by the mother for the last month.
- Seven months after fertilisation development is almost complete. Although there are still two months of pregnancy to go, there is a good chance of survival if there is a premature birth (Figure 12.5).

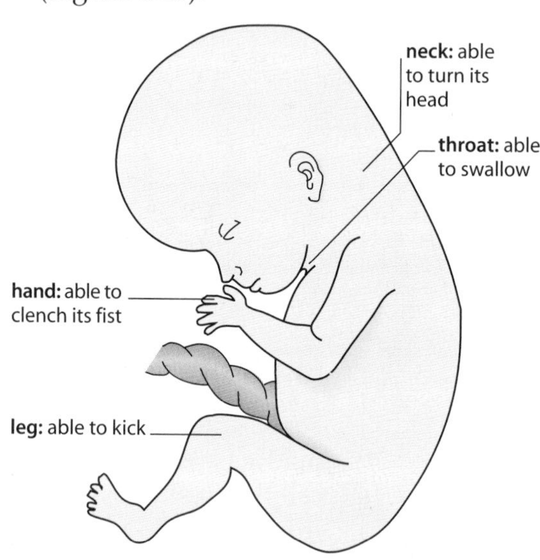

Figure 12.4 Fetus three months after fertilisation.

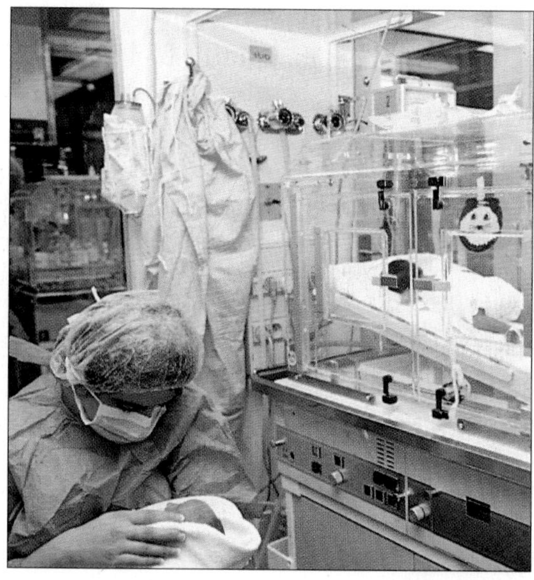

Figure 12.5 Nowadays many countries have specialised equipment to help babies born prematurely. Any baby with a mass of less than 2.5 kg at birth is defined as premature. Premature babies often have problems in keeping warm, breathing and sucking.

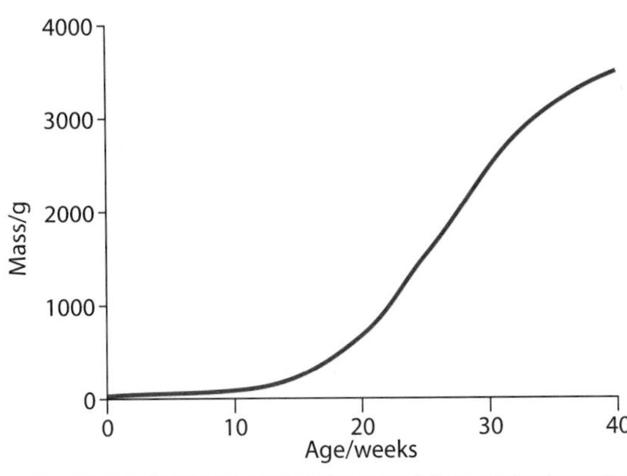

Figure 12.6 The growth curve of a typical fetus from conception to birth.

1 deoxygenated blood: eventually returns to the mother's heart to be oxygenated and receives food substances from the mother's hepatic portal vein

2 oxygenated blood: from the mother; also rich in sugars, amino acids, vitamins and antibodies

lining of uterus

capillary network of placenta

3 vein in umbilical cord: carries oxygenated blood and useful substances such as glucose and amino acids from the placenta to the fetus. Fetal blood contains a special type of haemoglobin called fetal haemoglobin. Fetal haemoglobin is better at picking up oxygen than normal haemoglobin. As a result oxygen molecules diffuse from the mother's red blood cells to the red blood cells of the fetus

4 blood space in uterus: contains the mother's blood. This comes very close to the fetus' blood but does not actually mix with it

5 umbilical cord: connecting the fetus to the placenta

6 artery in umbilical cord: carries deoxygenated blood and waste products such as urea from the fetus to the placenta

fetus

Figure 12.7 Structure of the placenta and umbilical cord. As the placenta develops it secretes a hormone called gonadotrophin. This causes the ovaries to continue to secrete oestrogen and progesterone. As a result, the lining of the uterus wall is maintained during pregnancy and production of FSH by the pituitary gland is inhibited. This ensures that ovulation does not occur during pregnancy.

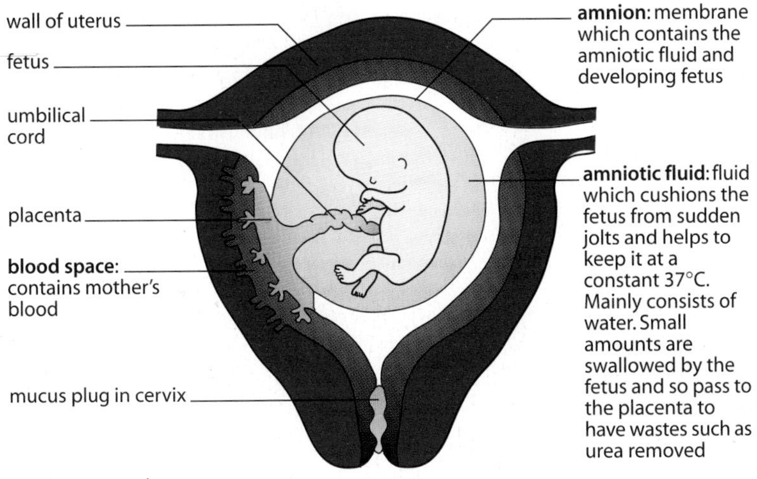

Figure 12.8 The fetus in its womb some eight weeks into pregnancy.

During pregnancy the fetus increases in mass enormously. At conception an egg weighs only a fraction of a gram. Most newborn babies have a mass of between 3 and 4 kg (7–9 lbs). Figure 12.6 shows how most mass is put on between weeks 16 and 36. A full pregnancy lasts, on average, some 38 weeks from conception to birth (equal to 40 weeks from the end of the previous menstruation to birth).

Q3: By what factor does the mass of the fetus increase between weeks 16 and 36?

The role of the placenta

As soon as the embryo implants into the lining of the uterus, some of the cells of the embryo, together with cells from the mother, form the **placenta**. The structure of the placenta a few months into pregnancy is shown in Figure 12.7. Note that the blood of the mother and fetus never actually mix, though they come very close to each other. This is because the mother and fetus are genetically different. The blood of the fetus and the blood of the mother often belong to different blood groups. When this is the case, the fetus might die if its blood mixed with that of its mother (see page 31).

Q4: By what process do you think oxygen moves into the capillary network in the placenta from the mother's blood?

Q5: By what process do you think urea moves from the fetus' blood to the mother's blood in the capillaries of the placenta?

Q6: Why are the fetus and its mother genetically different?

The relationship between the developing fetus, the placenta and the other structures in the uterus are shown in Figure 12.8. Note how the fetus is cushioned in **amniotic fluid**.

The needs of the mother and fetus

During pregnancy it helps if the woman's partner, family and friends are around, so as to provide both practical and emotional support. Many women find pregnancy deeply satisfying. Nevertheless pregnancy makes very considerable physical and mental demands on the mother. These may (but don't necessarily) include:

- nausea (feeling sick) as a result of 'morning sickness' caused by hormonal changes – especially in the early months of pregnancy
- tender breasts
- tiredness
- backache – most women put on around 12 kg during the pregnancy
- frequent visits to the toilet – due to pressure on her bladder from the enlarged womb
- a loss of sexual drive
- worries over money and the additional demands that a baby may make.

During her pregnancy a woman should go regularly to an **antenatal clinic**. Here a number of tests will be carried out during her pregnancy to check her health and that of the developing fetus.

What happens at an antenatal clinic?

A woman can expect the following things to happen at her antenatal clinic.

- She will be asked about her medical record, general health and personal circumstances.
- Her weight will be measured on each visit. After the first three months of pregnancy she can expect to put on between about 400 and 500 g per week as a result of her pregnancy. This is due to the increasing mass of the fetus, her growing uterus, the placenta, amniotic fluid and umbilical cord, and to fat reserves that may build up in anticipation of **lactation** (milk production).
- Her blood pressure will be taken regularly to check that it isn't too high. Too high a blood pressure may indicate that the mother's body is failing to cope with the extra demands made on it due to the pregnancy. This can result in a build up of proteins and waste substances in her blood. This condition is known as **toxaemia** which can be dangerous, or even fatal, for both mother and fetus if it is not treated.
- An internal examination of her vagina and cervix will be made to see that she has no infections such as thrush (a fungal condition). A **cervical smear** is taken to check whether the early stages of cervical cancer can be detected.
- Blood tests will be taken to see that she has enough haemoglobin and isn't developing **anaemia**. These tests also allow the woman's blood group to be noted, in case she needs an emergency blood transfusion. A doctor will also check to see that the woman has antibodies to German measles. She should have these antibodies as a result of the rubella injection given to practically all girls when aged about 12 years.
- Urine tests will be taken to see if sugar or proteins are present. Sugar may indicate diabetes while proteins suggest that the kidneys are not working normally and can indicate toxaemia.
- **Ultrasound scans** may be taken later in pregnancy. These allow the mother and the person operating the ultrasound scan to see the developing fetus (Figure 12.9). The fetus can be checked to see that its heart is beating normally and that there are no physical abnormalities. The sex of the baby can sometimes be identified, though many parents prefer to find this out only at the birth itself.

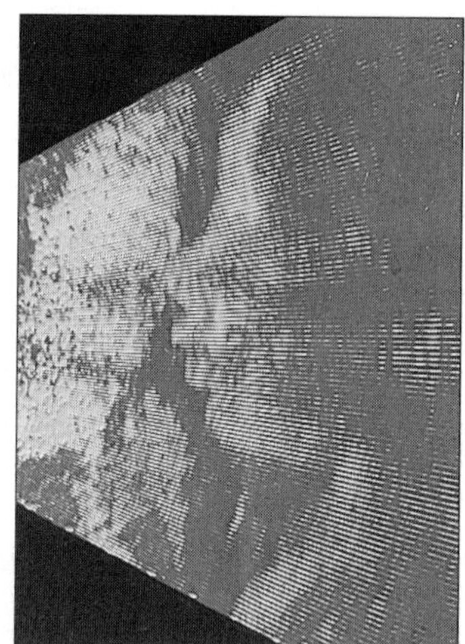

Figure 12.9 This ultrasound scan shows a healthy fetus 30 weeks into pregnancy. How many structures can you identify?

Q7: What effect would you expect anaemia in a mother to have on her fetus?

Birth

By the end of pregnancy the baby normally lies in the womb with its head towards the woman's vagina (Figure 12.10). The events that surround and include the birth can be divided into a number of stages. Together they are called **labour** – for reasons which are clear to any mother.

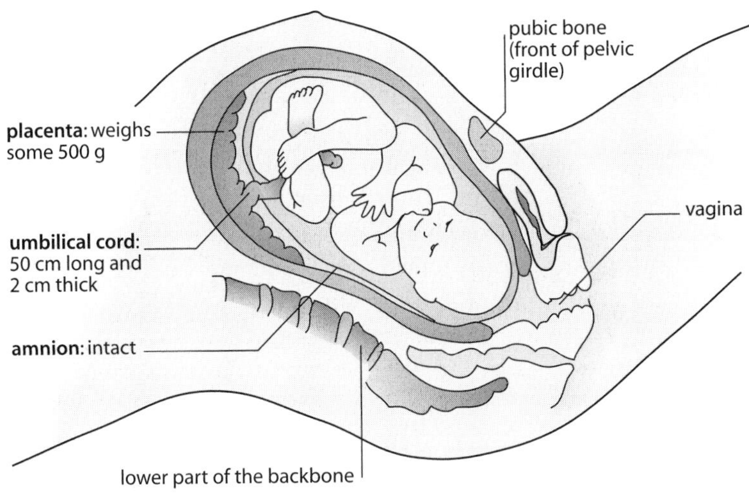

Figure 12.10 An early stage in labour.

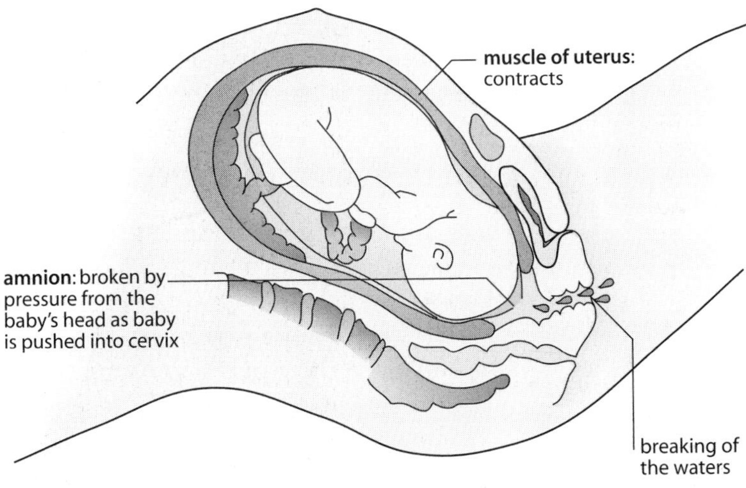

Figure 12.11 A later stage in labour after the amnion has broken.

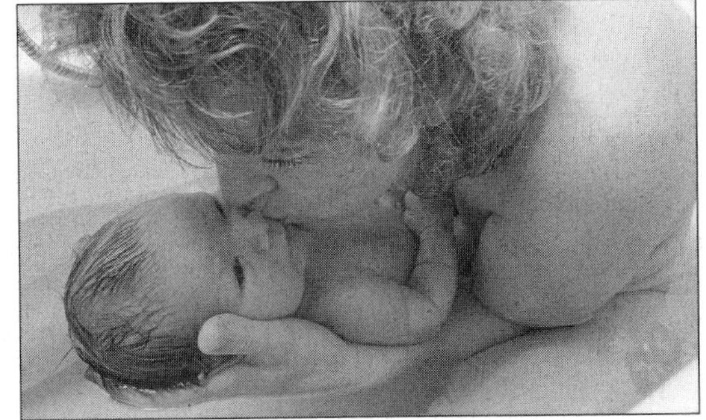

Figure 12.12 A mother cuddling her newborn baby a few minutes after delivery, which took place in a birthing pool.

First stage of labour

Labour begins when the mother feels the first **contractions**. These are the muscular contractions of the wall of her uterus. Eventually they will push the baby out through the vagina. At first they come approximately every 20 minutes. Later they become more frequent and are very intense. Contractions are caused by secretion of the hormone **oxytocin** from the mother's pituitary gland. At some point in labour the amnion breaks and the amniotic fluid is released. This is known as the **breaking of the waters** (Figure 12.11). During labour the cervix gradually dilates (becomes wider). The first stage of labour comes to an end once the cervix has dilated enough for the baby's head to begin to pass through. This is typically within 4–12 hours of the first contractions starting.

Delivery

The second stage of labour begins as the baby's head is pushed out of the cervix into the vagina. The uterus, cervix and vagina together now form a continuous **birth canal**. Strong contractions continue to push the baby along and within 10–60 minutes the baby's head emerges from the birth canal. The rest of the baby's body follows within minutes, helped by a **midwife** (a nurse who specialises in births) or **obstetrician** (a doctor who specialises in births).

Babies can get quite short of oxygen as they pass out through the birth canal. The skin of white babies may look bluish immediately after birth. A few breaths of air, often accompanied by cries, soon oxygenate the blood sufficiently for the red blood cells to develop their usual reddish colour (due to the presence of oxyhaemoglobin). Once the baby is breathing, the umbilical cord is clamped in two places (to prevent subsequent bleeding) and the cord between these clamps is cut. Mother and child are now two separate individuals (Figure 12.12).

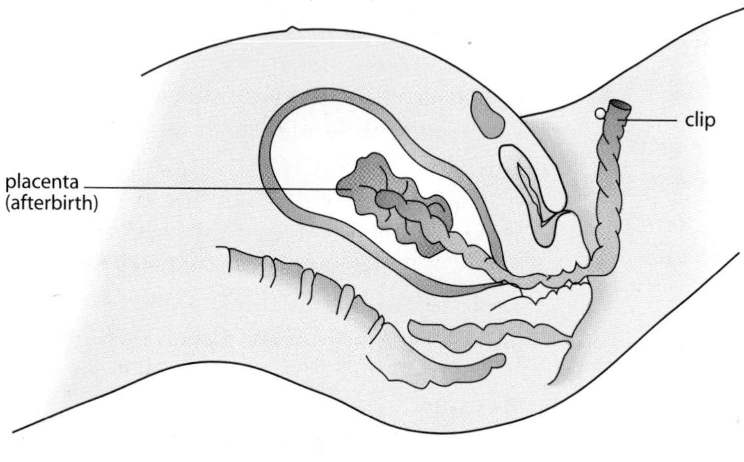

Figure 12.13 The final stage in labour is when the afterbirth emerges.

Afterbirth

Contractions of the muscular wall of the uterus continue after delivery and the placenta and umbilical cord are soon pushed out of the vagina (Figure 12.13).

Q8: Where is the umbilical cord attached on the fetus?

Complications at the end of pregnancy

Various things can happen to mean that the birth isn't quite as straightforward as we have indicated so far.

Breech birth

If the baby's bottom or feet emerge first the baby is said to be in the **breech position**. If detected early enough, a midwife or obstetrician may be able to turn the baby around so that it is born head first, as normal. If not, labour might take longer than usual. This could endanger the baby, so forceps may be used or a Caesarean section performed.

Forceps delivery

Forceps can be used to turn the baby around or help ease the baby out of the uterus if the mother's contractions are rather weak. Nowadays forceps are used less often than was once the case. This is because there is a slight risk that they might damage the baby's head.

Caesarean section

This is a surgical procedure in which the baby is 'born' through a cut in the mother's abdominal wall and uterus. It can be used when too long a pregnancy is thought risky for the health of the mother or baby. The mother is given an anaesthetic and needs to stay in hospital longer than usual until she has recovered.

Induction

This is when labour is started artificially, either by cutting the amnion – so releasing the amniotic fluid – or by giving the mother an injection of the hormone oxytocin to induce (start) the contractions. A baby may be induced if the health of the mother or baby is at risk or if the birth is overdue by more than a week or two.

Birth defects

The great majority – around 97% – of all babies are born strong and healthy. Sometimes, though, this is not the case. **Birth defects** may have genetic or environmental causes or both.

Genetic causes of birth defects

There are many genetic causes of birth defects. Some of the more common are as follows.

- **Down's syndrome** is when the baby has an extra copy of chromosome 21. This means that it has 47 chromosomes, instead of the usual 46, in each of its cells. People with Down's syndrome have almond-shaped eyes and a roundish face. They generally have severe learning difficulties and a reduced life expectancy. The older a couple are, the more likely they are to have a child with Down's syndrome. The mother's age is more significant than the father's.
- **Sickle cell anaemia** is a disease in which a person's blood is less efficient at carrying oxygen. Under the

microscope the person's red blood cells have a characteristic shape (see page 180). Life expectancy is often significantly reduced.

- **Cystic fibrosis** is a disease in which the person's lungs produce a very sticky mucus (see page 165). Life expectancy is significantly reduced though tremendous medical advances have been made in recent years in the treatment of cystic fibrosis. A nasal spray has been developed using genetic engineering and is helping to alleviate symptoms.

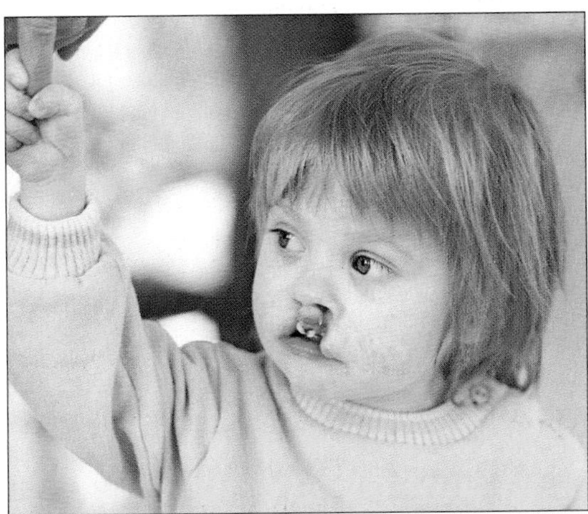

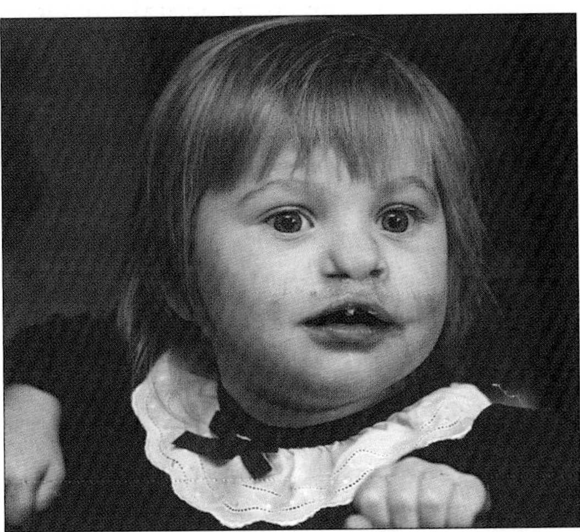

Figure 12.14 Top: A child with a cleft palate – an environmentally caused birth defect.**Bottom:** The same child after a successful operation to correct the condition.

Environmental causes of birth defects

Some of the more common environmentally caused birth defects are as follows.

- **Spina bifida** is a condition in which part of the spinal cord protrudes through (sticks out of) the vertebral column. The condition varies greatly in its severity: some people with spina bifida are paralysed; others lead normal, independent lives.
- The effects of a **cleft palate** can be seen in Figure 12.14 (Top). Figure 12.14 (Bottom) shows the same child after a successful operation to correct the condition.
- **Cigarette smoking** can have a serious effect on the fetus. If either parent smokes, especially the mother, the baby is likely to have a significantly reduced birthweight, to suffer more respiratory tract infections during its early life and to have a higher risk of dying from a cot death.
- If a mother drinks too much alcohol during pregnancy, her baby may be born with **fetal alcohol syndrome**. Such a baby has characteristic facial features and is likely to be significantly less intelligent than would otherwise have been the case.

To help ensure that both the woman and her fetus are as healthy as possible, a pregnant woman will be encouraged to:

- eat well and look after herself. Supplements of folic acid and other vitamins may be recommended as these are needed in extra amounts
- avoid cigarettes, illegal drugs and unnecessary medication (some medical drugs can be dangerous for an unborn child), and limit alcohol intake
- get enough exercise
- get enough rest and sleep
- go to **antenatal classes**.

Multiple births

Unlike most animals, humans normally only give birth to one offspring at a time. **Multiple births** are when two or more babies are born at the same time. Most multiple births are **twins**, when two babies are born together. However, **triplets** sometimes occur and, even more rarely, four, five or six children may be born together.

Two sorts of twins occur.

Monozygotic twins

Here just one zygote is involved. The twins result from the fertilisation of one egg by one sperm. However, for some reason, the zygote divides into two separate balls of cells before it implants. The two twins may share a placenta or may each have their own. Monozygotic twins are genetically identical and so are also known as **identical twins** (Figure 12.15a).

Dizygotic twins

Here two separate zygotes are involved. For some reason the mother releases two eggs from her ovary at the same time and both are fertilised, each by a different sperm. The two twins have separate placentas. Dizygotic twins are no more closely genetically related to each other than are normal siblings (brothers and sisters). For this reason dizygotic twins are known as **non-identical twins**.

Q9: Can monozygotic twins be of different sex? Explain your answer.

Q10: What is the chance of a pair of dizygotic twins being of the same sex?

Women who have difficulty ovulating can be given hormonal treatment to help them conceive. In the early days of such treatment (1970s and 1980s) the women sometimes produced as many as five or six eggs at once. Consequently as many as half a dozen embryos might result. The trouble with this was that the babies that were eventually born tended to be extremely underweight, sometimes weighing as little as 1–2 kg. As a result infant mortality was extremely high, and the babies that survived were sometimes very ill. Nowadays techniques have improved, so that women receiving these sorts of **fertility drugs**, or benefiting from *in vitro* fertilisation (page 93), only give birth to one or two babies at a time.

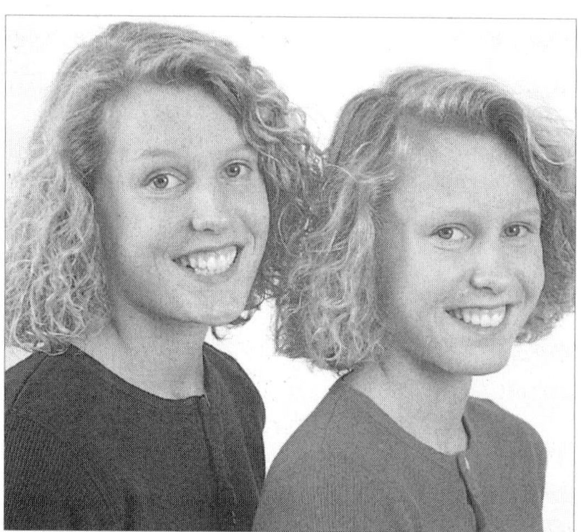

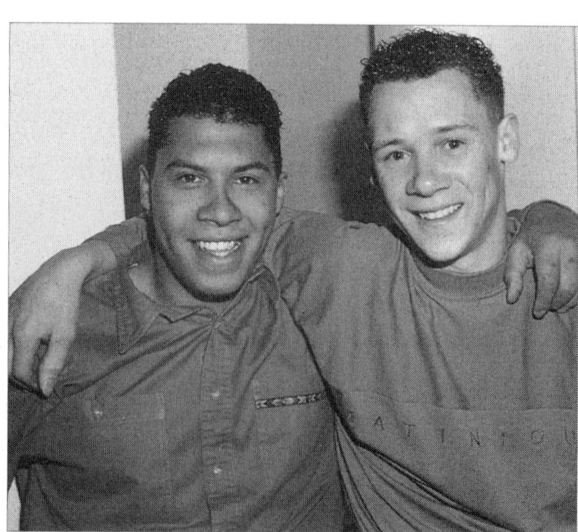

Figure 12.15 a) Identical twins not only look very similar, but often have similar personalities and behave like each other. **b)** Non-identical twins.

Checking for genetic abnormalities in the fetus

There are two main ways in which the fetus may be checked for genetic abnormalities early in pregnancy.

- In **amniocentesis** a sample of the amniotic fluid is taken about 14 to 16 weeks into pregnancy. Amniotic fluid contains cells from the fetus. After being grown in culture for three to four weeks, these cells can be tested for certain genetic abnormalities.
- In a more recent technique called **chorionic villi sampling**, a sample from the placenta is taken about 8 to 10 weeks into pregnancy. The sample can be tested within a couple of days to reveal the presence of certain genetic abnormalities.

In both amniocentesis and chorionic villi sampling, there is a small risk (about 0.5 to 2%) of the fetus being harmed or of a miscarriage resulting. In addition, neither technique can be used to help the fetus if it is found to be suffering from a genetic abnormality.

For these reasons the two techniques tend only to be offered to pregnant women where there is a significant chance that the fetus may be affected by a genetic abnormality. This might be because the mother is over the age of about 35 (as older women are more likely to give birth to children with Down's syndrome) or because a family member is already known to be affected by a serious genetic disorder such as cystic fibrosis.

Genetic counselling

Suppose a couple have had a child with cystic fibrosis and want to know the chances of another child of theirs having this condition. The couple can go to a **genetic counsellor**. Genetic counsellors need to have a good understanding of human genetics, to be able to explain things clearly and to help people make up their own minds. A woman may go to a genetic counsellor having had the results of a test such as amniocentesis. For example, she might know that if her child is born it will have Down's syndrome. The genetic counsellor will explore all the medical and legal options with her, which may include termination of the pregnancy (**abortion**).

Summary

- Implantation is when the ball of cells that results from fertilisation settles into the lining of the uterus at the beginning of pregnancy.
- From fertilisation to birth is typically about 38 weeks. During this time an embryo, later called a fetus, increases greatly in mass and develops all the different human tissues and organs.
- Most newborn babies have a mass of between 3 and 4 kg.
- The placenta is formed from cells from the embryo and cells from the mother.
- The placenta provides the embryo/fetus with oxygen, food and antibodies. It removes carbon dioxide and other waste products such as urea.
- The developing embryo/fetus is surrounded by amniotic fluid enclosed in the amnion.
- The health of a woman and her fetus can be monitored at an antenatal clinic.
- Labour starts with contractions of the uterus, caused by secretion of the hormone oxytocin, and the breaking of the waters. It ends with the expulsion of the afterbirth.
- Some 3% of babies are born with birth defects. These may be genetic or environmental in origin.
- Multiple births can result either from the release of more than one egg at a time, or from the division of a single zygote into two or more separate balls of cells before implantation.
- The possibility of genetic abnormalities in the fetus can be tested by amniocentesis or chorionic villi sampling.

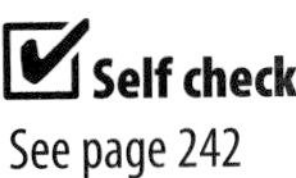

See page 242

CHAPTER 13

Childhood to old age

In this chapter you will learn how people grow and develop from the time they are born through childhood and puberty to adulthood and, eventually, old age and death.

Growth and development

Growth can be defined as an irreversible increase in the dry mass of an organism. The word 'irreversible' is included because, for example, we wouldn't want to include the small amount of weight one puts on during a meal as an example of growth. **Development** means a regular change in the structure and functioning of an organism as it ages. There are four main aspects to development:

- physical
- mental
- emotional
- social.

Growth and development are closely linked. Of the two, growth is easier to measure – you simply need to record a person's height or mass over the years. To measure a person's development, you need to record changes in such things as:

- **anatomy** – for example, have a baby's milk teeth started to come through the gums?
- **behaviour** – for example, can a baby walk unaided?
- **mental abilities** – for example, how large a vocabulary does a child have?

The first careful attempt to record the growth of a person was carried out by a Frenchman, Count Montbeillard, between the birth of his son in 1759 and his son's 18th birthday. The data are shown in Figure 13.1. At first sight this figure may not look very helpful. But now look at Figure 13.2. This shows the same data but this time instead of showing the boy's height each year, it shows how much the boy grew each year. The following four parts of the curve can clearly be distinguished:

- the boy's height increased most during the first couple of years of life – he grew over 20 cm in the first year of life
- between the ages of 3 and 13 the boy grew rather little, about 5 or 6 cm a year
- around the ages of 14 and 15 years-old, the boy put on a growth spurt, growing over 10 cm a year
- after the age of 15 the boy grew less and less each year.

Q1: What do you think caused the growth spurt around the age of 14–15 years?

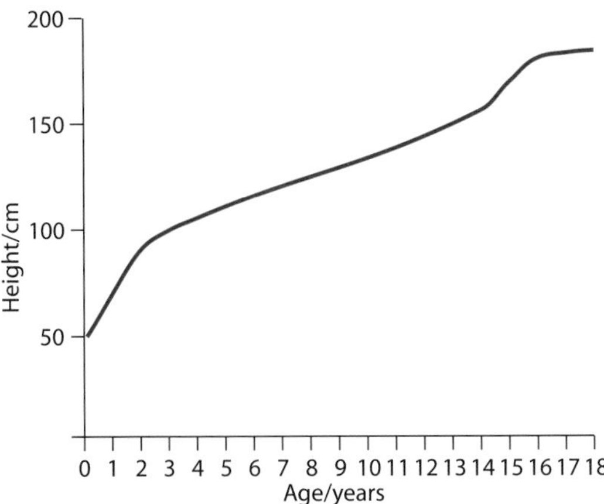

Figure 13.1 The height of Count Montbeillard's son from his birth in 1759 until he was aged 18 years.

Q2: The data shown in Figure 13.1 and 13.2 show postnatal (after birth) growth. By how much did the boy grow during the 38 weeks of pregnancy? Convert this to height gained per year. What do you notice about this figure?

There are two main differences between the growth curves of males and females.

- On average girls reach puberty, with an accompanying growth spurt, a couple of years before boys do. Puberty is typically around 10–14 years for girls in the UK compared with 12–16 years for boys.
- Boys have a bigger growth spurt at puberty than do girls. The result is that men are typically taller and heavier than women by the time both sexes have more or less finished their growth (around 18–20 years).

These two differences can be seen in Figure 13.3. Notice that girls are often taller than boys at the age of 12 or 13.

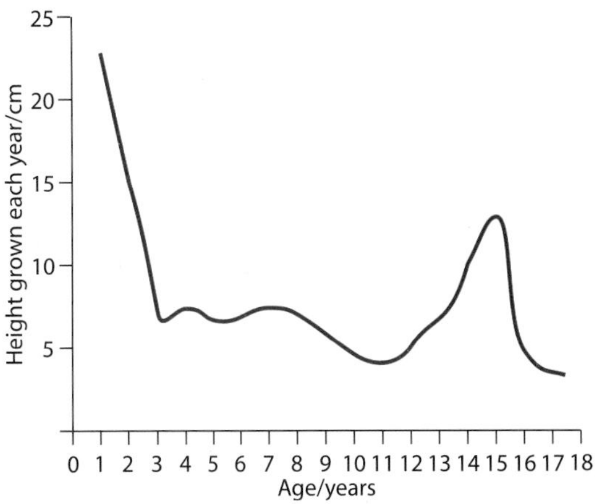

Figure 13.2 The gain in height, in cm, of Count Montbeillard's son each year.

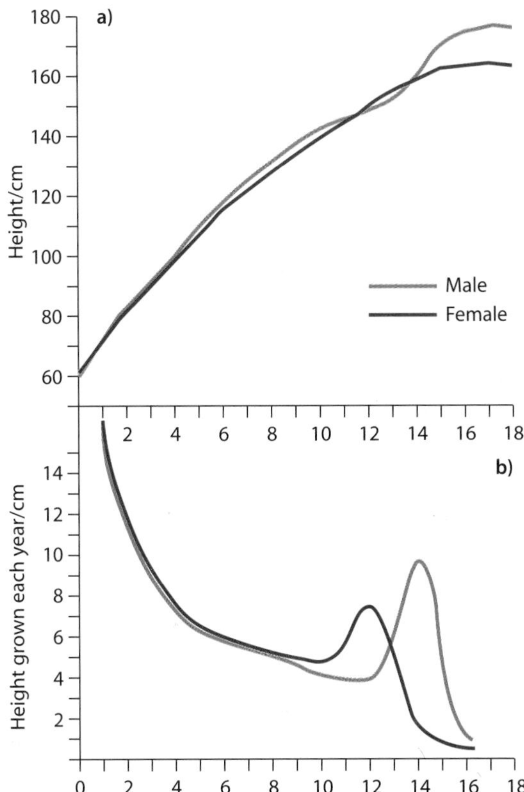
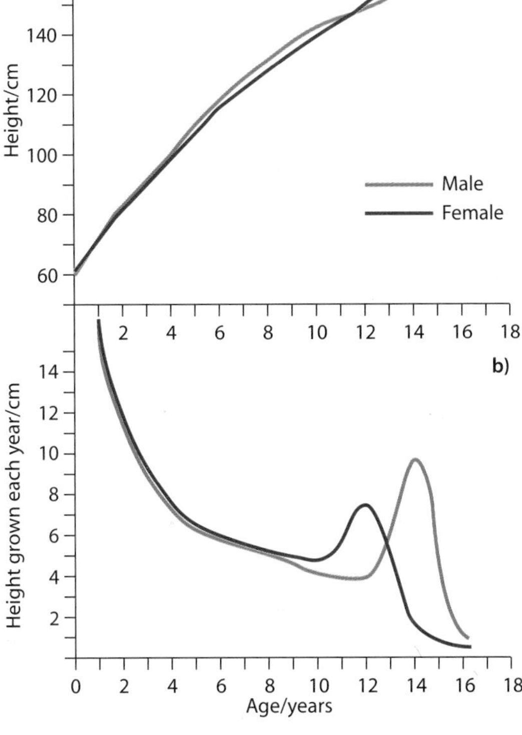

Figure 13.3 Growth curves for typical males and females. **a)** Height against age. **b)** Annual height gain against age.

Milk production

One of the defining characteristics of mammals is that adult females produce milk after their young are born. In humans, milk production begins within a couple of days of a baby being born. This is a result of the hormone **prolactin**. Prolactin is secreted by the pituitary gland once the baby is born. In the first few days after the birth of her child, before normal milk production has become established, a mother's breasts produce a yellowish, watery fluid called **colostrum**. Colostrum is of great value because it contains antibodies which help protect the baby against infections.

Between them, colostrum and breast milk are an ideal food for a baby for the first 4 to 9 months of its life. Of course, breast-feeding isn't essential for a baby's health. However, most studies suggest that if they are breast-fed, babies grow better, suffer from fewer diseases, cry less and form emotional bonds with their mothers more easily. Unfortunately, society doesn't always make it very easy for a mother to breast-feed her baby. Some people disapprove of breast-feeding in public. What do you think?

Childhood

Childhood can be defined as the period from birth to puberty. It can be considered as a number of overlapping stages.

From birth to our first birthday each of us is a **baby**. Many developmental changes take place in these 12 months:

- within a few days of birth most babies can recognise their mothers by their smell
- by three months of age a baby smiles a lot and reacts to different people in different ways
- by six months of age a baby can make a variety of different sounds, plays with objects and can sit up, if helped
- by their first birthday most babies are beginning to walk, can say a few words and understand some of what they hear.

From about the age of one to two we are **toddlers**. During this year most toddlers:

- learn to walk independently
- begin to feed themselves (Figure 13.4).
- start to show a preference for their left or right hand
- start toilet training
- may have temper tantrums
- begin to string words together into short sentences
- start to draw.

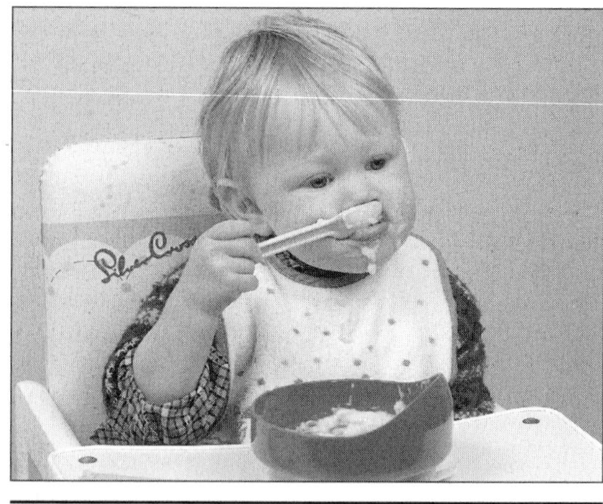

Figure 13.4 This little girl is learning to feed herself – often a very messy process for a young child!

By the time they are five, most children:

- can go to the toilet on their own
- enjoy playing with other children
- know their address
- are ready to go to school.

Between the age of 5 and puberty, developmental changes are more difficult to summarise, but include the following:

- an increase in vocabulary and powers of expression
- the development of insight into what other people think or feel
- an ability to think abstractly using ideas such as probability and concepts such as justice, truth and honesty.

Puberty

The period of time during which a person's sex organs (**genitals**) mature is called **puberty**. Puberty is the time at which we become able to have children. In a female it means that her periods (**menstruation**) start. In a male it means that he becomes able to ejaculate sperm.

When a girl starts to menstruate, her periods may be irregular, possibly occurring only once every few months. Within a year or two they tend to settle down, each typically lasting about 4 to 7 days. During periods, most women use either **tampons** (worn inside the vagina) or **sanitary towels** (worn outside the vagina) to absorb the blood that results from menstrual bleeding. Many women find that in the days or week before menstruation they suffer from **pre-menstrual tension (PMT)**. PMT is a result of the hormonal changes that occur before menstruation. Symptoms may include:

- headaches
- irritability
- weight gain due to fluid retention
- sore breasts.

If the symptoms of PMT are severe, it is worth seeing a doctor. Further details of the menstrual cycle and of sperm production are given on pages 88–89. The average age at which girls have their first period is shown in Figure 13.5. Notice how, in a number of different countries, it has fallen over the last 150 years.

Q3: Between 1860 and 1960, by how many years did the average age at which girls in northern Europe had their first period decrease?

Q4: Suggest why the average age at which girls have their first period has fallen considerably over the last 150 years.

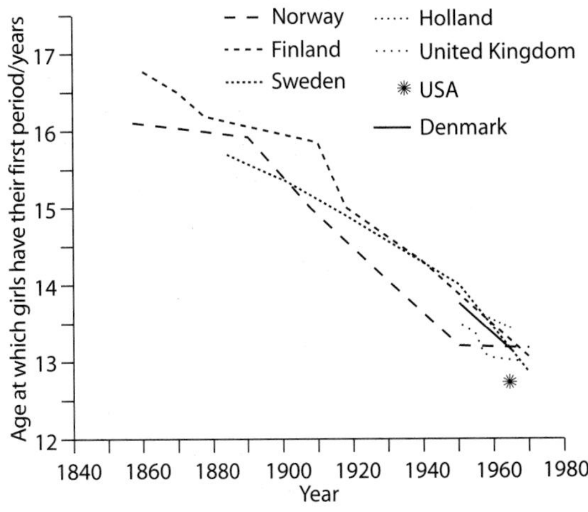

Figure 13.5 The age at which girls, on average, have their first period in various countries over the last 150 years.

Puberty is also the time when **secondary sexual characteristics** develop. Secondary sexual characteristics include such things as:

- growth of pubic hair (in both sexes)
- growth of breasts (in a female)
- widening of the hips (in a female)
- deepening of the voice (in a male)
- growth of facial hair (in a male).

In a female the events of puberty are triggered by the production of the hormone **oestrogen** by the ovaries. In a male the events of puberty are triggered by the production of the hormone **testosterone** by the testes.

The main physical changes that accompany puberty are summarised in Figures 13.6 and 13.7. During puberty muscular strength increases in males more so than in females (Figure 13.8). What Figures 13.6, 13.7 and 13.8 do not show you are the emotional changes that can occur at this time, during **adolescence** – 'the teenage years'. These emotional changes vary from person to person but may include:

- a belief that no-one, certainly not parents/guardians, has any idea how awful life can be
- worries about spots and about every other aspect of appearance, including clothes and friends (or lack of them)
- family rows as teenagers begin increasingly to exert their independence perhaps through such things as staying out late, wearing what they want to wear, or deciding that certain activities are beneath them.

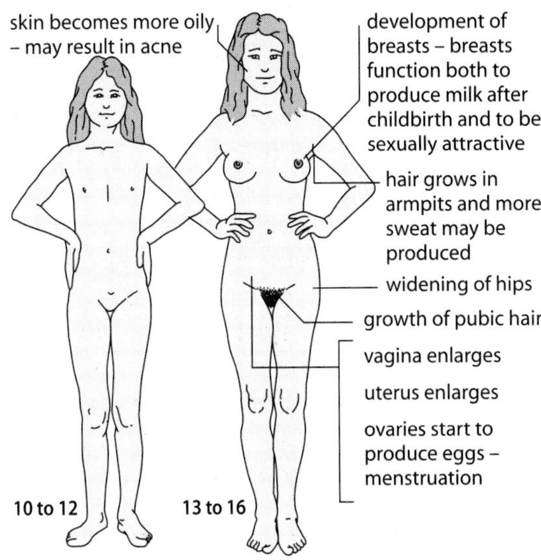

Figure 13.6 Changes in a girl's body at puberty.

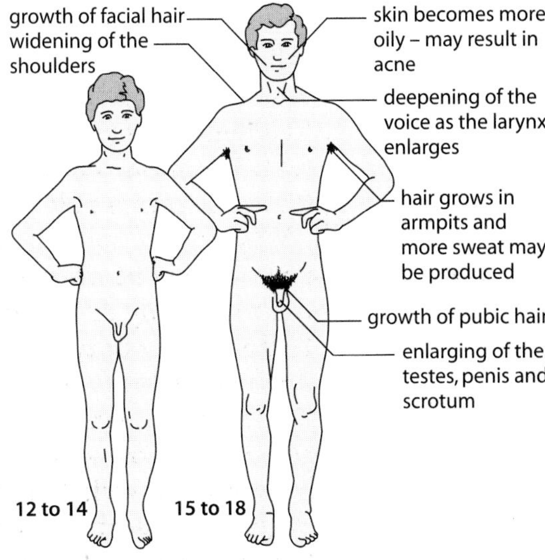

Figure 13.7 Changes in a boy's body at puberty.

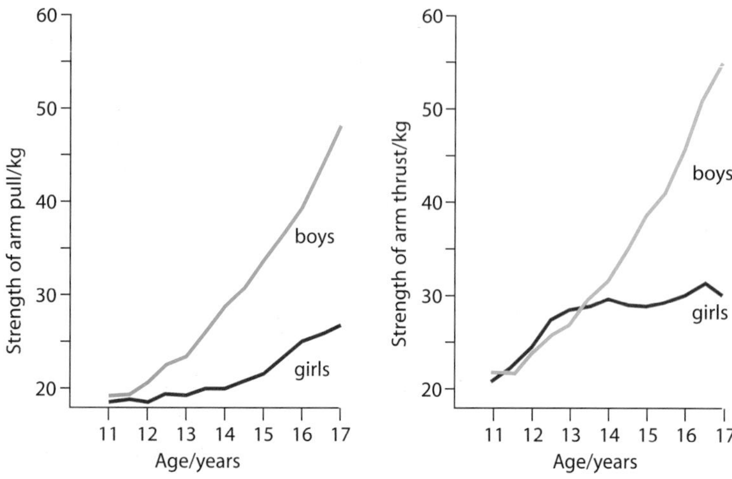

Figure 13.8 During adolescence boys usually become significantly stronger than girls.

Of course, people's experiences at adolescence vary greatly. At one extreme may be the person, usually female, who is sexually abused by a family member or 'friend' of the family. For some people life can simply not seem worth living. On the other hand, the great majority of people emerge from adolescence with:

- a better sense of their own identity
- hopes (and worries) about what life may have ahead of them
- a realisation that from now on life is largely their own responsibility now that they have embarked on adulthood.

Adulthood

Humans take longer to reach adulthood than any other animal. It is difficult to define precisely when we reach adulthood but it is more or less when:

- our physical growth and development are complete
- we are capable of living independently of our parents/guardians
- our formal education has largely come to an end.

As we grow towards adulthood, we don't just get taller and heavier. We also change in shape. Look at the outlines drawn in Figure 13.9. Although they have been drawn so that they are the same size, it is immediately obvious that these outlines show people of increasing age from left to right. As we get older our heads, though still becoming *absolutely* larger, become *relatively* smaller; that is, they form a smaller proportion of our overall bodies.

Figure 13.9 Drawings to show the typical body proportions, from left to right, of a male aged zero (i.e. newborn), two, six, twelve and twenty-five years.

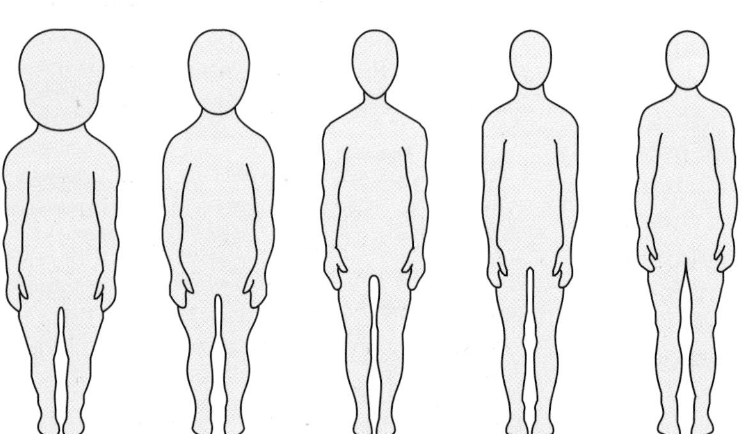

Q5: From Figure 13.9 work out (a) what percentage of a new born baby's height is due to its head; (b) what percentage of an adult man's height is due to his head.

It's not just our heads that change in size relative to the rest of our bodies. Figure 13.10 shows how each of the following grow from birth (defined as zero growth) to adulthood (defined as 100% growth):

- lymphoid system (thymus, lymph nodes and tonsils)
- brain, head and nervous system
- general (e.g. arms, legs, trunk)
- reproductive system (ovaries, oviducts, testes, epididymes, seminal vesicles).

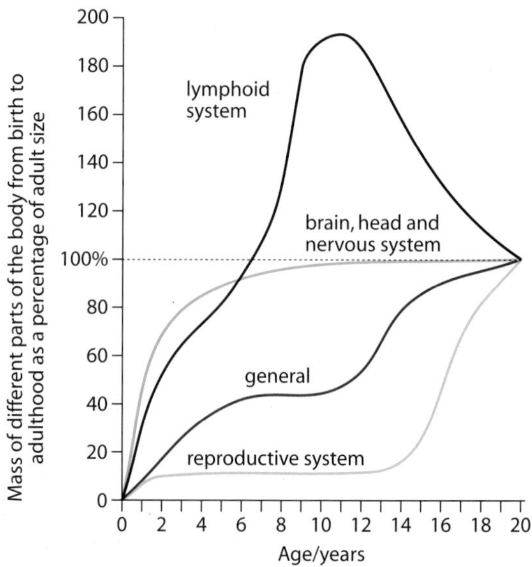

Figure 13.10 Growth curves of four different parts of a human from birth to adulthood.

The reason for the rather surprising curve shown by the lymphoid system is that, in most people, this reaches its maximum size in childhood when the body is developing immunity to a large number of infectious diseases. The curve for the brain and head confirms what we saw in Figure 13.9. The general curve is rather like the growth curve we saw in Figure 13.1, except that Figure 13.10 refers to mass, which shows more of a growth spurt at puberty than does height. The curve for the reproductive system, as one might expect, only takes off at puberty.

During adulthood the majority of people in the UK:

- leave the home in which they were brought up
- start full-time work
- form sexual relationships
- have children.

However, there are, of course, exceptions to all these generalisations. These exceptions may be the result of personal choice or other factors. For example, someone may choose not to have children or may be unable to, either because they never establish a sexual relationship with someone of the opposite sex or because they are infertile. Similarly, someone may choose not to work or be unable to get a job because of unemployment.

For a woman, one significant event during the second half of her life is the **menopause**. This is when her menstrual cycles stop permanently, usually between the ages of 45 and 55. Between puberty and the menopause a woman's periods may stop for a while because:

- she is pregnant
- she is breast-feeding
- her body mass has dropped considerably – something which can happen in top athletes or women with anorexia nervosa.

Q6: Suppose a woman reaches puberty at 12 and the menopause at 52. What is the maximum number of eggs she is likely to produce during her lifetime? Show your working.

Q7: Suppose the same woman actually had three children and breast-fed each of them for 4 months. Approximately how many eggs would she produce during her lifetime? Show your working and assume she doesn't ovulate while breast-feeding.

Old age and death

In one sense, old age begins soon after we enter adulthood. In most sports it is difficult for an athlete over the age of 35 to compete at the highest level. The decrease in the ability of a person to function as well as they did, due to their getting older, is called **senescence**.

Senescence in humans has the following main features:

- loss of muscle strength (including cardiac muscle strength)
- decrease in vital capacity of the lungs
- loss of performance of the nervous system (including a longer reaction time, loss of hearing, poorer eyesight, and poorer sense of taste and smell)
- loss of libido (sexual desire)
- stiffening of the joints and loss of flexibility
- weakening of the bones (**osteoporosis**)
- wrinkling of the skin
- greying and loss of hair
- loss of ability to control body temperature when the environment gets too hot or too cold
- loss of mental ability.

The changes in a person's external features mean that we can easily tell, even from a photograph, approximately how old someone is (Figure 13.11). As a person reaches old age, they become increasingly dependent on others for daily life.

Eventually death comes to us all, for death is a natural feature of all living organisms. Of course, not all people die of 'old age'. However, in a society such as ours, where infectious diseases are no longer the main killers, most people live to be over 70 and eventually die from heart disease, cancers, a stroke or some other result of the body weakening. In most cases it is obvious when a person has died, but the increasing sophistication of modern medicine means that, for example, a person may be kept alive on an artificial ventilator for years, even though they are unconscious. Doctors and legal experts now talk about different types of death and it can be difficult to define exactly when a person has died. Before a person's organs can be used for donations, at least two doctors must confirm that the person is, indeed, dead.

a) 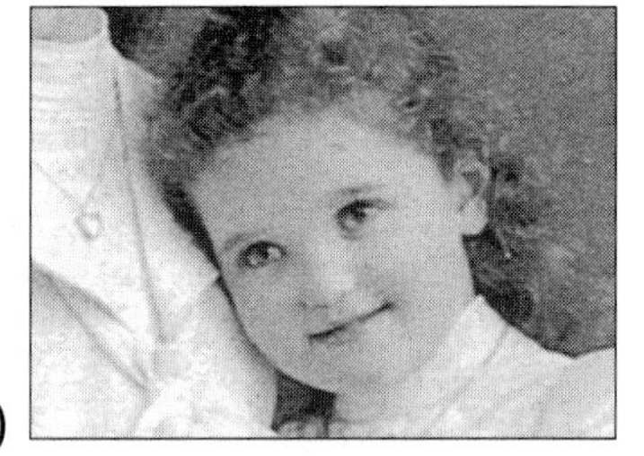

b) 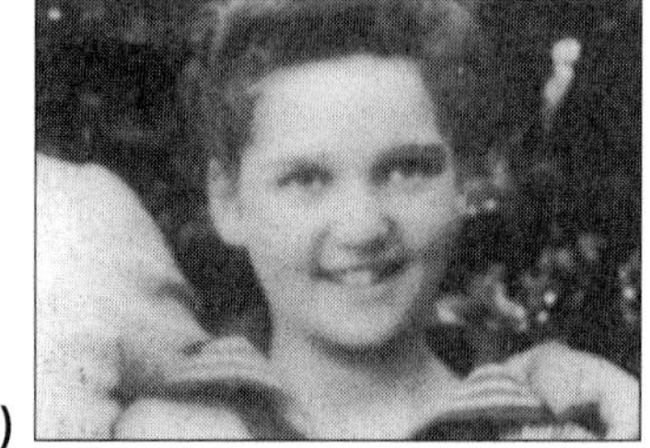

c) 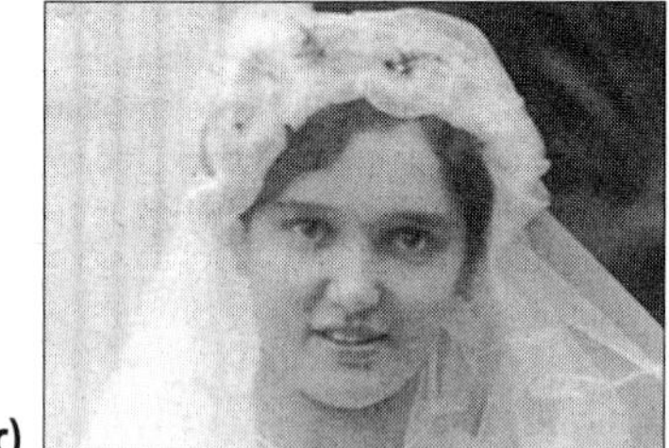

d) 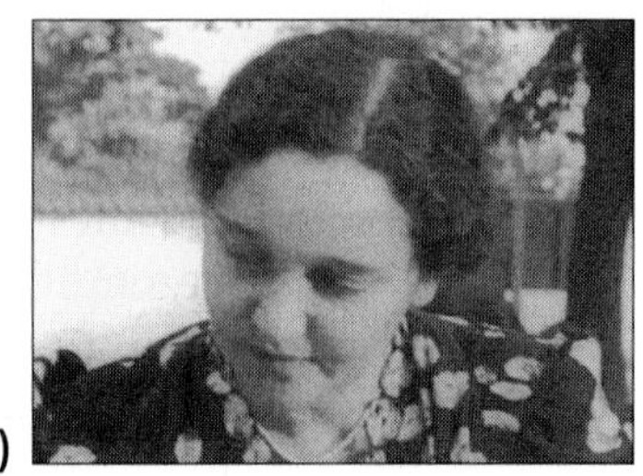

e) 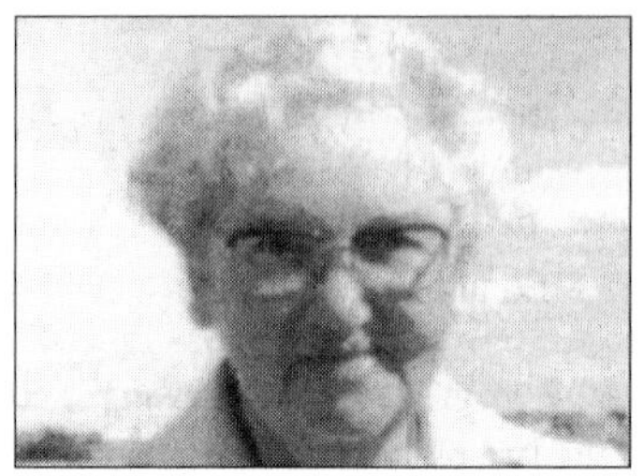

Figure 13.10 One person, F.S. (1899–1981) over the course of her life, aged. **a)** 3, **b)** 12, **c)** 21, **d)** 40 and **e)** 79 years.

Summary

- Growth is an irreversible increase in the dry mass of an organism.
- Colostrum and breast-milk are the ideal food for a developing baby.
- Development means a regular change in the structure and functioning of an organism as it ages. Development has physical, mental, emotional and social aspects to it.
- Girls generally reach puberty a couple of years earlier than boys while boys have a bigger growth spurt at puberty than do girls.
- A person's life after birth can be divided into the following stages: babyhood, being a toddler, childhood, adolescence, adulthood, senescence.
- Major developmental features during the first five years of life include walking and running, speech, toilet training, self-feeding, play and increasing independence.
- Puberty is the time during which a person's genitals mature and their secondary sexual characteristics develop.
- At puberty a girl starts to menstruate. Except for pregnancy, breast-feeding and certain medical conditions such as anorexia nervosa, a woman continues to menstruate roughly once a month until she reaches the menopause, somewhere between the ages of 45 and 55.
- Adolescence can be a difficult time, but the great majority of teenagers emerge from it with a better sense of their own identity.
- As we grow, some parts of our body (e.g. our brain) develop earlier than others.
- Senescence is accompanied by changes in physical and mental functioning.
- In the UK relatively few people die of infectious diseases. Most people live to be over 70 and die of heart disease, cancers or a stroke.

Self check
See page 244

CHAPTER 14

Health and the community

In this chapter you will learn what it is to be healthy. You will learn how such things as diet, exercise, smoking and the environment in which we live and work all affect our physical health, and see that health is more than the absence of physical injury or disease.

What do we mean by health?

There are two very different ways of answering the question 'What is good health?'.

- One way is to produce a sort of checklist – the ability to do a certain amount of exercise without getting over-tired, the absence of illness, etc.
- The other way is to ask people, 'What does it mean for you to be healthy?'

The first way might seem more *objective*, but health is increasingly seen as something we decide for ourselves. In other words, it is *subjective*.

When asked, 'What is good health?' people generally give the following sorts of answers:

- being free from disease
- living a long life
- being able to enjoy life
- having friends and family
- being free from pain
- not being tired or stressed all the time
- having a satisfying job or occupation.

The World Health Organisation defines health as 'a state of complete physical, mental and social well-being, and not merely the absence of disease or infirmity'. Health can be studied at various levels: at the level of the individual, the family, the community, the nation and internationally. It is important to realise that an individual's health is affected by the community in which they live. For example, a clean, dry, well-ventilated home that is warm when the weather is cold and which provides shelter against the elements significantly aids good physical health by, for instance, reducing the risk of infectious diseases. The importance of loving, caring, responsible adults for the physical, mental and emotional health of babies and children cannot be over-stressed.

Health workers and organisations

A large number of different workers and organisations play their part in the management of the good health of the community.

- **Health Practitioners** are consulted by us when we are concerned about our health or the health of close relatives (e.g. children and elderly dependants). The most familiar are **doctors** and **nurses**. Everyone in the UK is allocated to a **general practitioner** (**GP**) who looks after general aspects of our health. If need be, our GP can refer us to a specialist doctor, such as a surgeon, paediatrician (who specialises in children's health) or gynaecologist (who specialises in the reproductive health of women). In addition to doctors and nurses, we may see a **dentist** in connection with our teeth and gums, an **optician** for our eyes, a **pharmacist** to obtain drugs that have been prescribed for us by doctors, a **counsellor**, for example if we are depressed or having problems in relationships, or a **chiropodist** for our feet.
- **Health visitors** are qualified nurses who specialise in the health of babies and young children. They visit people, especially mothers with young children, in their homes and provide advice and guidance.
- **Environmental health officers** and **public health inspectors** are responsible for enforcing legislation that relates to health in the environment. For example, they check that restaurants comply with health and safety regulations to do with the preparing and selling of food, that permitted noise levels aren't exceeded, and that industries comply with requirements about the safe removal of waste matter from factories.
- The **Health Education Authority** is a UK organisation, largely funded by central government, responsible for the promotion of good health through education. Examples of **health education** campaigns are given in Table 14.1. Such campaigns vary in their effectiveness. Often they succeed in giving people *information* about what causes ill health, but this is a long way from enabling people to change their behaviour so that they become healthier! Another difficulty is that sometimes genuine controversy exists in health education. For example, many experts feel that it is still unclear whether cutting down on cholesterol in the diet significantly reduces the chance of getting a heart attack. For reasons such as these, health education campaigns are sometimes limited in their effectiveness.
- The **World Health Organisation** (**WHO**) is an international organisation that works to improve health, mainly through the prevention of disease. It was responsible for the elimination of smallpox, but has found other diseases, such as AIDS and malaria, much more difficult to tackle.

Table 14.1 Examples of health education campaigns run by the Health Education Authority and other organisations

Aim of campaign	Messages of campaign
Reduce the incidence of lung cancer and coronary heart disease	Smoke less; eat fewer saturated fats
Reduce gut complaints and bowel cancer	Eat more fibre
Reduce the incidence of AIDS	Slow the spread of HIV by avoiding contact with other people's body fluids (semen, vaginal secretions, blood) and not sharing needles
Prevent accidents	Wear seat belts; fires in the home can kill; take care with electrical appliances

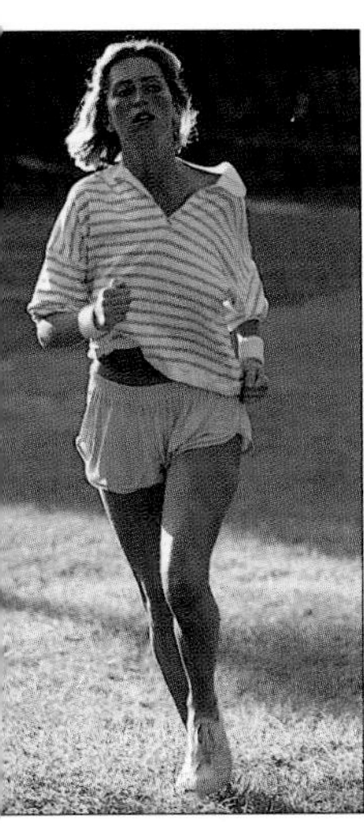

Figure 14.1 Jogging helps to build up stamina. Ensure you have good footwear and build up the amount you run gradually. Try to avoid doing all your running on hard surfaces, such as roads.

Fitness

The words 'fitness' and 'health' are sometimes used to mean the same thing. However, **fitness** generally refers to physical fitness. Physical fitness has three components:

- **stamina** – i.e. **endurance**, the ability to keep going without gasping for breath (see Figure 14.1)
- **strength** – i.e. **muscle power** (see Figure 14.2)
- **suppleness** – i.e. **flexibility**, having the maximum natural range of movement in your joints (see Figure 14.3).

Activities differ in the effects they have on stamina, strength and suppleness (see Table 14.2). If you take up a new sport or form of exercise, be prepared to exercise for several weeks before you can expect to see any significant improvement in your physical fitness. The important thing is to do something you enjoy, to start slowly and to take care. For any lasting improvement in stamina, you will probably need to do the activity so that you get *breathless* at least *three times a week* for *15 or more minutes on each occasion*.

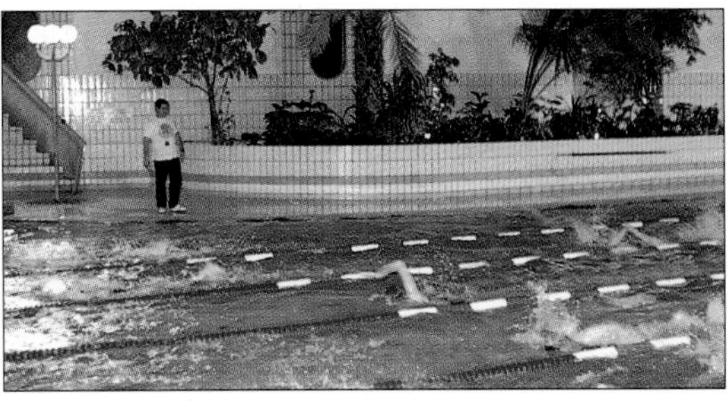

Figure 14.2 Swimming helps to build up strength as well as stamina and suppleness.

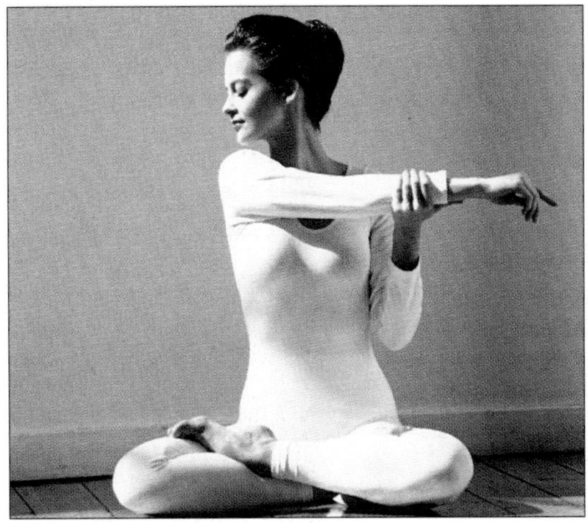

Figure 14.3 Yoga helps to increase suppleness.

Q1: Which activity in Table 14.2 is best for all round physical fitness?

Table 14.2 The consequences of different activities for physical fitness
* = no real benefit; ** = beneficial effect; *** = very beneficial effect; **** = excellent effect

Activity	Stamina	Strength	Suppleness	Activity	Stamina	Strength	Suppleness
Badminton	**	**	***	Housework	*	*	**
Canoeing	***	***	**	Jogging	****	**	**
Climbing stairs	***	**	*	Judo	**	**	****
Cricket	*	*	**	Rowing	****	****	**
Cycling (hard)	***	***	**	Sailing	*	**	**
Dancing (ballroom)	*	*	***	Squash	***	**	***
Dancing (disco)	***	*	****	Swimming (hard)	****	****	****
Digging	***	****	**	Tennis	**	***	***
Football	***	***	***	Walking (briskly)	**	*	*
Golf	*	*	**	Weightlifting	*	****	*
Gymnastics	**	***	****	Yoga	*	*	****
Hill walking	***	**	*				

Practical 14.1 To measure a person's recovery rate

A good way to determine someone's fitness is to measure their resting heart rate and see how long it takes to return to normal after a set amount of exercise. The fitter a person is, the quicker their heart beat returns to its resting level.

Requirements
Watch with second hand or electronic timer
Graph paper

1 Get the person to sit down quietly for 5 minutes.

2 Find their heart rate in beats per minute by counting their pulse for 30 seconds and multiplying by 2. The pulse can be felt either at the wrist or on the neck. Do not use your thumb when taking the pulse.

3 Wait 30 seconds and repeat step 2.

4 Get the person to undertake a fixed task – e.g. walking up and down a flight of stairs five times. If you intend to compare the recovery rates of different people, make sure they undertake the same task, and take the same amount of time to complete it.

5 Get the person to sit down and rest.

6 30 seconds after the end of the task, measure their heart rate by counting their pulse for 30 seconds and multiplying by 2.

7 Wait 30 seconds and then, again, measure their heart rate by counting their pulse for 30 seconds and multiplying by 2.

8 Repeat step 7 until their heart rate has returned to normal.

9 Plot a graph of heart rate against time.

10 Find out from your graph approximately how long it takes from the end of the exercise for the person's heart rate to return to normal (see Figure 14.4).

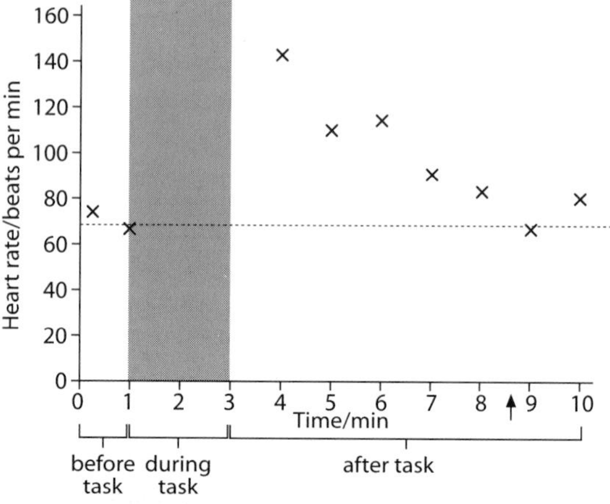

Figure 14.4 A graph showing what a person's heart rate might be before and after a period of exercise. Notice how the heart rate takes some time, in this case five and a half minutes, to recover after the exercise has ended.

Diet

In Chapter 3 we saw how the body needs the following components in the diet:
- proteins
- lipids (fats, oils)
- carbohydrates
- minerals
- vitamins
- dietary fibre
- water.

If eaten in the correct proportions, these components make up a **balanced diet** (healthy diet). Too much or too little of these components can have serious consequences.

Deficiencies in the diet

Our bodies can use lipids, carbohdrates and proteins as sources of energy. The energy provided by food is measured in kilojoules. The *approximate* amounts of energy needed by different types of people are listed in Table 14.3 on page 116. Note that these values are only approximate. Our energy needs are affected by:
- whether or not we are still growing
- our level of physical activity
- gender – males have an energy requirement about 10% more than females of the same size and activity
- environmental conditions – less energy is needed if it is warm
- clothing and other insulation
- individual variation – people vary considerably in their energy requirements depending on their physiology
- pregnancy and lactation
- age.

Practical 14.2 To measure the amount of energy in food

This is a very simple way of measuring energy in food. There are several alternative methods which give more accurate results.

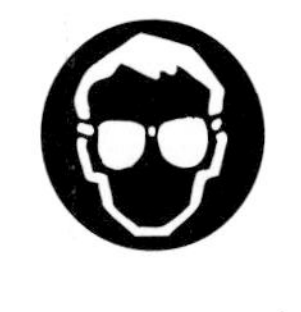

Wear eye protection

Requirements

- Pyrex© test tube
- Test tube rack
- Measuring cylinder
- Tongs
- Mounted needle
- Thermometer
- Bunsen
- Peanut
- Water

1 Measure 10 cm^3 water into a test tube.

2 Measure the initial temperature of the water (T_1°C).

3 Weigh the peanut (W) and secure it to the mounted needle.

4 Wear eye protection. Ignite the peanut in a Bunsen flame and immediately place it under the test tube of water held in tongs as in Figure 14.5.

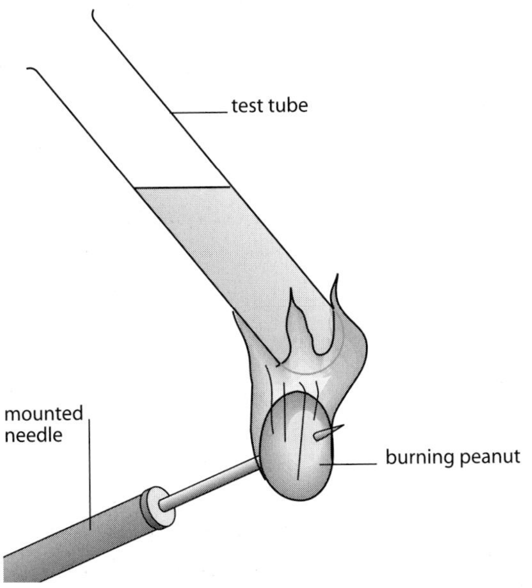

5 After the peanut has completely burnt out, measure the final temperature of the water (T_2°C).

6 Carry out the following calculation to find the energy value of the food in Joules. To do this, you need to know the following:

Mass of 10 cm^3 water = 10 g (1cm^3 water weighs 1 g)
4200 J raises 1 g of water by 1°C

Increase in temperature of water = $T_2 - T_1$°C

Energy in 1 g peanut = $\frac{4200 \times (T_2 - T_1 °C)}{W \times 10}$ J g^{-1}

Example calculation:

Initial temperature = 19°C

Final temperature = 45°C

Mass of peanut = 0.5 g

Volume of water = 10 cm^3

Energy in peanut = $\frac{4200 \times (45 - 19)}{0.5 \times 10}$ J g^{-1}

= $\frac{4200 \times 26}{5}$ J g^{-1}

= 21 840 J g^{-1}

= 21.84 kJ g^{-1}

7 The actual energy value of an average peanut is approximately 30 kJ g^{-1}. This method is very inaccurate because there are several ways in which the heat energy escapes. For example, some energy is lost when the peanut is ignited in the Bunsen flame. List three other ways in which heat energy is lost to the surroundings.

Figure 14.5 Apparatus for Practical 14.2.

Table 14.3 Approximate daily energy requirements for different types of people

Type of person	kJ per day	Type of person	kJ per day
Newborn baby	2 000	Office worker (adult female)	9 000
Child 1 year	3 000	Office worker (adult male)	11 000
Child 5 years	7 000	Heavy manual worker	15 000
Girl 12–15 years	9 500	Full-time athlete (female)	15 000 +
Boy 12–15 years	11 000	Full-time athlete (male)	20 000 +
Woman 16–19 years	10 000	Pregnant woman	10 000
Man 16–19 years	12 000	Woman breast-feeding	11 000

For an adult, consuming fewer than about 5000 kJ a day eventually leads to death by starvation. In the UK, the most common reason for adults to consume inadequate amounts of food is anorexia. **Anorexia nervosa** (**anorexia**) is a condition in which someone doesn't eat enough, even though they have access to food.

Q2: Using Table 14.3, work out (a) how many times more energy you would expect a 16–19 year-old woman to need from her food than a newborn baby; (b) by what percentage a woman who works in an office might expect to increase her food intake while lactating.

Anorexia

Approximately 90% of all people with anorexia are women, and most of them are in the 15–30 age bracket. If not treated soon enough, the condition can be extremely serious, even fatal. Even if not fatal, a person might spend many years obsessed by food and by their weight. Treatment usually combines counselling or psychotherapy to tackle the underlying problems and being encouraged by a doctor or dietician to eat enough to stay reasonably healthy while therapy is underway. Most experts agree that someone with anorexia often chooses, subconsciously, to eat very little as a means of exercising control over at least one area of their life. Therapy frequently involves encouraging the person to see why they are so strict about their food intake, while at the same time enabling them to explore what their life has been like to date.

Insufficient protein results in a disease called **kwashiorkor**. The person is weak and may have a swollen abdomen caused by the excessive retention of fluid in the tissues (**oedema**).

Vitamin and mineral deficiencies were considered in Chapter 3. A shortage of dietary fibre increases the risk of getting **bowel cancer**. Most people in the UK don't get enough fibre in their diet. Fruits, vegetables and cereals are all good sources of fibre.

Excesses in the diet

Excesses in the diet can cause as many problems as deficiencies.

- Too much **sugar** can result in tooth decay. This is because bacteria in our mouths turn the sugar into acids which attack the enamel of our teeth (Figure 14.6).
- Too much **salt** can cause high blood pressure, which in turn can cause health problems.
- Too much **animal fat** may increase the risk of **coronary heart disease**, though

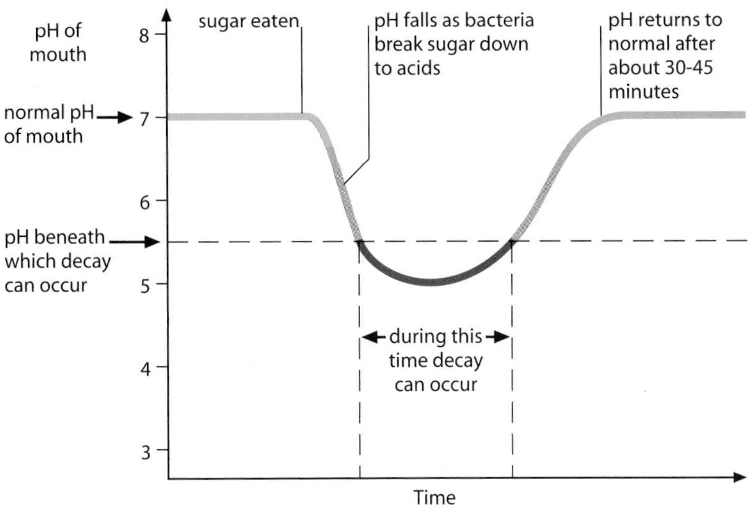

Figure 14.6 Eating sugar, or a food with a lot of sugar in it, results in a drop in the pH in our mouths. This is because bacteria in our mouths break down the sugar to acids. If the pH falls below about 5.5, the acids damage the enamel of our teeth. Too much damage eventually results in tooth decay.

the evidence for this is controversial. (Most animal fats are **saturated** with hydrogen and are usually solid at room temperature. Plant oils are **unsaturated** and are usually liquid at room temperature.) There is considerable evidence to suggest that if you don't get much exercise and are seriously overweight, eating animal fats may increase your chances of getting a **blocked artery** (see page 35). This occurs when fats, especially **cholesterol**, build up on the inside of certain arteries. This means that it is harder for the blood to be pumped through the arteries, which leads to a rise in blood pressure. If one of the arteries supplying the heart muscle with blood (i.e. one of the **coronary arteries**) becomes so filled with these fatty deposits that it becomes completely blocked, a **heart attack** results. Excess animal fats can also lead to **gallstones** which develop in the gall bladder and can cause pain (see page 25). They can be removed by surgery or broken down by ultrasound.

- Too high an **energy intake** can cause us to put on weight. Someone who is 30% overweight is said to be **obese**. If you are seriously overweight, your life expectancy and quality of life may be reduced due to increased risks of heart attack, damage to your joints, diabetes and varicose veins. However, in recent years feminists have criticised the notion of being 'overweight'. Rather than trying to stick to some ideal weight, it would probably be much healthier for all of us to get used to eating only when we feel hungry and making sure we take enough exercise. Certainly, going on a weight reduction diet almost never works. Over 99% of people who go on such a diet end up at least as heavy. The main reason is that the body becomes accustomed to surviving on less food. Once the diet is over, the person's weight soon goes up again.
- Some people are allergic to the protein **gluten**. Gluten occurs in wheat, and such people need to eat gluten-free products, otherwise they suffer from **coeliac disease**.

Some people try using laxatives or vomiting after a meal to keep their weight down. This can develop into an unhealthy repetitive cycle of eating abnormally large amounts of food very quickly, followed by induced (deliberate) vomiting. This condition is called **bulimia nervosa** (**bulimia**). It is accompanied by various health problems, can be dangerous, is expensive and time-consuming and may ruin your self-esteem.

Exercise

The immediate consequences of exercise, such as an increase in the rate and depth of breathing, were considered in Chapter 5. The long-term consequences of exercise are summarised in Figure 14.7 on page 118.

Q3: Suggest why exercise leads to the heart beating fewer times each minute when the person is at rest.

The effects of exercise shown in Figure 14.7 are all beneficial. However, excessive exercise can be bad for you. It can lead to injuries or to a feeling of perpetual tiredness. It can even weaken the immune system, making you more likely to become ill.

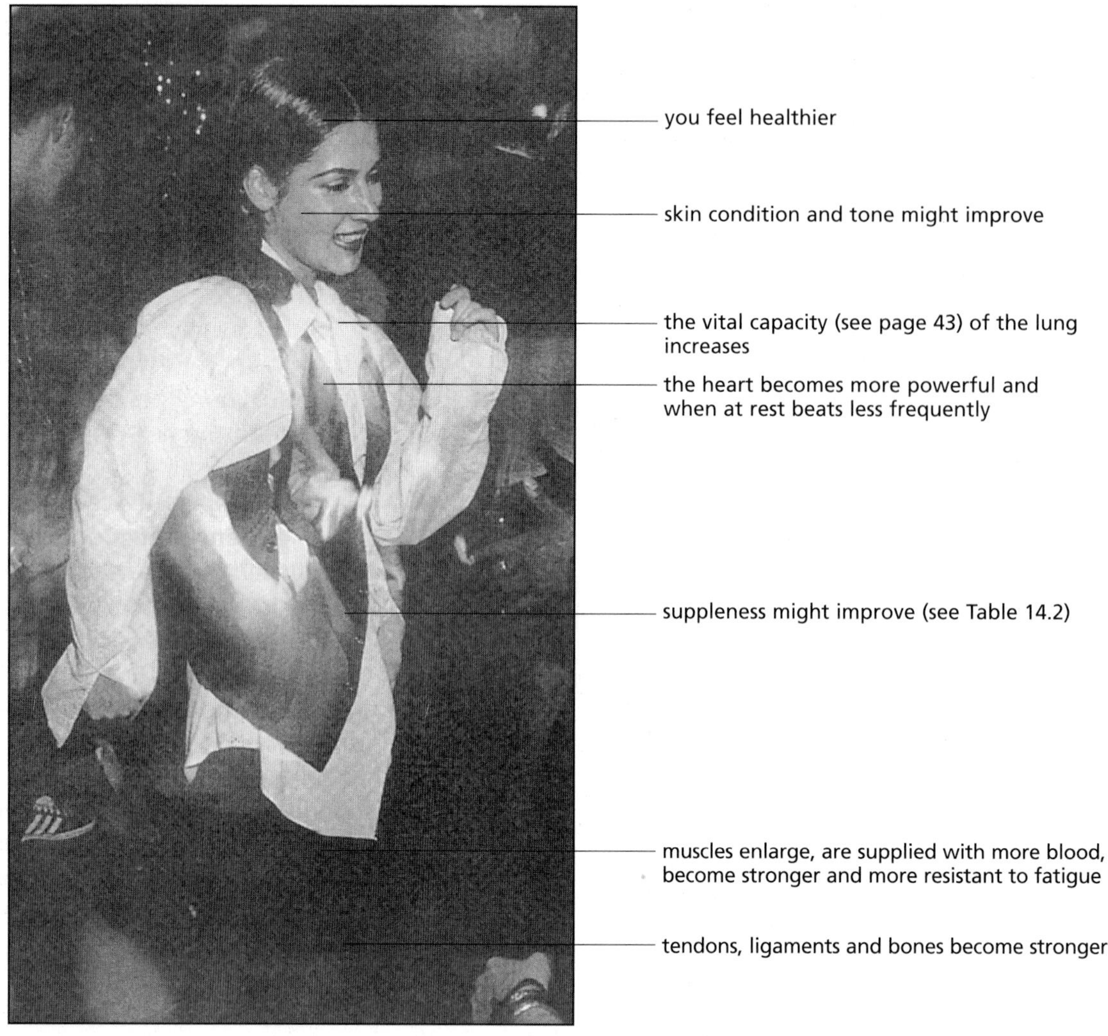

Figure 14.7 The long-term consequences of exercise are beneficial, unless the exercise is excessive.

Stress management

Many people find life stressful. A certain amount of stress is inevitable and may even be good for us, keeping us alert. However, too much stress can lead to anxiety, loss of sleep, unhappiness, irritability and poor physical health. **Stress management** is about managing your life so that you don't suffer from stress or its harmful consequences. Stress management can be achieved in two main ways.

- **Decreasing the amount of stress in your life.** For example, if you are stressed because you haven't enough time to fit everything in, you might decide to drop one of your commitments. If you are stressed because you feel members of your family don't listen to you, you might try taking some assertiveness classes or even writing to them explaining how you feel.
- **Coping better with the stress you experience.** For example, suppose you get stressed because you feel you aren't good enough at what you are doing. One possibility is to stop being so self-critical, admit that you can't be perfect, and set your sights a bit lower. Some people find that relaxation tapes help. Others find that simply talking about the problems are enough, whether to a friend or, if need be, to a counsellor. Still others find that treating themselves to something – such as new clothes or a night out – can help.

Substance abuse

Substance abuse occurs when someone takes drugs that aren't good for them. This definition *excludes* taking medication and non-excessive amounts of social drugs such as caffeine or alcohol. Drugs differ greatly in their effects, which last until the drug has either been **metabolised** (changed into another, less active substance, for example by enzymes in the liver) or **eliminated** from the body (usually in the urine).

Alcohol

Alcohol is the most commonly used and abused drug in the UK. Alcoholic drinks differ greatly in the amount of alcohol they contain (Table 14.4). In the UK, alcohol intake is measured in 'units'. One unit of an alcoholic drink contains 10 g of pure alcohol. This is the amount of alcohol a typical adult can break down in about an hour. The ethanol in alcohol is broken down to smaller molecules and most of these are then oxidised to carbon dioxide and water in respiration. On average, a medium strength half pint of beer contains one unit, as does a glass of wine or a single measure of spirits. In the UK, the maximum permitted legal level for someone driving is 80 mg of alcohol per 100 cm^3 of blood. Table 14.5 shows the blood alcohol levels expected for adult males and females of two different weights in relation to how much they have drunk.

Table 14.4 The strength of various drinks

Drink	Approximate % alcohol
Beers, ciders	1–8
Wine	10–20
Fortified wine (sherry, port, vermouth, etc.)	18–23
Spirits (rum, vodka, whisky, brandy, liqueurs, etc.)	35–50

Table 14.5 Average blood alcohol levels in relation to a person's weight, sex and how much they have drunk

Intake	Average blood alcohol level soon after consuming the drinks /mg per 100cm^3 of blood			
	Female 50kg	Female 75kg	Male 60kg	Male 90kg
1 unit	40	28	28	18
2 units	80	55	55	37
4 units	160	110	110	75
8 units	320	220	220	150

Q4: Using Table 14.5, suggest how many pints of average strength beer a woman of 75 kg could drink and still be legally permitted to drive.

Many people like alcoholic drinks, either because of their taste or because they may help them to relax. Alcohol reduces the activity of the brain and is classed as a **depressant**. For an adult female, consuming more than 21 units of alcohol a week is bad for your health; for an adult male, the figure is 28 units. Long-term consequences of consuming significantly more than this amount of alcohol each week can include:

- alcohol dependency (addiction)
- cirrhosis (damage to the liver)
- strokes (due to small blood clots in the blood vessels that supply the brain)
- cancers of the mouth, throat, oesophagus and liver
- being more prone to violence (as alcohol lowers self-control)
- hoarseness of the voice.

About 40 000 deaths in Britain each year are related to alcohol consumption. Alcohol can be **addictive** and **withdrawal symptoms** include:

- irritability
- shakiness
- insomnia (not being able to get to sleep)
- sweating

- nausea (feeling sick)
- panic attacks
- persistent shaking, a high pulse and even visual hallucinations – a condition known as **delirium tremens**.

Cannabis

Cannabis is the most widely used illegal drug in the UK. Approximately one in three people in the UK will have tried cannabis by the time they are 18. This compares with 98% of people who will have consumed alcohol by the time they are 18. The consequences to your health of using cannabis (also known as marijuana, hashish or grass – depending on how it is taken) are minor unless you take it regularly. Long-term consumption of cannabis has the same sort of health consequences as the long-term consumption of high tar cigarettes (see Smoking).

Heroin

Heroin is obtained from the opium poppy, along with other drugs such as **morphine** and **codeine**, both of which are used as pain relievers. Heroin is not a widely used drug – in part because of its expense. At 1995 prices, a typical year's supply costs around £10 000. In the UK, approximately 50 people a year die as a result of heroin use. The consequences of taking heroin are also serious for the following reasons:

- its expense means that its use is often associated with illegal means of obtaining money such as prostitution or theft
- it only takes a short time to become addicted compared to most other drugs
- the withdrawal symptoms can be quite severe, making it difficult for many people to give it up
- the fact that heroin is often injected means that its use is associated with the various problems associated with frequent injecting. These problems include the risk of transmitting HIV and other disease-causing pathogens.

Solvent abuse

Solvent abuse, sometimes referred to as **glue sniffing**, refers to the practice of inhaling the fumes released by a variety of household items including correcting fluids, hair lacquers, glues, hair sprays and even oven cleaners and de-icers. Approximately 120 people a year die in the UK as a consequence of solvent abuse. The main dangers come from suffocation, inhalation of vomit and drowning. Solvents are popular among some teenagers, in part because they are cheap to obtain.

Q5: Why do you think it is generally less dangerous if people abuse solvents in groups rather than on their own?

Smoking

Nicotine is the addictive ingredient in **tobacco**, used in cigarettes, cigars and pipes. About 100 000 people die in the UK each year as a result of smoking. Approximately one third of the adults in the UK regularly smoke cigarettes, though the number has fallen over the last 20 years. More men than women smoke, except in the 15–25 year-old age group, where the numbers are similar for both sexes.

Most people who smoke say they would like to give up. Unfortunately, nicotine is a powerful drug and people often find it very difficult to stop smoking. On the other hand, many people who smoke don't want to give up and get very irritated by what they see as increasing infringements on their personal liberty as smoking is banned in more and more public places.

Tobacco smoke contains **tars** and **carbon monoxide** in addition to nicotine. Tars eventually destroy the tiny hairs (**cilia**) that line much of our gaseous exchange system (see page 39). These hairs protect our lungs by carrying mucus, with trapped dust and bacteria, from the air passages into the throat, where it is swallowed. Without this

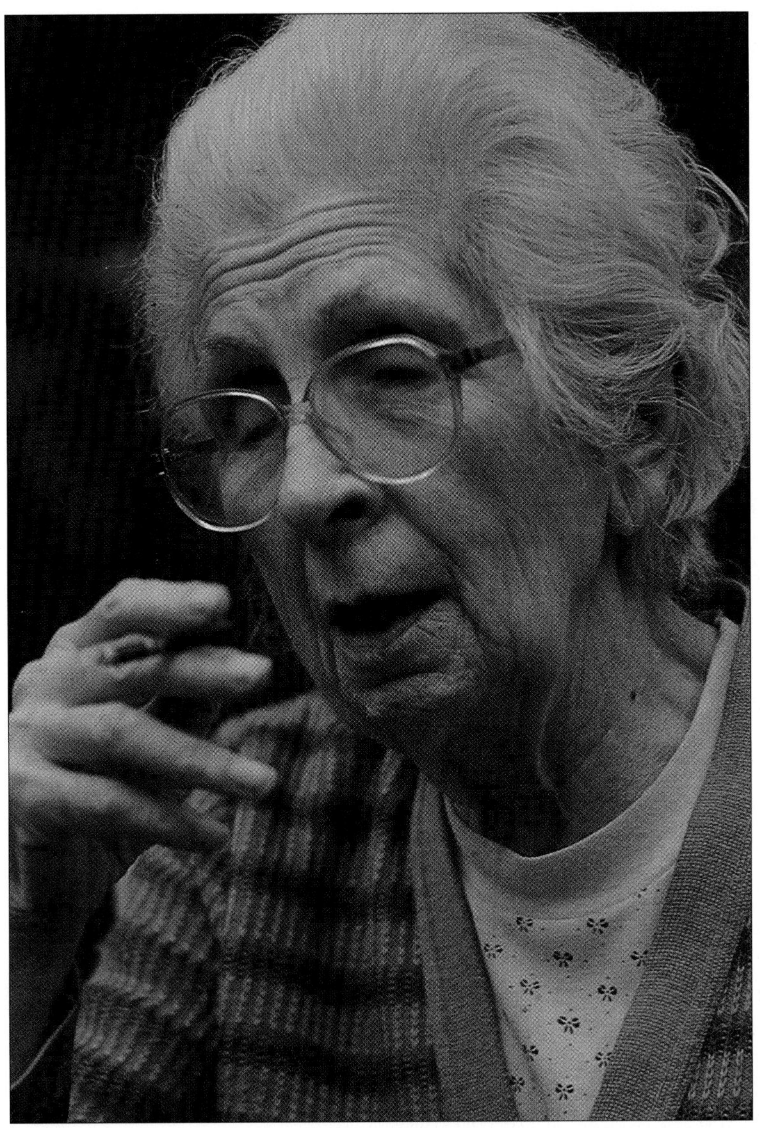

Figure 14.8 Cigarette smoking increases the chances of your getting bronchitis, which results in painful coughing. Other substances can cause bronchitis and damage the lungs. For example, exposure to industrial dusts, including coal dust, can result in bronchitis and other so-called occupational diseases.

protection, the alveoli in the lungs can become damaged, eventually resulting in **emphysema**, a condition in which a person is permanently breathless. Many smokers also develop **bronchitis**, a condition in which the bronchi and bronchioles become inflamed. The consequences of bronchitis are:

- heavy coughing (Figure 14.8)
- greater risk of developing **pneumonia** and certain other diseases.

The tars also cause **lung cancer** which is the most common cancer in the UK. Over 99% of the people who die from lung cancer have smoked cigarettes.

The carbon monoxide in tobacco smoke leads to heart disease and kills more people than lung cancer.

Few, if any, health benefits are associated with smoking, except that many smokers says it calms them. There is some evidence that smoking may, in some people, delay the onset of **senile dementia** resulting from **Alzheimer's disease**. In recent years it has been found that even if you don't smoke yourself, inhaling other people's smoke (**passive smoking**) can damage your health.

Freedom and responsibility

The issue of health often brings into focus the tension between freedom and responsibility. Take drug misuse, for example. One can argue that someone should be free to decide, for example, to take cocaine. This is the argument from the perspective of individual privacy and personal liberty. On the other hand, experience shows that people can very quickly become addicted to cocaine. Cocaine is so expensive that illegal methods are often used to finance its acquisition. So by passing laws to ban the sale or use of cocaine and other hard drugs, society attempts to protect itself.

Similar issues are raised by the use of socially acceptable drugs such as alcohol and nicotine and by sexually transmitted diseases. Should it, for example, be illegal for someone knowingly infected with HIV to have unprotected sexual intercourse with someone else without telling them of the fact?

Cancer

There are many different sorts of cancer. All cancers involve the uncontrolled growth of cells, which often results in a **tumour**. A tumour is a mass of abnormal cells which continue to multiply even though the body does not need extra cells. Cells from **malignant** tumours invade surrounding healthy tissues or enter the blood system and are carried to other parts of the body. Here they form secondary tumours which are themselves cancerous.

There are many causes of cancer including:

- tars in cigarette smoke which may cause lung tumours
- a shortage of dietary fibre which increases the risk of getting bowel cancer
- chemical **carcinogens** (cancer-causing substances) such as asbestos which may cause lung tumours
- **ionising radiation** which may cause cancer of the bone marrow, resulting in **leukaemia**
- **ultraviolet light** which may cause **skin tumours**.

Cancers can often be successfully treated by surgery, radiotherapy or chemotherapy.

Occupational hazards to health

Each working day, two people in the UK are killed and about 6000 are injured at work. There are many ways in which our working environment can be hazardous to our health. Think of your school or college laboratory. There are many rules you are expected to follow to reduce any dangers. A *selection* of these is as follows:

- do not run
- do not eat
- if you have long hair, tie it back
- keep benches and floor areas tidy
- follow your teacher's/lecturer's practical instructions
- report accidents immediately to your teacher/lecturer
- mop up minor spills; report others to your teacher/lecturer
- wear goggles/eye protection when heating substances or using acids and alkalis
- hold test tubes at an angle when heating them, heat the tube gently about one-third of the way from the bottom and don't point it at anyone.

To help reduce the chance of accidents in science laboratories and elsewhere, hazardous substances are marked with hazard warning symbols (Figure 14.9).

Safety at work and in educational settings is helped by a number of legal requirements. Two sets of these are of particular importance.

- The 1974 **Health and Safety at Work Act** controls the making, acquisition, storage and use of potentially dangerous materials and equipment. In particular, employers have a duty to provide a safe working environment and to train and inform staff about safe working practices.
- The 1988 **Control of Substances Hazardous to Health Regulations** ('COSHH Regulations') specify that a **risk assessment** arising from the use of hazardous substances (including organisms) must be made before the substances are used. For example, ethanol is highly flammable. For this reason it is stored in bottles marked

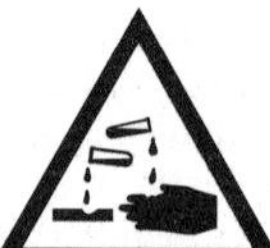
Corrosive

Highly flammable

Risk of electric shock

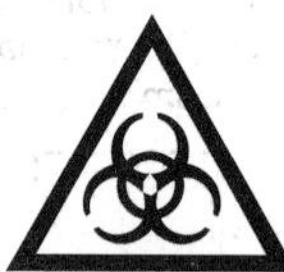
Biohazard

Danger

Oxidising

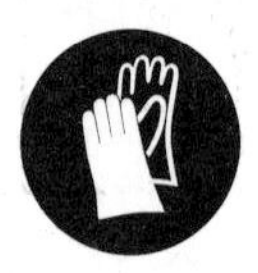
Gloves should be worn

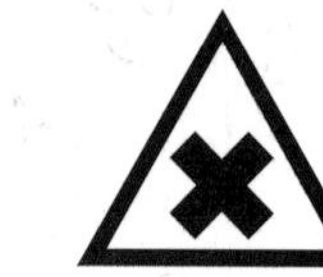
Harmful or irritant

Wear eye protection

Toxic

Figure 14.9 Hazard warning symbols used in science laboratories and elsewhere.

with the 'Highly flammable' symbol indicated in Figure 14.9. Before your teacher/lecturer allows you to use ethanol, he/she is required to assess the risk involved, and take the appropriate action. For example, if using ethanol to decolourise a leaf, you will be told to make certain that all Bunsen burners have been extinguished.

First aid

It is, of course, best if accidents can be prevented. However, if they do occur, prompt first aid can be invaluable. First aid cannot be learned just from a book. If you are interested in learning about first aid, you should attend a suitable training course, for instance one run by the St John Ambulance, the British Red Cross or the St Andrew's Ambulance Association.

Artificial resuscitation (artificial respiration/the kiss of life) was described on page 42. Other first aid procedures everyone should know are as follows.

- **Chemicals in the eye** This should be treated quickly as indicated in Figure 14.10.
- **Minor burns and scalds** These should be treated as indicated in Figure 14.11. Do *not* touch the affected area (or break blisters). Do *not* apply any creams, ointments or lotions to the affected area. Do *not* use adhesive dressings.
- **Bleeding** If necessary, remove clothing to expose the wound. Unless it contains broken glass or other sharp debris, press firmly over it, preferably using a clean dressing or pad. Maintain the pressure, raising and supporting the injured part. Get appropriate medical help.

For further guidance about emergency first aid procedures at home, at work and at leisure, see *First Aid Manual*, the authorized manual of St John Ambulance, St Andrew's Ambulance Association and British Red Cross, published by Dorling Kindersley.

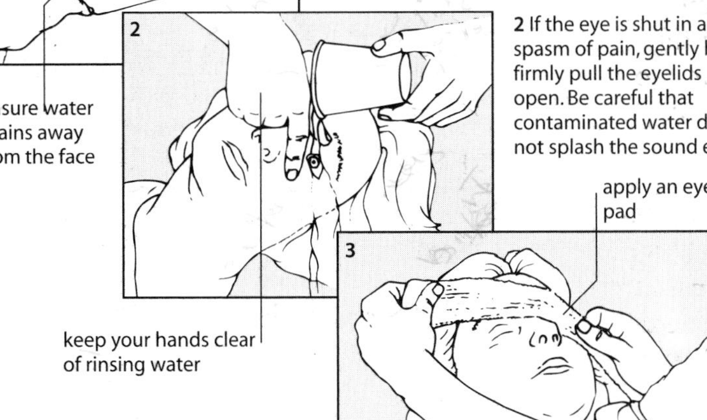

Figure 14.10 First aid for chemicals in the eye. Note that laboratories often have special eye-wash bottles.

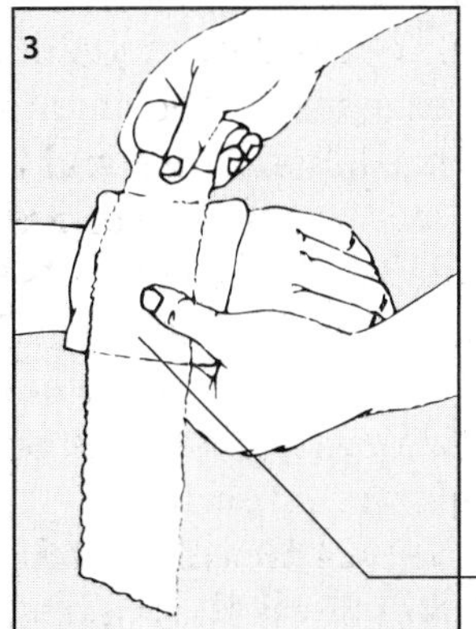

Figure 14.11 First aid for minor burns and scalds.

Mental health

Mental health is something we don't think much about when we have it. A number of different things can lead to a loss in mental health:

- inborn mental disability – such as Down's syndrome
- neuroses – such as obsessions (e.g. repeated hand-washing), phobias (e.g. fear of open spaces) and some forms of depression
- psychoses – such as schizophrenia.

Recent UK government policy has been to move away from the long-term treatment of mental illness in hospitals, out into the community. Most people agree that this is a good idea in principle, but that it needs proper funding, otherwise patients who are mentally ill don't get the treatment they need and, on very rare occasions, may be dangerous to members of the public.

Summary

- Different people may mean different things when using the word 'health'.
- Health practitioners, heath visitors, environmental health officers/public heath inspectors, the Health Education Authority and the World Health Organisation all play a part in the management of the good health of the community.
- Health education aims to enable people to improve their health through teaching them about what results in good or bad health.
- Physical fitness has three components: stamina, strength and suppleness.
- If eaten in the correct proportions, the components of our food provide us with a balanced diet.
- Different people need different amounts of energy supplied by their diet.
- Poor health can result from deficiencies or excesses in the diet.
- The long-term consequences of exercise are beneficial, unless the exercise is excessive.
- Stress management can be achieved either by decreasing the amount of stress in your life or by learning to cope better with the stress you experience.
- Alcohol and nicotine are the most commonly used and abused drugs in the UK.
- Other drugs that are abused include cannabis, heroin and solvents.
- More people die in the UK as a result of nicotine addiction than from all the other drugs added together.
- Cigarette smoking often results in heart disease, cancers or other diseases.
- Various pieces of legislation, including the Health and Safety at Work Act and the Control of Substances Hazardous to Health Regulations, help to protect people against occupational hazards to health.
- If accidents do occur, first aid can reduce suffering and save lives. First aid courses are run by a number of voluntary organisations.
- Cancers can result from a number of causes, including harmful substances, ionising radiation and ultraviolet light.

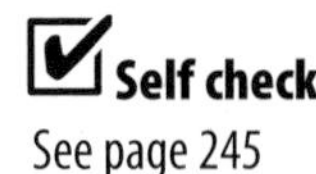

See page 245

CHAPTER 15

Infection

In this chapter you will learn about a range of human diseases caused by infectious organisms. The prevention and treatment of disease is covered in Chapter 16.

The spread of pathogens

Organisms that cause disease are called **pathogens** or, in everyday speech, germs, though this is not a scientific term and it should not be used in examinations. Different pathogens spread in different ways, the principle ways being by:

- airborne infection
- droplet infection
- contaminated food and water
- physical contact with an infected person
- animal vectors.

Sexually transmitted diseases

Each year **sexually transmitted diseases (STDs)** affect about one million people in Britain, more than any other infectious disease. As the term suggests, a sexually transmitted disease can be transmitted by sexual contact, normally sexual intercourse. However, some STDs can also be transmitted in other ways, for example from mother to fetus across the placenta.

Most STDs are not life-threatening if treated early. However, they can cause discomfort, embarrassment and in some cases sterility if not dealt with quickly enough. Treatment, whether by a GP or at a Special Clinic (Figure 15.1), is always confidential.

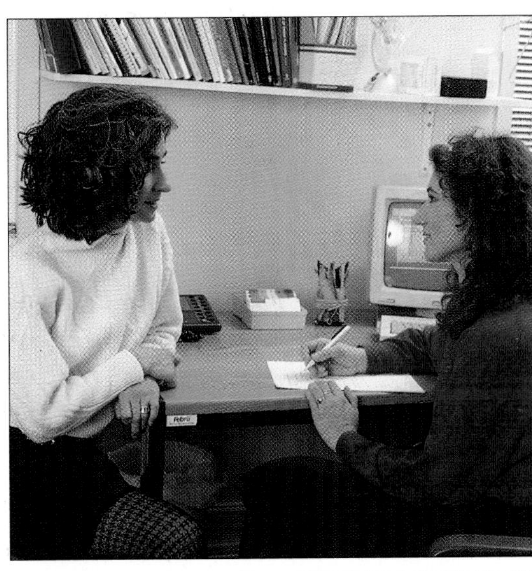

Figure 15.1 A patient discussing her case with a nurse in a Special Clinic. If you go to a Special Clinic your GP doesn't need to know about it, and the treatment is free and confidential. Special Clinics used to be known as Genito-urinary Clinics.

STDs are caused by a wide variety of organisms including:

- **viruses** – cause genital herpes, genital warts and AIDS
- **bacteria** – cause chlamydial infection (the most common STD in the UK), syphilis (which is now rare in the UK) and gonorrhoea
- **fungi** – cause thrush
- **protozoa** – cause trichomoniasis
- **arthropods** (pubic lice, also known as 'crabs').

Gonorrhoea

Gonorrhoea is caused by a bacterium which lives in the cervix, urinary tract, mouth and rectum. In women, the disease can spread to the ovaries and oviducts, causing **pelvic inflammatory disease**. This can result in infertility.

The early symptoms of infection with the bacterium are mild and may include a burning sensation on urination and a discharge from the vagina or penis. However, many people have no symptoms at first which makes the disease very hard to control. Treatment is relatively straightforward and involves a course of antibiotics. However, some strains of the bacterium are resistant to a number of the most commonly used antibiotics.

In common with other STDs, gonorrhoea cannot be caught from toilet seats or by kissing. However, pregnant women can transmit the bacterium to their unborn children.

AIDS

AIDS (Acquired Immune Deficiency Syndrome) is caused by a virus called **human immunodeficiency virus (HIV)**. The structure of the virus is shown on page 144. HIV was only identified in 1983. By 1995 there were approximately 20 million people world-wide infected with HIV. Unlike a number of other diseases caused by viruses, there is no vaccination available as yet to protect against infection.

HIV can only be spread:

- by sexual intercourse with someone infected with HIV
- by receiving blood from someone infected with HIV (e.g. through a cut, sharing needles for drug injection, or by receiving blood for medical reasons)
- from a mother with HIV to her offspring (either across the placenta, at birth or, rarely, in milk).

In the UK, most people with AIDS are men who became infected with HIV by having sexual intercourse with other men (Table 15.1). However, this pattern is changing. More and more cases of HIV transmission in the UK are due to heterosexual intercourse. Indeed, world-wide, most of the people infected with HIV have acquired the virus as a result of heterosexual intercourse.

Ways of preventing the spread of HIV are discussed on page 134.

Table 15.1 The causes of HIV infection among the 8529 people with AIDS in the UK by 1 January 1994

Cause of infection	Number of people with AIDS
Sexual intercourse between men	6318
Sexual intercourse between men and women	936
Blood/tissue donation – mainly to haemophiliacs	484
Injecting drug use (IDU)	438
IDU or sexual intercourse between men	134
Other/undetermined	117
Mother to infant	102

Q1: From the data in Table 15.1, what percentage of people with AIDS became infected as a result of mother to infant transmission?

Other pathogenic diseases

Rubella

If a woman catches **rubella (German measles)** during the first three months of pregnancy, the virus can cause serious damage to the nervous system of the fetus.

For an adult the disease is much less serious, and has the symptoms of a slight rash and a raised temperature. Rubella is spread by droplet infection (in tiny droplets of moisture). Vaccination against rubella is described on page 134.

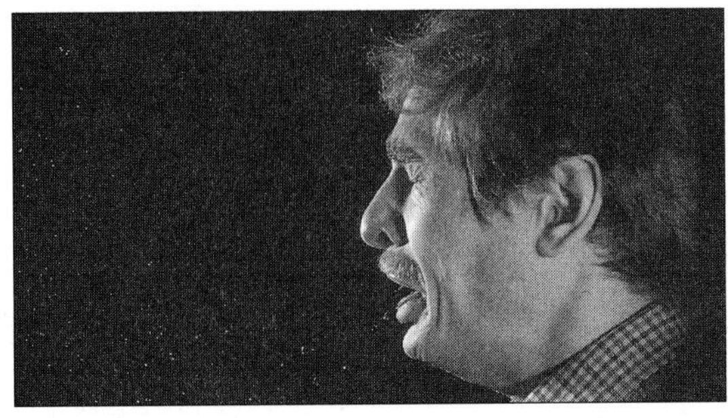

Figure 15.2 The influenza virus is transmitted in tiny droplets of moisture. Sneezing increases the chance that the virus infects other people.

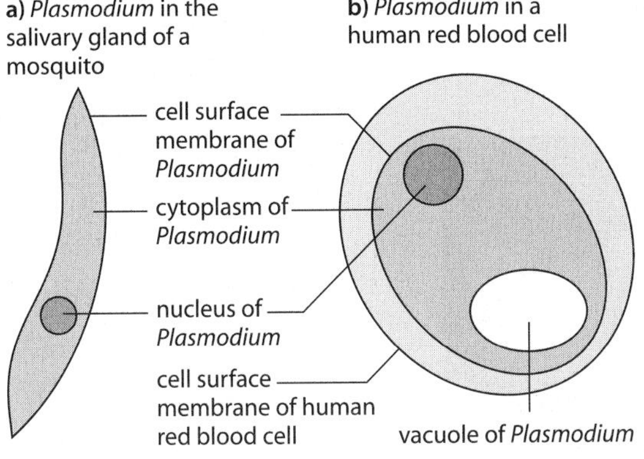

Figure 15.3 The protozoan, *Plasmodium*, which causes malaria, has a structure which varies depending on the stage of its life cycle.

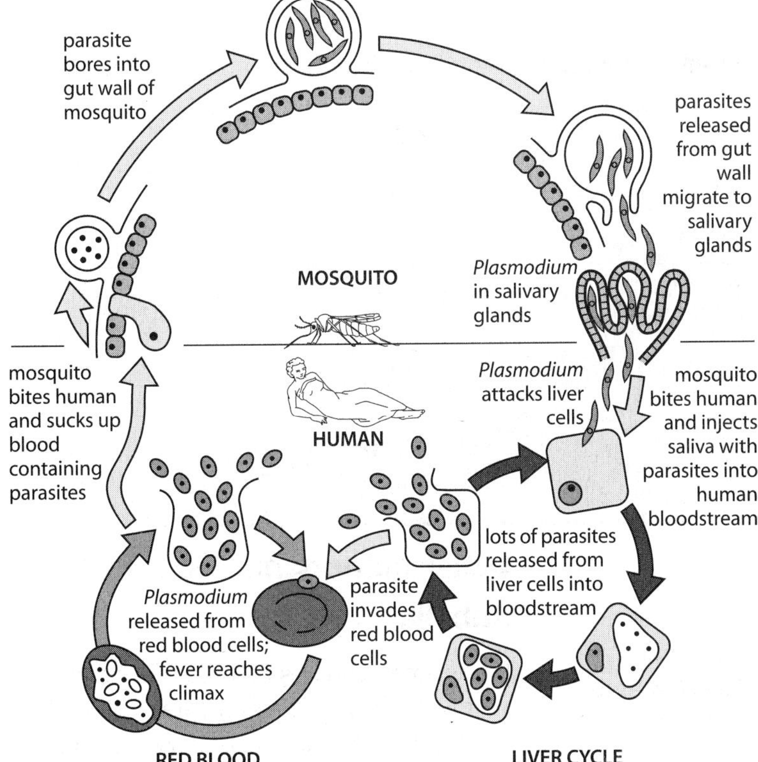

Influenza

The influenza virus (page 145) attacks the lining of the throat and gaseous exchange system. Like rubella, it is spread by droplet infection (Figure 15.2), so overcrowded or badly ventilated conditions make it easier for the disease to spread. In a healthy person the symptoms generally last 2 to 4 days and consist of a raised temperature, headache and weakness. The best treatment is to retire to bed and, if adult, take aspirins. However, the disease can be serious enough to require medical attention. The damage it causes may allow bacteria to enter and cause a secondary infection. Many elderly people die from 'flu'. Once a person has had influenza they are immune to that strain for several years. However, many different strains of the virus are known, so you may become infected many times.

Q2: Influenza is much more common in some years than others. Can you suggest why this might be?

Malaria

Malaria is a tropical disease caused by a protozoan called *Plasmodium* (Figure 15.3). The parasite needs a female mosquito called *Anopheles* to act as a vector and carry it from person to person. The life cycle of *Plasmodium* is complicated and is summarised in Figure 15.4. Notice the following stages:

- female mosquito bites a person and injects saliva with *Plasmodium* into them
- *Plasmodium* attacks and multiplies both in human liver cells and in human red blood cells
- another female mosquito bites the person and this mosquito becomes infected with *Plasmodium*
- *Plasmodium* reproduces within the mosquito.

The main symptom of malaria is bouts of fever. The affected person's temperature

Figure 15.4 Life cycle of the parasite which causes malaria. The mosquito needs water in which to breed.

shoots up from its normal value of 37°C to around 40 or even 41°C. These bouts of fever recur every few days. Among children they can often be fatal. Whilst adults rarely die, they continue to suffer periodic attacks of fever and weakness for years.

The prevention of malaria is discussed on page 135.

Athlete's foot

Athlete's foot is caused by a fungus which attacks the skin between the toes, causing itching and redness (Figure 15.5). It is passed on by walking barefoot on wet changing room floors or by sharing towels. Control of athlete's foot is described on page 135.

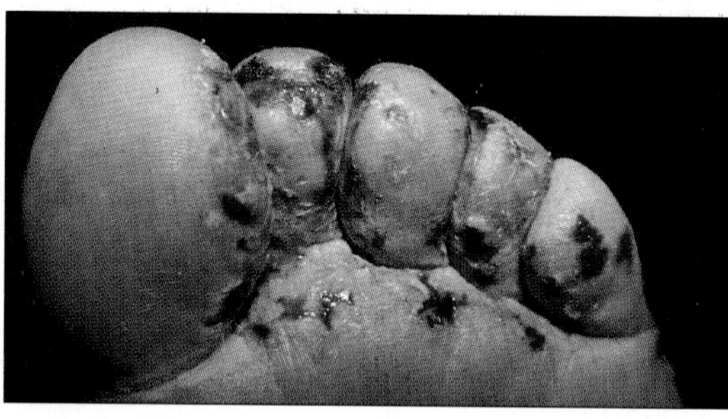

Figure 15.5
A severe case of athlete's foot.

Tuberculosis

Tuberculosis is caused by a bacterium which enters the body through the gaseous exchange passages. Recently it has been discovered that a surprisingly high proportion of people have the bacteria in their bodies, but do not suffer from the disease. However, if their immune system is weakened, through having a poor diet, living in overcrowded conditions or being infected with the human immunodeficiency virus, then they may develop the disease.

Cholera

Cholera is caused by a bacterium. It is spread through drinking water that has become contaminated with infected faeces. Because of this, cholera can be a problem in large refugee camps or in cities where the sewage system has broken down, for example in the aftermath of an earthquake. The bacteria infect the large intestine where they cause severe diarrhoea. This can be so bad that the patient, especially if a child, dies from dehydration. Vaccination usually only lasts for around six months and the key is prevention, or treatment with antibiotics and the transfusion of a saline solution to prevent serious dehydration.

Deer may help cure athlete's foot

A chemical found in a deer's sweat glands may one day be a treatment for such diseases as athlete's foot, tooth decay and acne. In 1995, William Wood, a scientist who works in California, published his finding that the sweat glands that lie close to the hooves of black-tailed deer contain large amounts of a particular chemical.

Scientists had always assumed that such chemicals were used for marking trails and sending messages to other deer. However, Wood found that the chemical seems to have no effect on the behaviour of other deer. But when Wood, 'on a whim', tested the chemical on a number of bacteria and fungi, he found that many of them were killed by the chemical. Microorganisms affected by the chemical include those responsible for athlete's foot, tooth decay, acne and dandruff. Wood suggests that the natural function of the chemical may be to help prevent the deer from developing infections on their feet.

Rabies

Rabies is caused by a virus which attacks a number of mammals including dogs, foxes and humans. It can be transmitted to humans when someone is bitten by an infected animal. The virus invades the nervous system and causes a fatal illness. Fortunately a good vaccine is available and it is hoped that the disease may soon be eliminated from mainland Europe. At present, no animals in the UK are known to be infected with rabies, thanks largely to the very strict quarantine laws which prevent infected animals from entering the country (Figure 15.6).

Food poisoning

Bacteria called *Salmonella* are found in the intestines of most vertebrates, for example cattle and chickens. If they succeed in infecting humans, they can rapidly multiply and cause **food poisoning** with its symptoms of vomiting and diarrhoea. Precisely how many people suffer from food poisoning in the UK each year is unclear, as most people with it never go to their doctor. In Chapter 16 we shall look at the ways in which food poisoning can be avoided.

Q3: Antibiotics are only effective against bacteria. Which diseases discussed in this chapter could be treated by antibiotics?

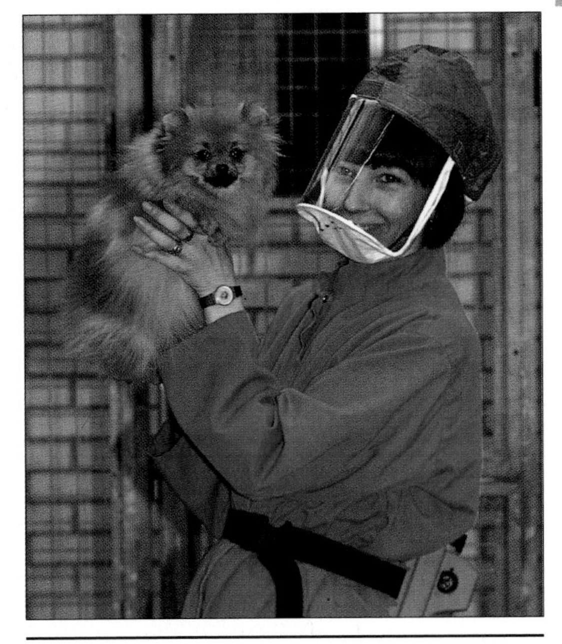

Figure 15.6 Any pet mammals brought into the UK have to be quarantined, at the owner's expense, for six months. This is long enough to ensure that they haven't become infected with rabies. Many people think that these regulations are too stringent, but they have helped prevent rabies from entering Britain for over half a century.

Summary

- Disease-causing organisms are called pathogens. They can be passed from person to person in a number of ways, including direct contact.
- A number of different organisms cause sexually transmitted diseases (STDs).
- STDs can be treated by a GP or at a Special Clinic.
- Gonorrhoea is caused by a bacterium and can result in infertility in women. Treatment is by antibiotics. Gonorrhoea can be spread by sexual intercourse or from mother to fetus.
- AIDS (Acquired Immune Deficiency Syndrome) is caused by a virus called human immunodeficiency virus (HIV). HIV can spread by sexual intercourse, by receiving infected blood or from mother to child.
- German measles (rubella) is caused by a virus which can seriously damage the nervous system of a fetus during the first three months of its mother's pregnancy.
- Influenza ('flu') is caused by a virus which attacks the lining of the throat and gaseous exchange system.
- Malaria is a tropical disease caused by a protozoan which also needs a mosquito to complete its life cycle.
- Athlete's foot is caused by a fungus which attacks the skin between the toes.
- Tuberculosis is caused by a bacterium and develops in people with a weakened immune system.
- Cholera is caused by a bacterium and is spread through contaminated drinking water.
- Rabies is caused by a virus which attacks a number of different mammal species.
- *Salmonella* bacteria can cause food poisoning.

Self check
See page 246

CHAPTER 16

Disease control

In this chapter you will learn how infectious diseases can be controlled. See Chapter 14 for details of non-infectious diseases.

Natural defences against disease

The human body has a wide range of defences against infections:

- the **skin** prevents many disease-causing microorganisms (pathogens) from entering the body
- the rapid formation of **scabs** prevents pathogens from getting into the blood system through cuts (see page 29)
- a pH in the **stomach** of about 1.5 kills many pathogens (the environment in the **vagina** is also acidic, though to a lesser extent)
- the enzyme **lysozyme** in **tears** kills pathogens that might otherwise enter through the eyes
- pathogens that are breathed in may be trapped in the **mucus** that lines the **trachea**, **bronchi** and **bronchioles** and then carried by **cilia** up to the throat where they are swallowed
- **white blood cells** destroy many of the disease-causing organisms that do get into the body
- our **brain** helps us to behave so as to reduce the chances of catching diseases; for example, we might keep our distance from someone with an infectious disease.

As we saw earlier, some white blood cells – called **monocytes** and **neutrophils** – are able to ingest (eat) bacteria and other pathogens (page 29). Other white blood cells, called **lymphocytes,** destroy disease-causing microorganisms in a different way. They produce special proteins called **antibodies.** The job of an antibody is to attach to molecules called **antigens.** Antigens are protein-based substances which lie on the outside of the disease-causing microorganisms as indicated in Figure 16.1.

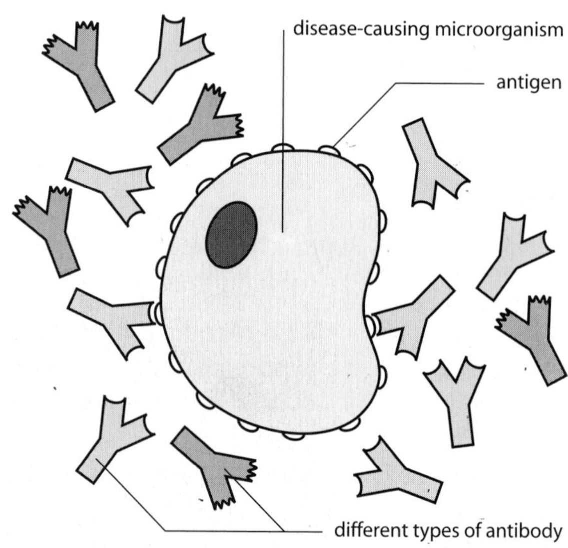

Figure 16.1 Diagram of a disease-causing microorganism covered with one type of antigen. Notice how only one shape of antibody binds to the antigens.

The presence of foreign antigens triggers the appropriate lymphocyte to multiply to form clones of cells, which produce the corresponding antibodies. Once antibodies of the right shape have been made in sufficient numbers, the invading microorganism is killed in one of a variety of ways. The antibody may:

- cause the microorganism's cell surface membrane to collapse
- cause the microorganisms to **agglutinate** (clump together). These clumps of cells are then more easily destroyed by neutrophils
- detoxify the poisons produced by certain pathogens.

Although our antibodies help protect us from disease, they can cause problems. For example, our antibodies recognise transplants (e.g. of kidneys) as foreign. For this reason, the donor and recipient need to be closely matched with respect to their antigens and to their blood groups, and the recipient may need to take immunosuppressive drugs to stop their immune system from rejecting the transplant. A related problem is that sometimes our bodies over-react to foreign substances. An **allergy** to pollen, for example, causes hayfever.

Q1: A few people are unable to produce antibodies. Sometimes these people are kept in large plastic containers from birth and become known as 'bubble children' (Figure 16.2). Explain why the plastic containers are needed.

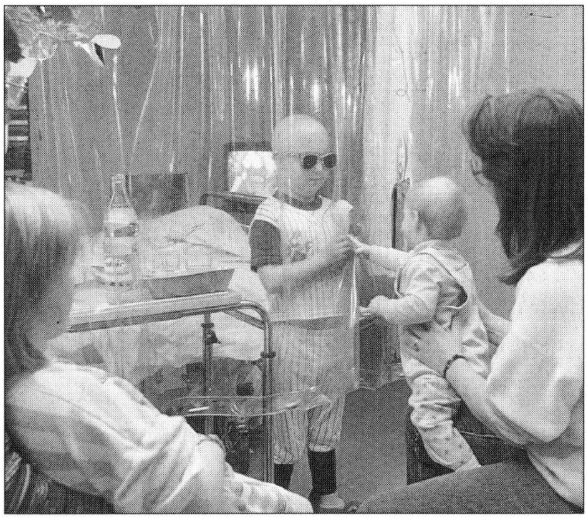

Figure 16.2 A few people are unfortunate enough to be born without functioning lymphocytes. They may be kept in plastic containers in an attempt to keep them alive. Thankfully, a treatment based on genetic engineering is now being developed which should help such people to lead normal, independent lives.

Natural immunity

It takes our bodies about a week or so to produce antibodies in response to a new antigen. This is why it takes about a week or so between becoming infected with a disease and beginning to recover from it. Once a person produces a particular sort of antibody, the body is able to respond so quickly to repeated infections that the person may never again suffer from the disease. The person is said to be **immune** and to have developed **natural immunity**.

Our bodies are capable of producing millions of different types of antibodies. This is vital because of the huge number of different antigens. For example, the antigens on the outside of a chicken pox virus differ in shape from those on the outside of, say, a measles virus. This means that different antibodies have to be made in response to all the different antigens. The problem is made worse by the fact that some diseases, such as influenza, can be caused by over a hundred different strains of virus. Each strain has its own characteristic antigens. This is why you may catch 'flu' several times during your life. Each infection is by a different strain of 'flu' virus.

A different way in which someone might develop natural immunity is by obtaining antibodies from their mother. These antibodies can be obtained:

- across the **placenta** before birth
- in **breast-milk** after birth.

Antibodies obtained in this way only protect a newborn baby for a few months, before the baby's own lymphocytes have 'learnt' how to produce the right sort of antibodies. In effect, the baby relies on its mother's antibodies. The few months of protection obtained in this way can save a baby's life.

Vaccination programmes

One problem with developing natural immunity is that you have to catch the disease first. In the case of a dangerous disease, such as smallpox, this is risky. Over a thousand years ago the Chinese successfully developed the practice of **inoculation** against smallpox. From here the technique spread to other countries.

Inoculation is an example of **acquired immunity**. The person gets (acquires) immunity through being given a small amount of the disease-causing micro-organism. It is known as **active immunity** as the person makes their own antibodies. Various techniques have been devised to ensure that the inoculation results only in a mild form of the disease, or in no disease whatsoever:

- the killed organism may be used, e.g. whooping cough
- a live non-virulent (non-dangerous) strain of the organism may be used. This is usually derived from many generations of selective sub-culturing in the laboratory, e.g. tuberculosis, rubella
- the antigens may be separated from the organism and used as a vaccine, e.g. influenza
- the toxin (poison) produced by the organism may be chemically modified so that it is no longer toxic, but is still sufficiently similiar to the toxin to result in manufacture of the appropriate antibodies
- genetically engineered bacteria may be used to mass-produce the relevant antigen, e.g. hepatitis B.

Inoculations can be used to help prevent many diseases including **cholera, polio, rubella, tetanus, tuberculosis, typhoid** and some strains of **influenza**. Sometimes they need to be helped, after a number of years, by giving the person a **booster** injection. Nowadays the terms 'vaccination', 'inoculation', and **immunisation**, are used to mean the same thing. Vaccinations/inoculations/ immunisations have been tremendously successful, saving the lives of many millions of people. They have even led to the complete eradication of smallpox as a result of a programme organised by the **World Health Organisation (WHO)**. Unfortunately, vaccines have not yet been successfully developed against a number of major diseases including malaria and AIDS.

There is one other way in which

The history of inoculation and vaccination against smallpox

Inoculation against smallpox was popularised in Britain by Lady Mary Wortley Montagu who went to Turkey with her husband in 1716. The next year, in a letter to a friend, she described what she had seen.

'The smallpox, so fatal, and so general amongst us, is here entirely harmless ... the old woman comes with a nut-shell full of the matter of the best sort of smallpox, and asks what veins you please to have opened. She immediately opens that you offer to her with a large needle (which gives you no more pain that a common scratch), and puts into the vein as much venom as can lie upon the head of her needle ... The children or young patients play together all the rest of the day, and are in perfect health to the eighth. Then the fever begins to seize them, and they keep their beds two days, very seldom three. They have very rarely above twenty or thirty in their faces, which never mark; and in eight days' time they are as well as before their illness ... There is no example of any one that has died in it; and you may believe I am very well satisfied of the safety of the experiment, since I intend to try it on my dear little son.'

Vaccination against smallpox was pioneered by the English doctor Edward Jenner. It had long been known that people who milked cows were unlikely to develop smallpox. Jenner wondered if this might be because people who milked cows often developed cowpox, a minor disease. Perhaps, he suggested, getting cowpox protected you against smallpox. In 1796 he carried out a famous experiment which produced evidence to support this theory. He injected a boy with cowpox and sure enough, the boy developed cowpox. Then, once the boy had recovered, Jenner injected him with smallpox. The boy did *not* develop smallpox. (Note: medical research is carried out rather differently nowadays!)

Jenner's approach became known as **vaccination** ('vacca' being the Latin for cow). The twentieth century smallpox vaccines that led to the eradication of smallpox were based not on live cowpox virus but on a weakened strain of the smallpox virus.

immunity may be acquired artificially, and that is by injecting a person with antibodies against a particular disease. This is known as **passive immunity**, to distinguish it from active immunity – in which the person makes their own antibodies once they have been artificially brought into contact with the microorganism's antigens.

Passive acquired immunity is useful when there is an *urgent* need to ensure that a person does not develop a dangerous disease. For example, someone who suffers a deep and dirty cut and has not recently been inoculated against tetanus, should be given anti-tetanus antibodies. Similarly, if you are bitten by a rabid dog or other animal while abroad and go to a doctor, you will be given anti-rabies antibodies. This is because both tetanus and rabies can be fatal – indeed, rabies always is. The differences between the various types of immunity are summarised in Figure 16.3.

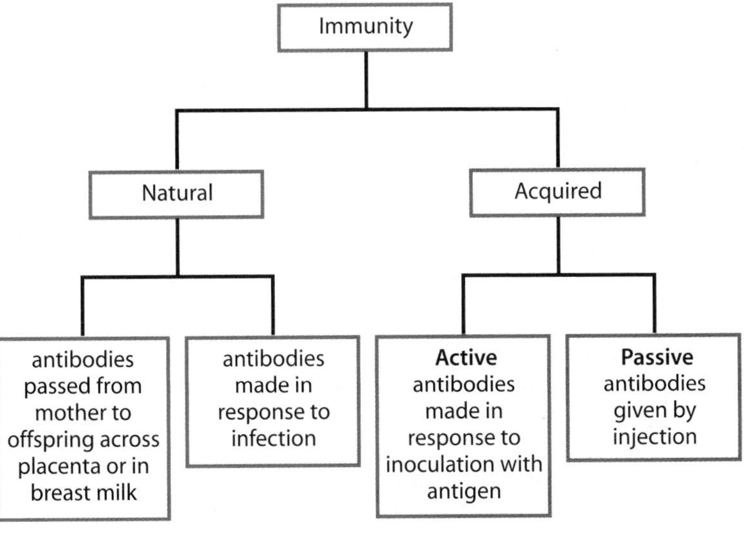

Figure 16.3 The various types of immunity.

Q2: Which protects a person more quickly against a disease: active or passive immunity? Explain your answer.

Q3: Which protects a person for longer against a disease: active or passive immunity.? Explain your answer.

Preventing the spread of diseases

Infectious diseases can be prevented by a variety of means. We shall concentrate on diseases of humans, but the same principles apply to diseases of non-human animals and of plants.

- **Eliminate the disease-causing organism**. On a world-wide basis this has only been done to date with the virus that causes smallpox, though the WHO has a plan to eliminate the polio virus. However, local exterminations may be possible, as we shall see when we consider ways of tackling malaria. On a smaller scale, every time you use soap to wash your hands you are killing disease-causing organisms.
- **Avoid coming into contact with the infectious organism**. Condoms, for example, can reduce the spread of sexually transmitted diseases by greatly reducing the chances of the disease-causing organisms passing from one person to another during sexual intercourse.
- **Boost the body's natural defences**. As we have seen, this is most notably done by vaccinations. However, simply maintaining a balanced diet, getting enough sleep and avoiding too much stress can significantly reduce the chances of developing diseases. Think about the times you most often get colds. Is it when your natural defences are low?
- **Treat the disease in its early stages**. Fungicides, for example, can be used to cure diseases such as athlete's foot and ringworm which are caused by fungi. Similarly, antibiotics kill bacteria and so can be used to treat disease such as gonorrhoea, tuberculosis, cholera and typhoid. Unfortunately, viruses are very difficult to destroy once they have succeeded in getting into a person, so recovering from a viral disease often means waiting until the body's natural defence system overcomes the infection through the production of antibodies.

Rubella

Rubella can be controlled by vaccination. Because it is so dangerous to a young fetus, it is especially important that girls are inoculated before they are likely to become pregnant. In many countries, including the UK, all girls are vaccinated against rubella by the time they are 12 years old (Figure 16.4).

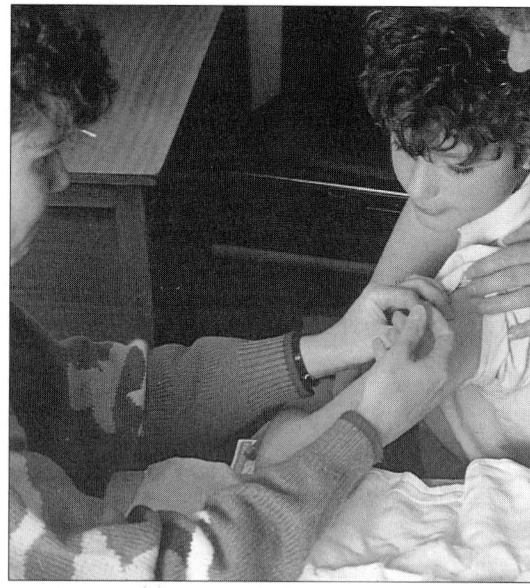

Figure 16.4 Rubella can be prevented by inoculation.

AIDS

Unfortunately there is still no vaccination against HIV, nor can drugs prevent HIV infection progressing to AIDS, though some drugs, including AZT, can help reduce the symptoms of AIDS and may slow the progression from HIV infection to AIDS. Other drugs are used to treat the various diseases which someone with AIDS tends to develop through having a damaged immune system.

The key to the prevention of HIV infection is educating people to change their behaviour. The spread of HIV in a country can be prevented by a combination of some or all of the following:

- encouraging people to have fewer sexual partners
- encouraging more people to use condoms, which serve as a barrier to HIV
- reducing the chances of people coming into contact with infected blood through such measures as getting dentists to wear gloves and getting sportspeople with cuts to come off the field of play
- reducing the sharing of needles among people who inject drugs (Figure 16.5).

It typically takes several years for someone infected with HIV to develop the first symptoms of AIDS. Unfortunately this means that someone infected with HIV can infect many other people without realising it. Someone infected with HIV but not showing any symptoms is known as a **carrier**. A person knowingly infected with HIV generally finds it impossible to get life insurance or a mortgage. Some people stigmatise (blame and avoid) people infected with HIV.

Q4: State two ways in which getting dentists to wear protective gloves can help slow the spread of HIV.

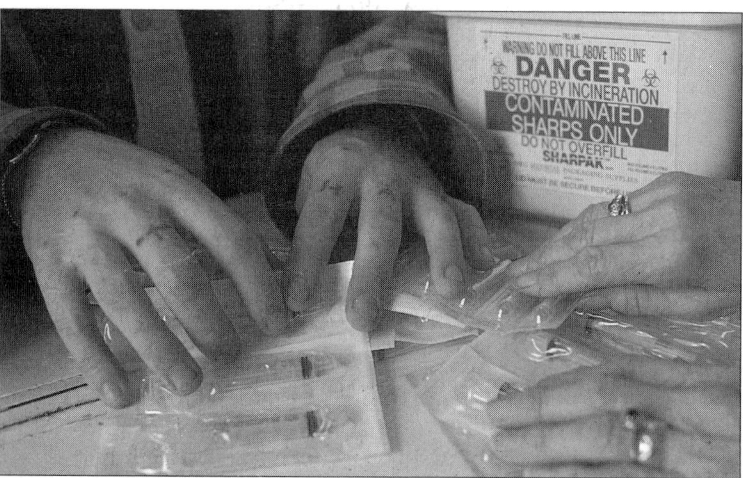

Figure 16.5 The spread of HIV can be slowed by encouraging drug misusers not to inject and ensuring that those who do are supplied with clean needles, as at this needle exchange scheme.

Malaria

As we have seen, malaria is caused by a protozoan carried by a mosquito (page 127). Despite the spending of countless millions of pounds, malaria is still one of the world's most serious diseases. However, the following measures have helped to control it, at least in part:

- spraying the breeding grounds (marshes and stagnant waters) of the mosquito with oils – this kills the mosquito larvae
- draining the breeding grounds of the mosquito
- using insecticides to kill the mosquito – unfortunately the mosquito often evolves resistance to the pesticides, which also kill many other insects including some that are beneficial to humans
- using biological control by introducing a predator, such as guppies (a fish) to eat the mosquito larvae
- preventing the female mosquito from biting people, e.g. by the use of mosquito nets over individual beds.

A number of drugs have been developed against malaria, the longest used being quinine, obtained from the bark of the conchona tree.

Athlete's foot

Athlete's foot can be controlled by:

- thoroughly drying yourself, especially your feet, after bathing
- not sharing towels for drying
- using disinfectants in swimming pools and communal showers
- treating the condition promptly with fungicides.

Food poisoning

Human food needs to be protected from two types of microorganisms:

- **disease-causing microorganisms**, such as the bacteria *Salmonella enteritidis*, *Campylobacter*, *Clostridium* (some forms of which produce a toxin which can cause **botulism**) and *Staphylococcus* (the toxin produced by *Staphylococcus aureus* causes food poisoning)
- **decomposers** which spoil food by causing it to decay, e.g. the moulds that grow on bread.

Many techniques are used to protect foods from microorganisms including:

- **refrigeration**, in which food is cooled to between 0°C and 5°C, thus causing microorganisms to grow only very slowly (regular defrosting is needed to ensure that these temperatures are not exceeded)
- **deep freezing**, in which food is cooled to below –18°C (in a three star freezer) or below –24°C (in a four star freezer), thus preventing the growth of microorganisms, but not killing them
- **dehydration**, in which water is removed from the food, e.g. by drying fish in sunny climates and by freeze-drying many foods, a process in which the food is frozen and then dried in a vacuum
- **pickling**, in which the addition of ethanoic (acetic) acid lowers the pH resulting in an acidity at which many microorganisms cannot reproduce
- **osmotic preservation**, in which sugar or salt is added to food, so making it impossible for most microorganisms to reproduce because they lose water from their cells by osmosis
- **pasteurisation**, in which liquids such as milk or beer are heated to 72°C for 15 seconds, and then rapidly cooled to 10°C, thus killing most bacteria, including *Salmonella*, without affecting the taste
- **ultra-heat treatment** (**UHT**), also known as **sterilisation**, in which food, most commonly milk, is heat to 132°C for 1 minute, and then rapidly cooled, thus killing virtually all microorganisms and their spores
- **cooking**, in which microorganisms are killed by heat
- **canning** or **bottling**, in which food is (usually) cooked and then sealed in sterile containers
- **vacuum packaging**, which means that there is no oxygen to support aerobic respiration
- **irradiation**, which kills most microorganisms, but is rarely used because many people feel uncomfortable about it.

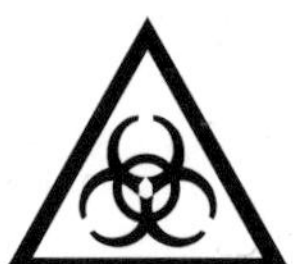

Biohazard

Wear eye protection

Practical 16.1 To investigate ways of keeping milk fresh

In this practical it is suggested that you devise a number of ways of keeping milk from going off and then test them to see how well they work.

Requirements

Milk, 250 cm^3

Various other items of equipment may be required, e.g. pyrex test tubes, Bunsen burner, tripod and gauze, thermometer, access to a freezer, access to a refrigerator, resazurin (dye)

1 Decide how you could detect when a sample of milk has gone off (Smell? Thickness when you try to pour it? Change in colour of resazurin dye which goes from blue to pink to white as oxygen is removed from any solution in which it is present? Another method?).

SAFETY: Do not taste any of your samples at any stage. Wash your hands with soap/detergent after completing each stage of the practical.

2 Obtain a sample of fresh milk.

3 Divide the sample of fresh milk into a number of smaller volumes (e.g. ten pyrex test tubes).

4 Decide on a number of different treatments (e.g. freezing; refrigeration; heating to 70°C for 30 seconds followed by refrigeration; heating to boiling for 30 seconds followed by refrigeration; mixing with a bactericidal mouthwash followed by refrigeration). Ensure that each treatment has at least two replicates.

5 Every 12 or 24 hours use the method you identified in step 1 to decide if the milk is still fresh in each treatment.

6 Attempt to interpret your results.

7 Suggest further experiments to test any explanations you have come up with.

Much of the treatment of food is done not to prevent the growth of micro-organisms but to enhance its appeal to the purchaser. A number of **additives** may be added to foods for a variety of purposes. Additives which are recognised as safe by the European Union are given an E-number.

- **Colourants** (E100–E180) are used to make food look 'more natural'. For example, they may be added to tinned peas to make them greener or to margarine to make it yellower.
- **Anti-oxidants** (E300–E320) prevent oxygen in the air from reacting with the food. For example, vitamin C may be added to cut fruit to stop it going brown.
- **Stabilisers** (various E numbers) prevent oil and water from separating out again. They may be used to thicken foods and can disguise the amount of fat or water that the food contains.

Q5: Supermarkets that display fresh foods under transparent wraps often ensure that the atmosphere that surrounds the food under the wrap is high in nitrogen gas and low in oxygen gas. Why do you think this is?

Q6: The atmosphere that surrounds steaks kept in supermarkets under transparent wraps is often deliberately made high in oxygen gas. Suggest the reason for this.

The 1995 **Food Safety (General Food Hygiene) Regulations** relate to the preparation and sale of food, whether this is by the owner of a five-star restaurant or by someone fund-raising in a village hall. They require anyone in charge of a food business to:

- make sure food is supplied and sold in a hygienic way
- identify food safety hazards
- know which steps are critical for food safety
- ensure safe controls are in place, maintained and reviewed.

The chances of food poisoning can be virtually eliminated by carrying out the appropriate food preservation procedures and by:

- ensuring that those involved in the preparation of food regularly wash their hands

- keeping flies, cockroaches, rodents and other animals away from food
- keeping raw meat separate from cooked meat – so as to prevent the raw meat from cross-infecting the cooked meat (Figure 16.6)
- thoroughly cleaning working surfaces and kitchen equipment before and after use
- thoroughly cooking meats and meat products
- thoroughly thawing frozen food before cooking
- excluding known carriers of food poisoning microorganisms from the food industry
- motivating kitchen staff by a good working environment and adequate wages.

Figure 16.6 *Salmonella* food poisoning often results from eating chicken eggs or meat which has been inadequately cooked. Notice how food can be contaminated by pathogens through animal feed and abattoir practice. Chickens kept in battery cages are more likely to be infected with *Salmonella* than are free range chickens. *Salmonella* food poisoning can also result from drinking unpasteurised milk.

BO, spots and hair care

The skin has two kinds of gland:

- sweat glands produce **sweat** which helps cool the body when it evaporates
- oil glands produce an oily substance called **sebum** which helps keep the skin from drying out.

Sweat itself has no smell. However, some bacteria can feed on sweat and produce substances which result in body odour (BO). BO can be reduced by regular washing, paying particular attention to the armpits, groin and feet. Some people find that anti-perspirants help, but they can be expensive.

During adolescence, sebum production reaches a maximum. If the glands become blocked with sebum, spots (pimples) can result. Spots can be controlled by regular washing and avoiding the over-use of cosmetics. Squeezing spots really doesn't help and can lead to scarring. Bad cases of spots (**acne**) can be treated by your GP free of charge, or you can try buying one of the many commercial treatments, some of which contain **antiseptics** to kill the bacteria found in spots.

If the scalp produces too much sebum, the hair may become greasy. Dandruff is a mixture of dead skin cells and sebum. Nowadays there are plenty of good shampoos that can tackle dandruff and greasy hair.

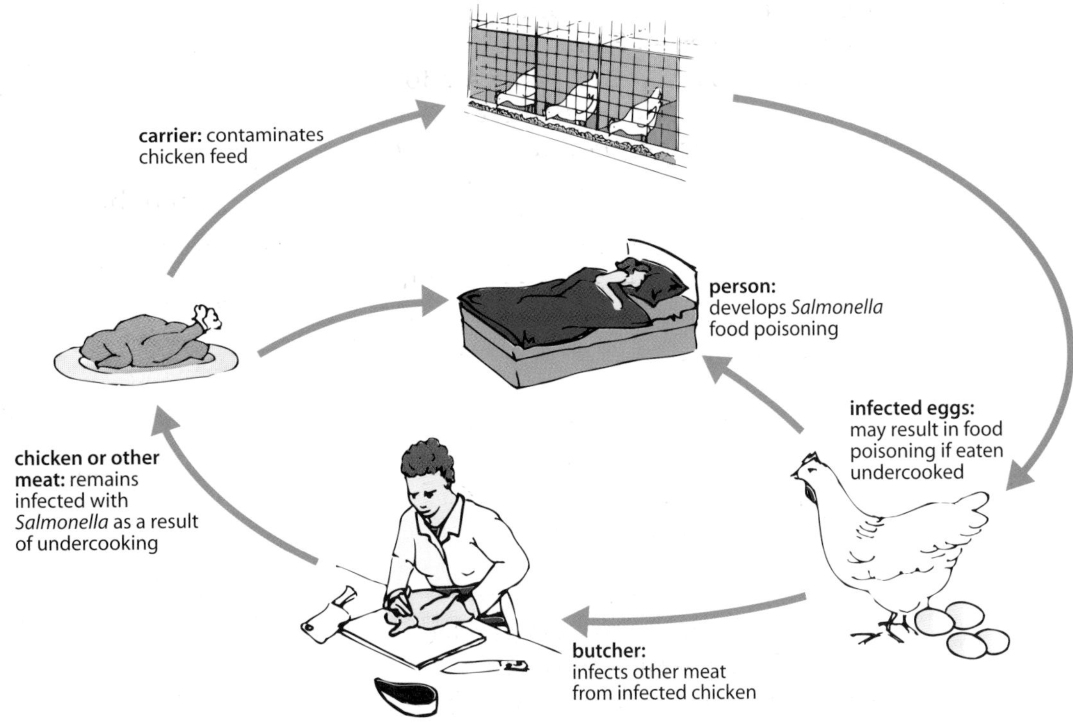

Summary

- Protection against infectious disease is provided by our skin, the formation of scabs, low stomach pH, lysozyme in tears, mucus and cilia in the gaseous exchange system, white blood cells and our behaviour.
- Some white blood cells ingest bacteria. Others, called lymphocytes, produce antibodies which react with antigens on the surface of disease-causing micro-organisms.
- Natural immunity occurs when a person produces antibodies in response to an infection, or when they receive antibodies from their mother.
- Vaccinations/inoculations are examples of acquired immunity.
- Vaccinations/inoculations rely on active immunity. Passive acquired immunity is when a person is artificially given antibodies against a disease.
- Infectious diseases can be prevented by eliminating the disease-causing organism, avoiding coming into contact with it, boosting the body's natural defences and treating the disease in the early stages.
- Rubella can be controlled by vaccination.
- The key to the prevention of HIV-infection is education.
- Malaria can be prevented by such measures as insecticides, draining the mosquito's breeding grounds and using mosquito nets.
- Athlete's foot can be prevented by thorough drying of the skin, by not sharing towels and by the use of disinfectants in swimming pools and communal showers.
- A range of measures is used in food preservation. These measures, together with hygienic precautions when preparing food, can prevent food poisoning.

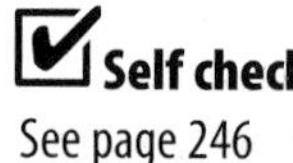

See page 246

CHAPTER 17

Variety of living organisms

In this chapter you will learn about the differences between living and non-living things. You will be introduced to the main features of the five kingdoms as well as using identification keys. Finally you will look at human characteristics and the evolution of humans.

Characteristics of living organisms

All living organisms show the following features.

- **Respiration** – the breakdown of food, e.g. sugar, to give energy.
- **Nutrition** – the gaining of raw materials for the activities of organisms. Animals obtain their food by eating other organisms. Plants manufacture their food from simple molecules.
- **Growth** – an increase in size at some stage of their life cycle.
- **Reproduction** – the production of new organisms sexually or asexually.
- **Excretion** – the removal of the waste products produced by the hundreds of chemical reactions (metabolism) going on inside organisms.
- **Irritability** – the ability to respond to stimuli, e.g. plants may respond to the stimulus of light; animals may respond to temperature.
- **Movement** – a change in position of parts of an organism or of the whole organism (**locomotion**).

Q1: Will material like wood, that was once living, show the features of living organisms or of non-living material, such as rock?

Five kingdom classification system

Living organisms are grouped into five kingdoms (See Table 17.1). The members of one kingdom, the Prokaryotes, do not have a membrane around their nucleus nor membrane-bound organelles in their cytoplasm. All the other kingdoms do have these structures and are termed **eukaryotic** ('true nucleus').

Viruses

Viruses cannot be placed in the above classification system. You do not need to know how they are classified, only that they:

- are variable in shape
- have an outer coat of protein
- have nuclear material that could be either DNA or RNA
- have no cytoplasm
- are all obligate parasites, i.e. need a host in order to survive.

Table 17.1 Features of the five kingdoms into which living organisms are grouped

Kingdom	Characteristics
Prokaryotes	Unicellular; have cell walls but no membrane-bound nucleus or membrane-bound organelles
Protoctists	Eukaryotic organisms that are neither animals, plants nor fungi; this kingdom includes photosynthetic algae as well as non-photosynthetic organisms like *Amoeba*
Fungi	Basic unit is usually a thread-like hypha; collection of hyphae makes up a mycelium; eukaryotic cells with cell walls that are not made of cellulose; no chlorophyll so cannot photosynthesise
Plants	Multicellular; feed by photosynthesis; do not show locomotion; eukaryotic cells having cellulose cell walls and fluid-filled vacuoles
Animals	Eukaryotic and multicellular; feed on other living organisms; usually show locomotion and have nervous systems

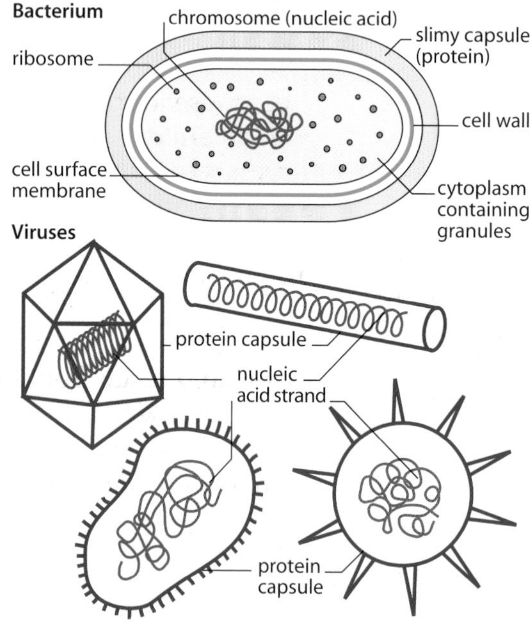

Figure 17.1 Bacteria and viruses compared.

Q2: Figure 17.1 shows a bacterium and four different viruses. Give three ways in which the bacterium shown is different in structure from all the viruses.

Classification groups

All organisms can be arranged into groups, called **taxa**. The smallest group (taxon) is the **species**. This can be defined as 'a group of organisms which share many common features and can normally interbreed to produce fertile offspring'. Figure 17.2 shows the other taxa and how they are arranged in a hierarchy:

- similar species are grouped into a **genus**
- similar genera are grouped into a **family**
- similar families are grouped into an **order**
- similar orders are grouped into a **class**
- similar classes are grouped into a **phylum**
- similar phyla are grouped into a **kingdom.**

A simple way of remembering this hierarchy is to use the first letter of each taxon, starting with the kingdom: KPCOFGS – **K**ing **P**eter **C**ame **O**ver **F**or **G**inger **S**naps.

To avoid confusion, all organisms are referred to by the name of their genus and species. Because this involves two names, it is called a **binomial** system. The name of the genus always takes a capital letter whilst the name of the species does not. Both are written in italics (or underlined in hand-written notes). For example, humans are called *Homo sapiens* and dogs are called *Canis familiaris*.

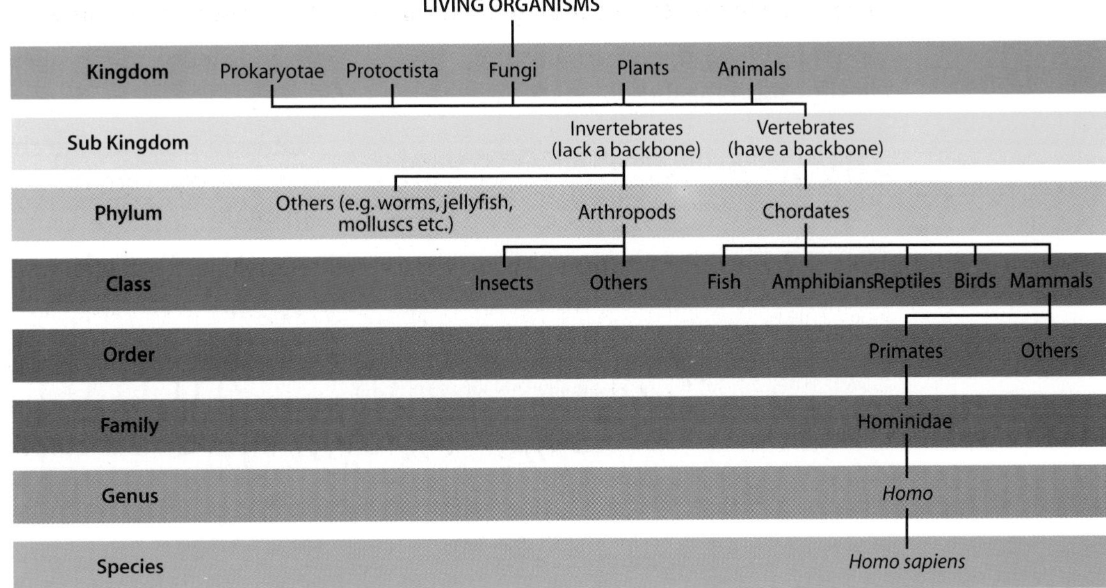

Figure 17.2 Classification of living organisms (simplified).

Identification keys

These are used to identify organisms. Figure 17.3 shows some organisms that affect humans. They are not drawn to scale. To make a key that could be used to identify these organisms, we must first select a characteristic which will separate the organisms into two groups. A suitable feature could be whether the body is divided into segments or not divided into segments. This would separate organisms V, U and Y from organisms X, W and Z.

- To separate Y from V and U we could use presence or absence of bristles.
- To separate U and V we could use presence or absence of body coiling.
- To separate Z from X and W we could use presence or absence of jointed legs.
- To separate X and W we could use the number of pairs of legs.

Figure 17.4 shows an identification key that would result from the above. Because the key always separates organisms into two groups, it is called a **dichotomous key**. Keys such as this are commonly used to identify unknown organisms.

Figure 17.3 Some organisms that can affect humans.

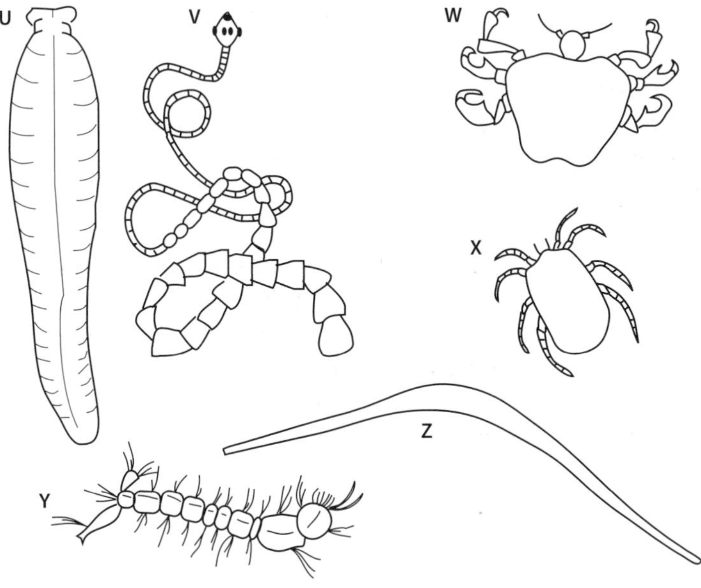

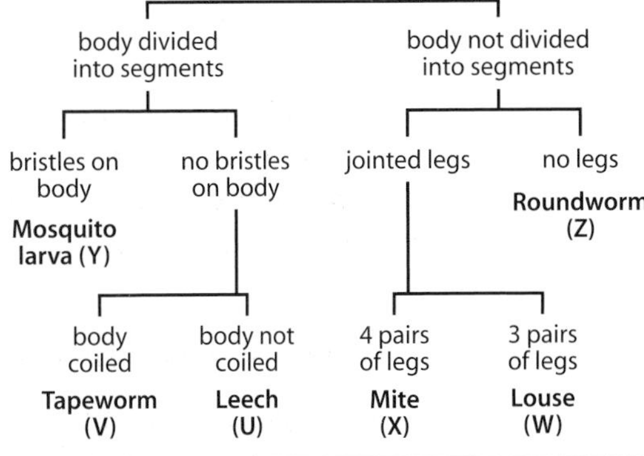

Figure 17.4 Identification key for the organisms in Figure 17.3.

Humans as special animals

On page 140 you learned about classification groups.

Q2: What do the initials KPCOFGS stand for?

Q3: Use Figure 17.2 and your own knowledge to classify a human.

Table 17.2 shows the characteristics of a human as a vertebrate, mammal and primate.

Table 17.2 The characteristics of a human as a vertebrate, mammal and primate

Group	Key characteristics
Vertebrates	Backbone made of vertebrae
Mammals	External ears; fur/hair; sweat glands and sebaceous glands (produce waxy sebum); some sebaceous glands modified to form mammary glands; most possess a placenta during pregnancy; endothermic; whiskers; diaphragm separates thorax from abdomen; eyelids protect eyes; seven vertebrae (cervical) in the neck
Primates	Excellent eyesight; eyes at the front of the head giving good judgement of distance; a large brain; opposable thumb gives ability to grasp objects, so allowing the full use of tools; finger nails rather than claws; few offspring produced
Human	Lack of body hair; large cerebral hemispheres allowing learning, reasoning and language development; ability to walk on two legs (bipedalism) .

Main stages in human evolution

Most of what is known about human evolution is based on incomplete evidence. However, fossil remains suggest that several humanoid (human-like) groups existed throughout Europe, Asia and Africa during the last four million years or so (Table 17.3). Evidence from anatomy (e.g. bone structure), serology (studies with antibodies), biochemistry and behaviour suggests that our closest living relatives are probably chimpanzees and gorillas. This does not mean that humans are descended from them but that they may all have had common ancestors about ten million years ago.

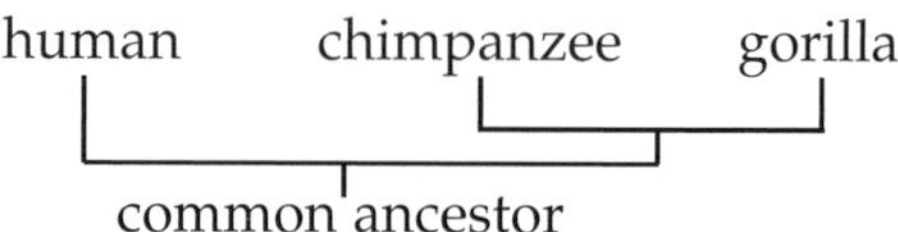

Note that the term 'Man' in Table 17.3 does not imply gender or male dominance but is the name commonly used in biology for the species *Homo sapiens*.

Table 17.3 Various stages in human evolution

Name	Estimated age of fossils	Features of interest
Australopithecus	1.5 to 4 million years	Walked upright; ape-like skull with small brain
Homo erectus (Java Man, Peking Man)	1 million years	Walked upright; larger brain than *Australopithecus*
Homo neanderthalis (Neanderthal Man)	350 000 to 500 000 years	Walked upright; brain about the size of that of people living today
Homo sapiens (modern Man)	less than 500 000 years	See characteristics of humans (Table 17.2)

Summary

- Living organisms all have the following seven characteristics: respiration; nutrition; growth; reproduction; excretion; irritability; movement.
- Living organisms are grouped into five kingdoms: prokaryotes; protoctists; fungi; plants; animals.
- Each kingdom is further divided into groups called taxa (singular taxon). In decreasing order of size, these taxa are: phylum; class; order; family; genus; species.
- Keys are used to separate organisms from one another using various specific characteristics.
- Humans can be distinguished from other primates by their ability to walk on two legs, lack of body hair and the presence of large cerebral hemispheres.

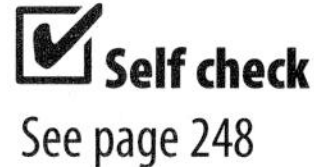
Self check

See page 248

CHAPTER 18

Helpful and harmful organisms

In this chapter you will learn about some of the many organisms with which humans interact. You will learn about how their structure enables them either to benefit or to harm us. Parts of this chapter should be read in conjunction with the relevant sections of Chapter 15 on infection, Chapter 16 on disease control and Chapter 17 on variety of living organisms.

Viruses

Viruses are so simple that many scientists don't even classify them as organisms. All viruses are parasites: they cannot live on their own. They must infect a **host** in order to reproduce and complete their life cycle. Some viruses attack bacteria, others attack animals and still others attack plants. Viruses are very small, ranging in size from 10 to 300 nm (nanometres). (There are a million nanometres in a millimetre.) Antibiotics are ineffective against viruses. However, antibiotics may be used if an initial viral infection is followed by a secondary bacterial infection.

HIV

HIV is the **Human Immunodeficiency Virus** (Figure 18.1). It is so-called because it often causes a human's immune system to become deficient, and thus unable to fight off disease-causing microorganisms. When this happens, the person becomes ill and eventually develops **AIDS (Acquired Immune Deficiency Syndrome)**. HIV attacks human lymphocytes, thus weakening our immune system. Once inside a lymphocyte, HIV takes it over and turns it into a factory for HIV production. Eventually the lymphocyte breaks open, releasing hundreds of new viruses. These travel to uninfected lymphocytes, attacking and infecting them in turn.

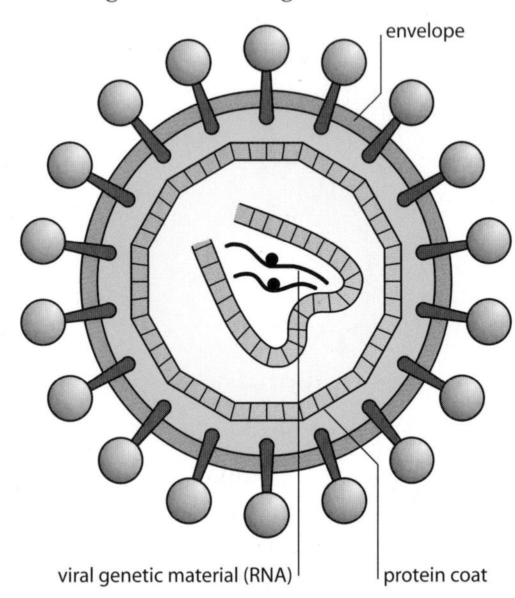

Figure 18.1 HIV. The virus uses its genetic material, RNA, to make more copies of itself inside human cells.

Influenza virus

Influenza (**'flu'**) is caused by the influenza virus (Figure 18.2).

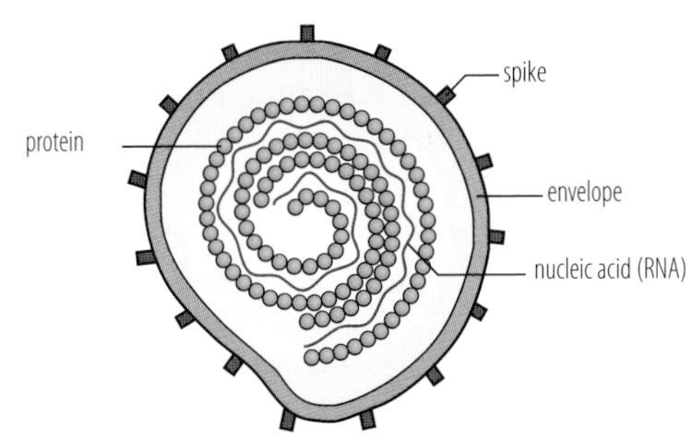

Figure 18.2 The influenza virus. As many people died from the influenza epidemic in Europe in 1918 as from both World Wars put together.

Rubella virus

As mentioned on page 134, practically all girls in the UK are given a vaccination against **rubella** (**German measles**) when aged about 12. This is because infection with the rubella virus during the first three months of pregnancy can cause the fetus to be severely damaged or even die.

Bacteria

Bacteria, including **blue-green bacteria**, are **prokaryotes**. This means that they have simpler cells than other organisms. They *do* have cytoplasm and ribosomes (unlike viruses which have neither) but they *lack* a nucleus, mitochondria and most of the cell structures possessed by all other organisms. Unlike viruses, bacteria are large enough to be seen under a good light microscope, where they are visible, either singly or in groups, often as spherical or rod-shaped structures (Figure 18.3). Under an electron microscope, their structure is visible in more detail (Figure 18.4). A typical bacterium is about 1 µm (one micrometre) in diameter. (There are a thousand micrometres in a millimetre.) Bacteria often reproduce by **binary fission**, as is the case, for example, in *Bacillus*, a rod-shaped bacterium with a structure like that shown in Figure 18.4. Binary fission is an example of asexual reproduction, though many bacteria also show sexual reproduction in which there is transfer of genetic material from one cell to another.

Bacteria show tremendous variety in terms of how they obtain their food. Most bacteria require a carbon source, a nitrogen source, mineral ions and certain growth factors (vitamins). In the right environment, growth of a bacterial colony is rapid and results chiefly from asexual reproduction. Precisely what the right environment is may differ greatly from one bacterium species to another. Each will have an optimum temperature, pH and oxygen level.

Figure 18.3 Different bacteria as seen under the light microscope.

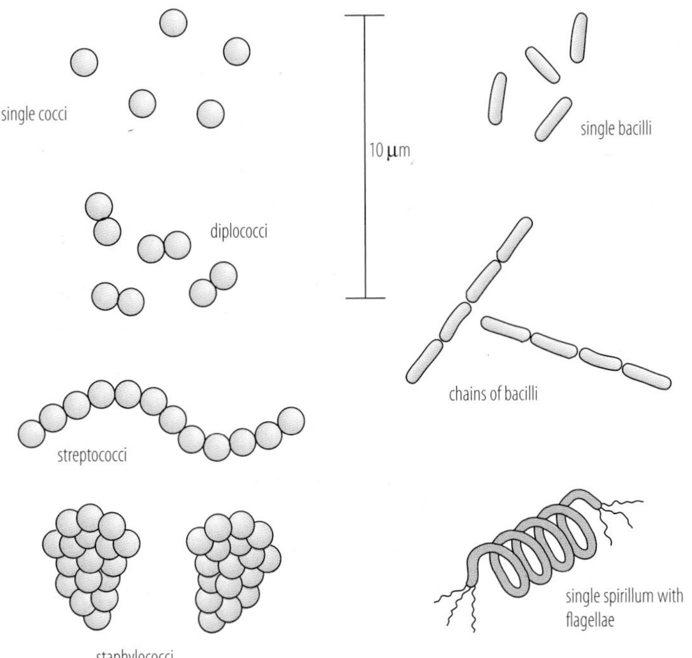

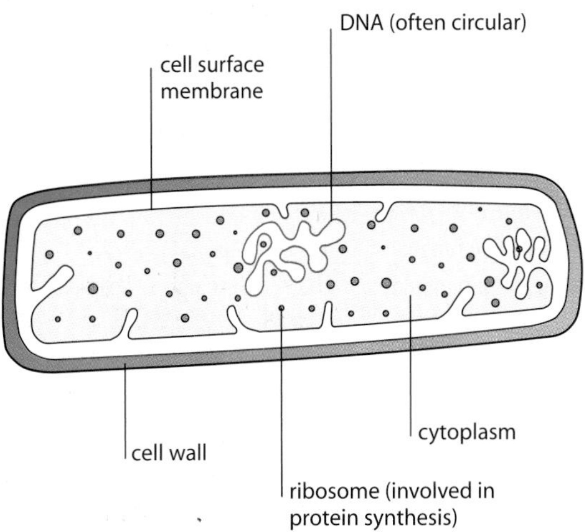

Figure 18.4 A drawing of a rod-shaped bacterium (a bacillus) based on photographs taken with the electron microscope.

Food-spoilage bacteria

Bacteria are so small and light that they are carried by air currents almost everywhere. Any food soon becomes colonised by bacteria (and fungi). These start to break down the food by releasing their enzymes onto it. This spoils the food for us.

Salmonella

Although the low pH in our stomachs kills many of the bacteria we ingest with our food, some bacteria can cause **food poisoning**. One such is *Salmonella*. Ways of avoiding infection with *Salmonella* are considered on pages 135–137.

Decomposers

Not all bacteria are harmful to us. Many are decomposers, breaking down dead organisms and their waste products in soil and water. Some bacteria play a vital role in the nitrogen cycle (page 207). Bacteria, along with protozoa and certain other organisms, also play an important role in the treatment of sewage (see page 226). A compost heap demonstrates the effectiveness of decomposers.

The vital roles played by bacteria in the biotechnology industry are considered on page 165.

Q1: Why is the inside of a compost heap often significantly hotter than the surrounding air temperature?

Q2: How would you expect the volume of a compost heap, left on its own for a few weeks, to change?

Q3: What would happen to food webs if there were no decomposers, and why?

Fungi

Fungi, along with plants and animals, are **eukaryotes**. This means that their cells possess a nucleus. Most fungi consist of thread-like structures called **hyphae** which form a **mycelium** (Figure 18.5). All fungi possess a cell wall, in common with bacteria and plants and unlike animals. However, fungi, unlike plants and some bacteria, cannot make their own food. Fungi are either parasites – feeding on living organisms – or decomposers – feeding off dead organisms or their waste products.

Athlete's foot

Athlete's foot is one of the small number of human diseases caused by fungi. The fungus usually lives in the skin between the toes. Here it causes itching and cracking of the skin.

Edible fungi

Many soil-living fungi produce fruiting bodies in autumn. Some of these are poisonous, but others, such as the edible mushroom, can be eaten (Figure 18.6). A number of edible fungi are now grown commercially indoors.

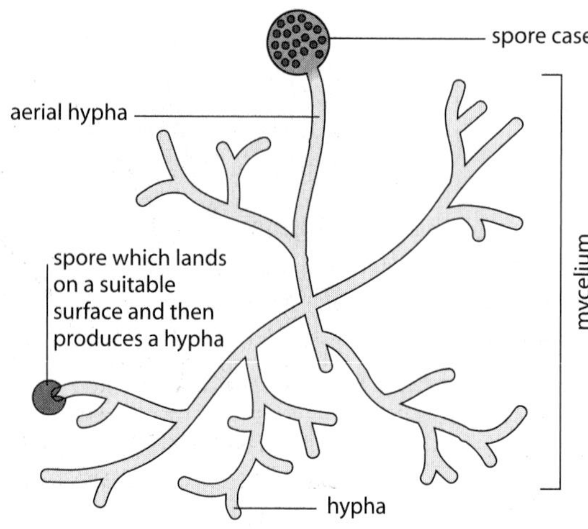

Figure 18.5 The structure of a typical fungus. The fungus shown is pin mould (*Rhizopus*), which is often seen if damp bread is left out for a few days. The spore production illustrated here is asexual, though *Rhizopus* can also reproduce sexually.

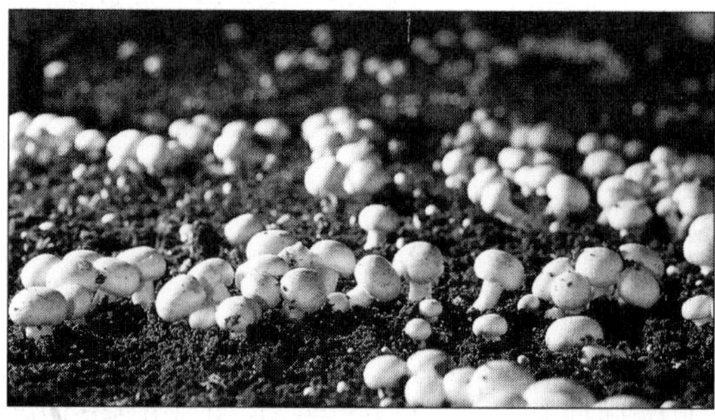

Figure 18.6 These edible mushrooms are grown commercially.

Q4: Do growers of edible mushrooms need to provide artificial lighting? Explain your answer.

Decomposers

Many fungi are decomposers, breaking down dead organisms and their waste products in the soil.

Yeast

Yeast is a fungus, yet is unicellular (Figure 18.7). As we saw on page 38, yeast is of great economic importance. It is used to make bread and other products from dough, as well as all alcoholic drinks. The importance of fungi in the biotechnology industry is discussed further on page 170.

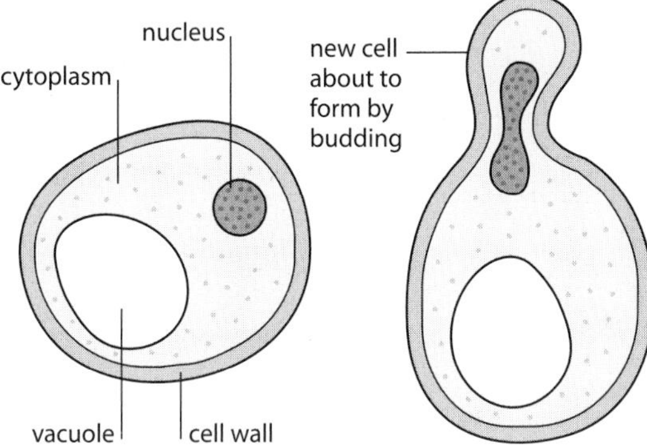

Figure 18.7 Yeast cells. One cell is in the process of dividing into two by an asexual process known as budding.

Protozoa

Protozoa are one-celled organisms that are rather like tiny animals. In common with animals, they are heterotrophs, so they cannot make their own food. They are usually a few micrometres in diameter. Some protozoa cause diseases such as sleeping sickness and malaria. Many protozoa are harmless. Some are beneficial, for example those found in sewage treatment works where, along with bacteria, they help to digest the organic matter in sewage (page 226).

Entamoeba

One form of the disease **dysentery** is caused by a protozoan called *Entamoeba* (Figure 18.8). *Entamoeba* is a parasite which lives in a person's gut and feeds on the cells that line the large intestine. It can cause internal bleeding, diarrhoea, vomiting and fever. The parasite passes out in the person's faeces and if it gets into drinking water or food, other people may become infected.

Q5: Explain why dysentery may be a problem if a city's sewage system is damaged, for example in an earthquake.

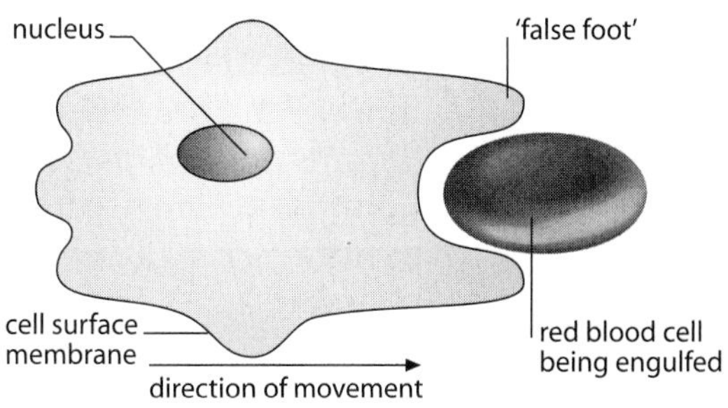

Figure 18.8 *Entamoeba*, the protozoan that causes dysentery, ingesting a human red blood cell.

Plasmodium

Malaria is a disease from which approximately two million people still die each year. It is caused by a protozoan called *Plasmodium*. However, on its own *Plasmodium* is unable to infect humans. It needs a **vector** (carrier) to get it into us. This vector is a female mosquito called *Anopheles* (Figure 18.9). The female mosquito needs blood in order to get enough protein to make her eggs. She gets this blood by biting people. If a mosquito is herself infected with the protozoan parasite, she may inject it into the person she bites.

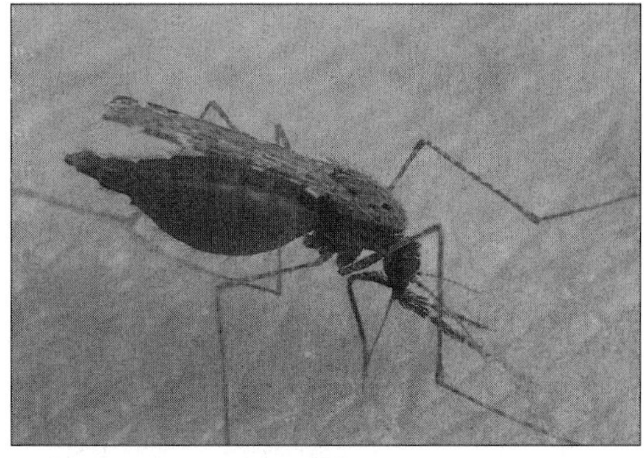

Figure 18.9 A female mosquito of the genus *Anopheles* biting a person. This mosquito can carry the protozoan that causes malaria.

Plants

It is impossible to overstate the importance of plants to us. Without plants there would be no animals and probably little or no oxygen in the atmosphere. Not only that, but plants form the majority of human foods. Plants are multicellular autotrophs with cell walls (see page 140). They vary greatly in structure but almost all plants of economic importance possess **flowers** and are called **flowering plants** (Figure 18.10). This distinguishes them from those plants, such as mosses and ferns, which lack flowers.

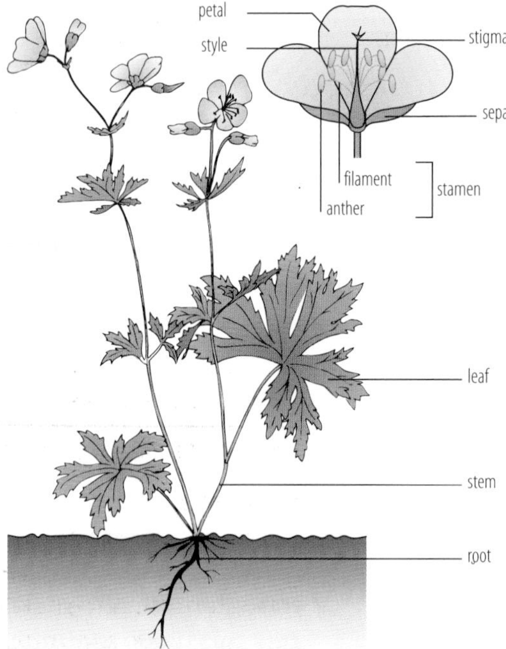

Figure 18.10 The structure of a wild geranium.

Q6: Why would there probably be little or no oxygen in the atmosphere in the absence of plants?

Flowering plants may be:

- **wind-pollinated** – in which case, like grasses and conifer trees, they have very small flowers and produce huge amounts of light pollen
- **insect-pollinated** – in which case, like most familiar garden plants, they have colourful flowers and produce smaller amounts of sticky pollen.

Q7: Why do wind-pollinated plants produce huge amounts of light pollen?

Q8: Why do insect-pollinated plants have coloured flowers and often produce nectar?

Crops

A **crop** is a plant that is grown for human benefit. Most crops are edible and the range of foods we obtain from plants is tremendous:

- vegetables such as peas and beans (seeds in a pod), cabbages and lettuces (leaves), carrots and cassava (roots) and potatoes (tubers)
- fruits such as apples, pears, plums, tomatoes, coconuts and dates
- cereals (technically, fruits) such as wheat, rice and maize
- sugar from the root of sugar beet or the stem of sugar cane.

Other useful products obtained from plants include:

- medicines – a quarter of all prescriptions in the UK contain ingredients derived from plants
- paper, today made mainly from conifer or *Eucalyptus* trees
- wood for furniture and the construction of houses, etc.
- dyes such as indigo
- rubber from the rubber tree
- natural insecticides such as pyrethrins
- alcohol made from sugar cane and used as a fuel in some countries
- fibres such as linen from flax and cotton from the cotton plant (Figure 18.11).

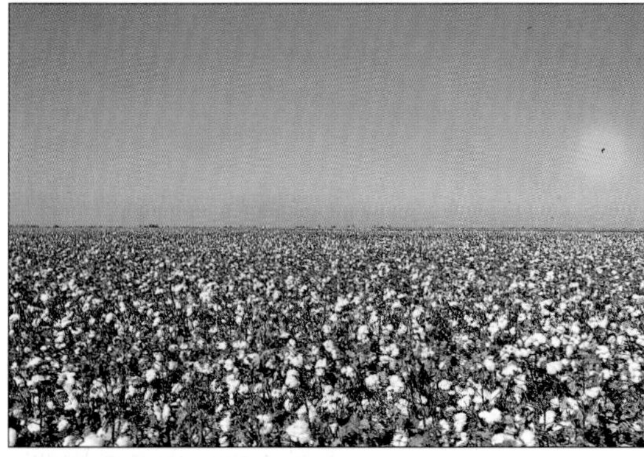

Figure 18.11 A field of cotton, one of the world's most economically important crops. Cottons are now being genetically engineered to improve the quality of their fibres and to produce a range of colours naturally.

Weeds

A **weed** is a plant that is growing in the wrong place. To many farmers, any plant except the crop plant is a weed (Figure 18.12). For this reason, **weedkillers** (also known as **herbicides**) are often extensively used. The main problem with weeds is that they compete with crop plants for sunlight, water, space and mineral ions. In addition, some weeds are poisonous or interfere with harvesting. In many industrialised countries such as the UK, herbicides are so efficient that much of the countryside is covered with large areas of aesthetically unattractive **monocultures** in which just one species of crop plant covers many hectares.

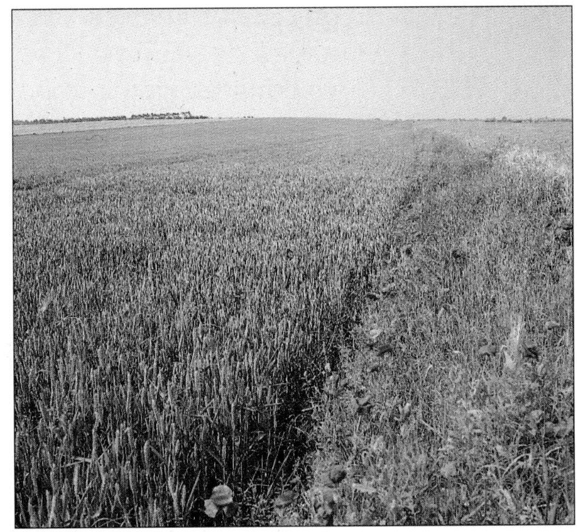

Figure 18.12 Many people like poppies, but to a cereal farmer poppies are weeds.

Animals

Animals are multicellular heterotrophs which lack cell walls and are usually mobile. Humans, of course, are animals.

Insects

It is easy to assume that all insects are pests. In reality, though, many are very beneficial.

- Many insects are needed for the pollination of flowering plants. Without insects there would be, for example, no apples, pears, plums, peas, beans or cabbages. **Honeybees** not only pollinate many crops but also produce honey.
- Some insects keep down the numbers of pests. For example, **ladybirds** eat aphids.
- Many insects are eaten by animals which are of value to us, either economically or aesthetically. For example, birds like titmice, woodpeckers and thrushes, and mammals like shrews and bats, are insectivores. Not only do such animals consume vast quantities of harmful insects, they are also very beautiful.

Housefly

The common housefly (Figure 18.13) can carry a number of disease-causing organisms including the bacteria which cause food poisoning.

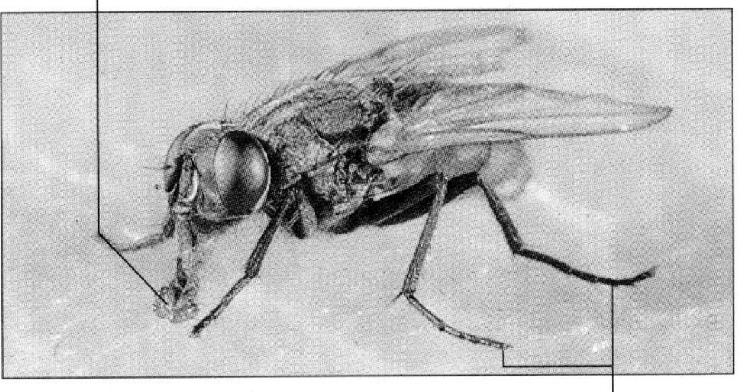

Figure 18.13 Houseflies can transmit diseases.

Mosquito

In some countries mosquitoes can carry malaria and other diseases. As we mentioned on page 127, when a female mosquito bites someone, she may inject the protozoan which causes malaria. The female locates her victim using her eyesight and sense of smell. She then flies towards them. Settling on them, she attempts to insert her piercing mouthparts through their skin. If she is successful, she is able to obtain a meal of blood. At the same time, though, she may inject micro-organisms living inside her into her victim.

Farm animals

A small number of farm animals provide us with many valuable products. In the UK only mammals and birds are of any economic importance:

- **Sheep** produce wool and meat (lamb and mutton)

- **Cattle** produce milk (from cows), meat (veal and beef) and leather
- **Pigs** produce meat (pork, bacon and ham) and leather
- **Chickens** produce eggs and meat.

Farm animals are increasingly kept using intensive farming methods. Many pigs and chickens spend their entire lives indoors, in overcrowded conditions and subject to artificial light regimes designed to maximise productivity (Figure 18.14). Farmers often feel they have been pushed into introducing such housing: the alternative being bankruptcy. Not surprisingly, increasing numbers of people feel that these conditions are unacceptable and now avoid meat or pay more for free range chickens or 'organic' meat.

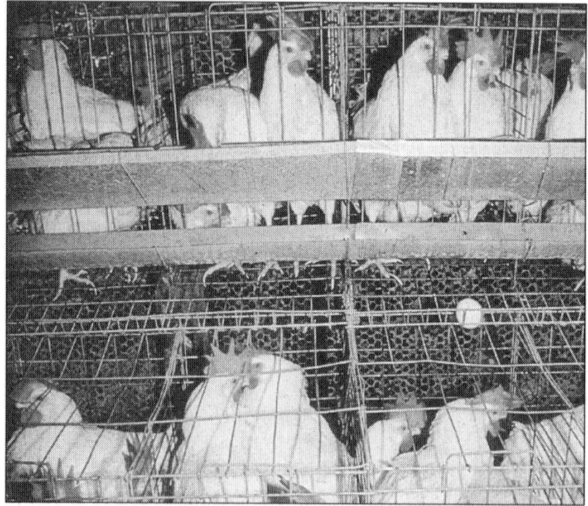

Figure 18.14 Most of the chickens in the UK are kept in conditions such as these.

Companion animals

The final group of animals of benefit to us are **companion animals**. Most familiar to us are **pets**. Benefits from keeping pets include:

- pleasure from watching them
- relaxation through playing with them or stroking them
- exercise if they are taken for walks
- educational benefits for children such as learning how animals grow up, reproduce and, sadly, die.

Scientific research shows that the health benefits from keeping and looking after a pet can be very significant. People recover quickest from heart operations if they have a dog as a pet. The exercise from walking the dog is good for them, while stroking a pet may reduce their blood pressure.

Some companion animals are even more important. For example, thousands of people with impaired sight rely on guide dogs. Similarly, monkeys can be trained to help severely disabled people in wheelchairs to lead a more independent life. The monkeys can be taught to fetch small objects, such as cups, on command.

Summary

- Viruses are very small parasites.
- HIV infection often leads to AIDS.
- Bacteria have cytoplasm and ribosomes, but lack a nucleus, mitochondria and most of the other cell structures possessed by other organisms.
- Some bacteria cause diseases; some are decomposers; some are used in the biotechnology industry.
- Most fungi consist of hyphae which form a mycelium. Yeast, though, is a unicellular fungus.
- Some fungi cause diseases; others are used in the biotechnology industry.
- Some protozoa cause diseases, such as malaria and one form of dysentery.
- Plants make the oxygen we breathe and provide us with most of our food.
- Other useful products from plants include medicines, paper, wood, dyes, rubber, natural insecticides and clothes fibres.
- A weed is a plant that grows where it is not wanted.
- Some insects are beneficial to humans, for example those that pollinate insect-pollinated crops.
- Other insects cause or carry diseases.
- Sheep, cattle, pigs and chickens are important farm animals in the UK, providing food and other valuable products.
- Some animals, such as pets, are important as companion animals.

Self check
See page 249

CHAPTER 19

Variety in humans

In this chapter you will learn about inherited and non-inherited variation. In addition you will study mitosis and meiosis before learning about the various genetic mechanisms that control human features.

Inherited and non-inherited variation

All the organisms within a single, sexually reproducing species are different from one another, i.e. there is variation in any population. These differences may be due to:

- environmental conditions, e.g. diet
- genes that have been inherited from the parent, e.g. genes for growth rate.

Q1: (a) What would you expect to happen to a person's physique if he/she took up weight-lifting on a regular basis? (b) Would these changes be due to the environment or due to genes?

You will study the causes of variation in greater detail in Chapter 21. In the rest of this chapter you will look at genes and their inheritance.

DNA, genes and chromosomes

Cells behave the way they do because of the enzymes they contain. These enzymes are made of proteins. Each protein in a cell is made according to the genetic code that the cell inherits. The material that makes up the genetic code is known as **deoxyribonucleic acid** (**DNA**). Each part of the DNA which codes for an individual protein is known as a **gene**. Genes are carried on long thin structures called **chromosomes**. Occasionally during cell division, each chromosome can be seen to be made up of two **chromatids** (Figure 19.7 on page 155).

Diploid and haploid cells

The genetic information needed to control a human body is carried in twenty three different chromosomes. Human body cells are **diploid**. This means that they contain two copies of each of these chromosomes. Human egg cells and sperm cells (gametes) are **haploid**. This means that they contain only one copy of each of these chromosomes (Figure 19.1).

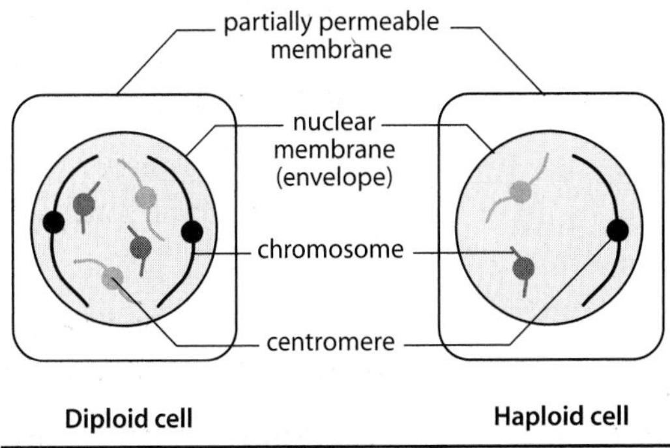

Figure 19.1 Diploid and haploid cells.

To understand this, imagine what happens during sexual reproduction (Figure 19.2). One egg cell, containing one copy of each of the twenty three human chromosomes, fuses with a sperm cell that also contains one copy of each of the twenty three human chromosomes. The fertilised egg cell now has two copies of each chromosome, one from the egg cell and one from the sperm cell. During development, this fertilised egg cell divides to form a fetus containing millions of cells. During division, each of these cells obtains an exact copy of the chromosomes present in the fertilised egg cell. Thus, all the body cells in a human are identical and carry two copies of each chromosome.

We commonly represent diploid as **2*n*** and haploid as ***n***, as shown in Figure 19.2.

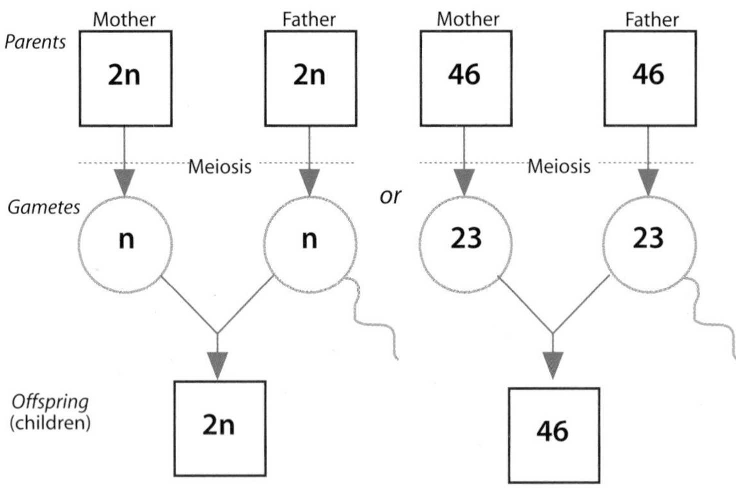

Figure 19.2 Maintenance of the diploid number.

Q2: What is (a) the diploid; (b) the haploid number in the cells in Figure 19.1?

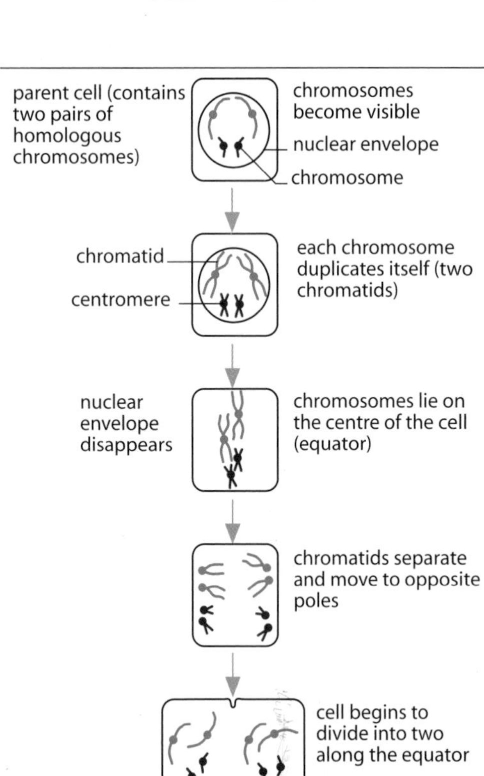

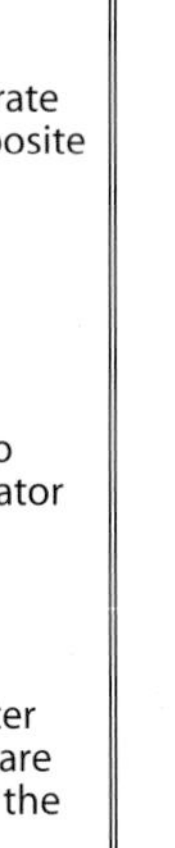

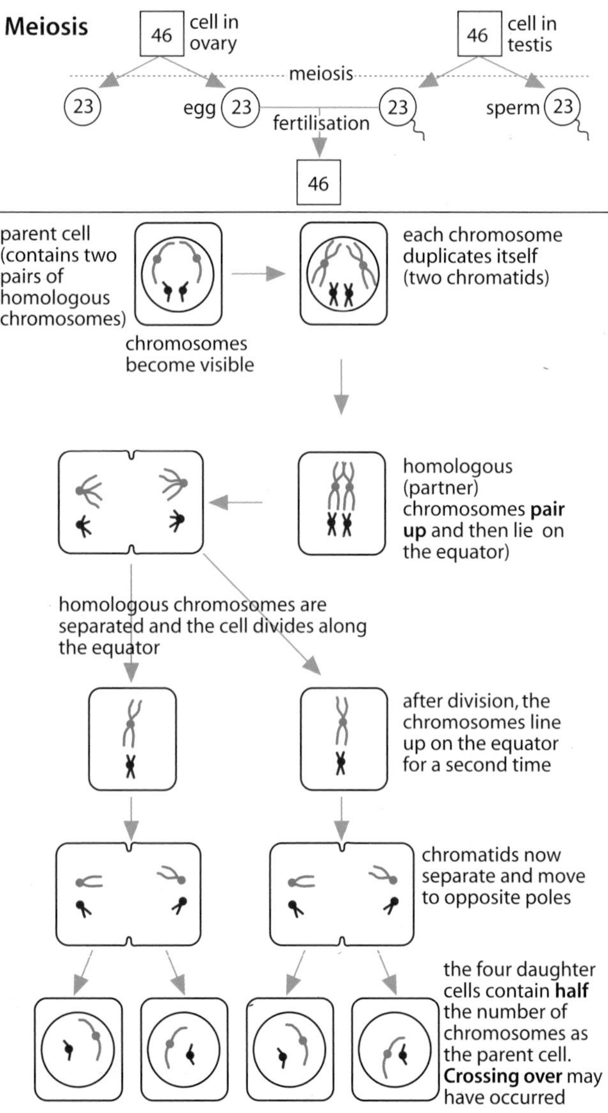

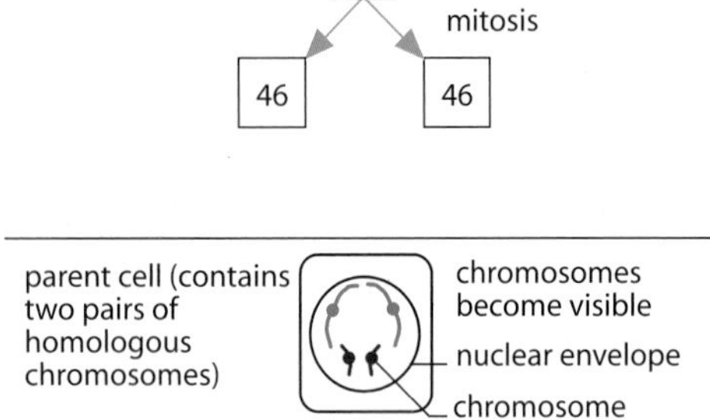

Figure 19.3 Comparison of mitosis and meiosis (greatly simplified).

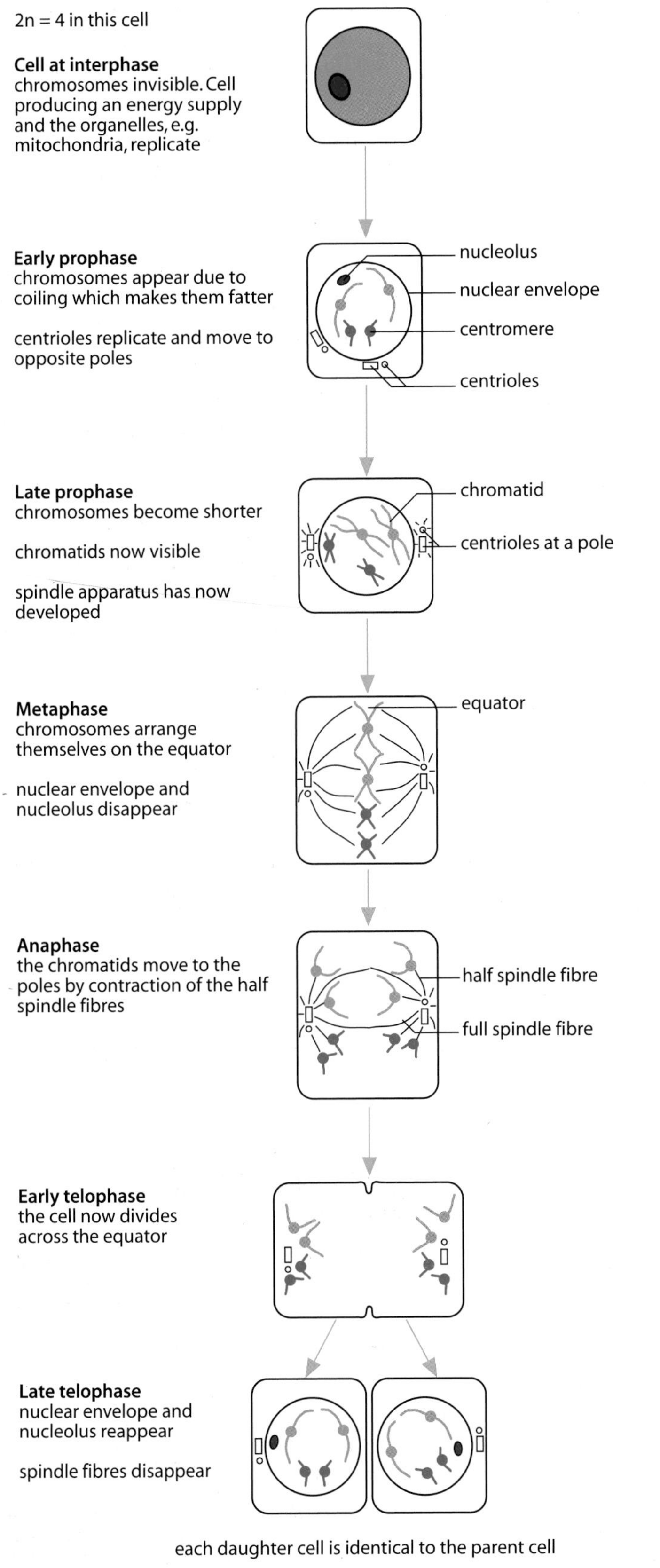

Mitosis and meiosis

Cell division occurs in all types of cell. During this process the nucleus divides by one of two processes:

- mitosis
- meiosis.

The differences between these two types of division are summarised in Figure 19.3.

Mitosis

The cells produced by mitosis contain a copy of every chromosome that was present in the parent cell (Figure 19.4). This type of cell division occurs in the body cells, particularly when cells are replaced or when growth is occurring. Figure 19.5 shows cells in a root tip undergoing mitosis. See if you can identify the different stages.

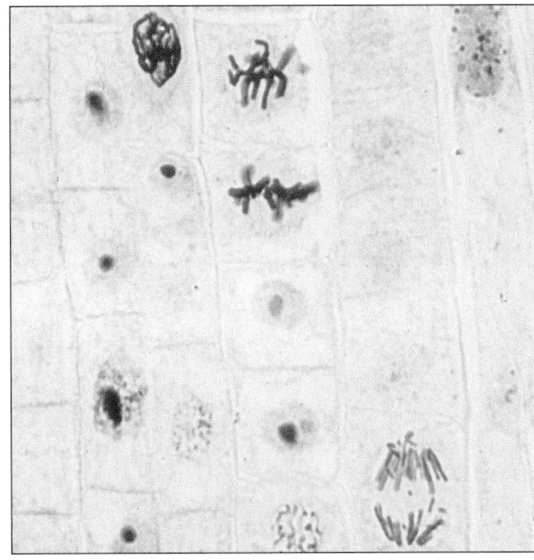

Figure 19.5 Photograph of cells from the root tip of onion undergoing mitosis.

Q3: Suggest a part of the body in which mitosis occurs.

Q4: A diploid cell divides to form two new diploid cells. What must have happened to the DNA in the original cell?

2n = 4 in this cell

Cell at interphase
chromosomes invisible. Cell producing an energy supply and the organelles, e.g. mitochondria, replicate

Early prophase
chromosomes appear due to coiling which makes them fatter

centrioles replicate and move to opposite poles

nucleolus
nuclear envelope
centromere
centrioles

Late prophase
chromosomes become shorter

chromatids now visible

spindle apparatus has now developed

chromatid
centrioles at a pole

Metaphase
chromosomes arrange themselves on the equator

nuclear envelope and nucleolus disappear

equator

Anaphase
the chromatids move to the poles by contraction of the half spindle fibres

half spindle fibre
full spindle fibre

Early telophase
the cell now divides across the equator

Late telophase
nuclear envelope and nucleolus reappear

spindle fibres disappear

each daughter cell is identical to the parent cell

Figure 19.4 Mitosis.

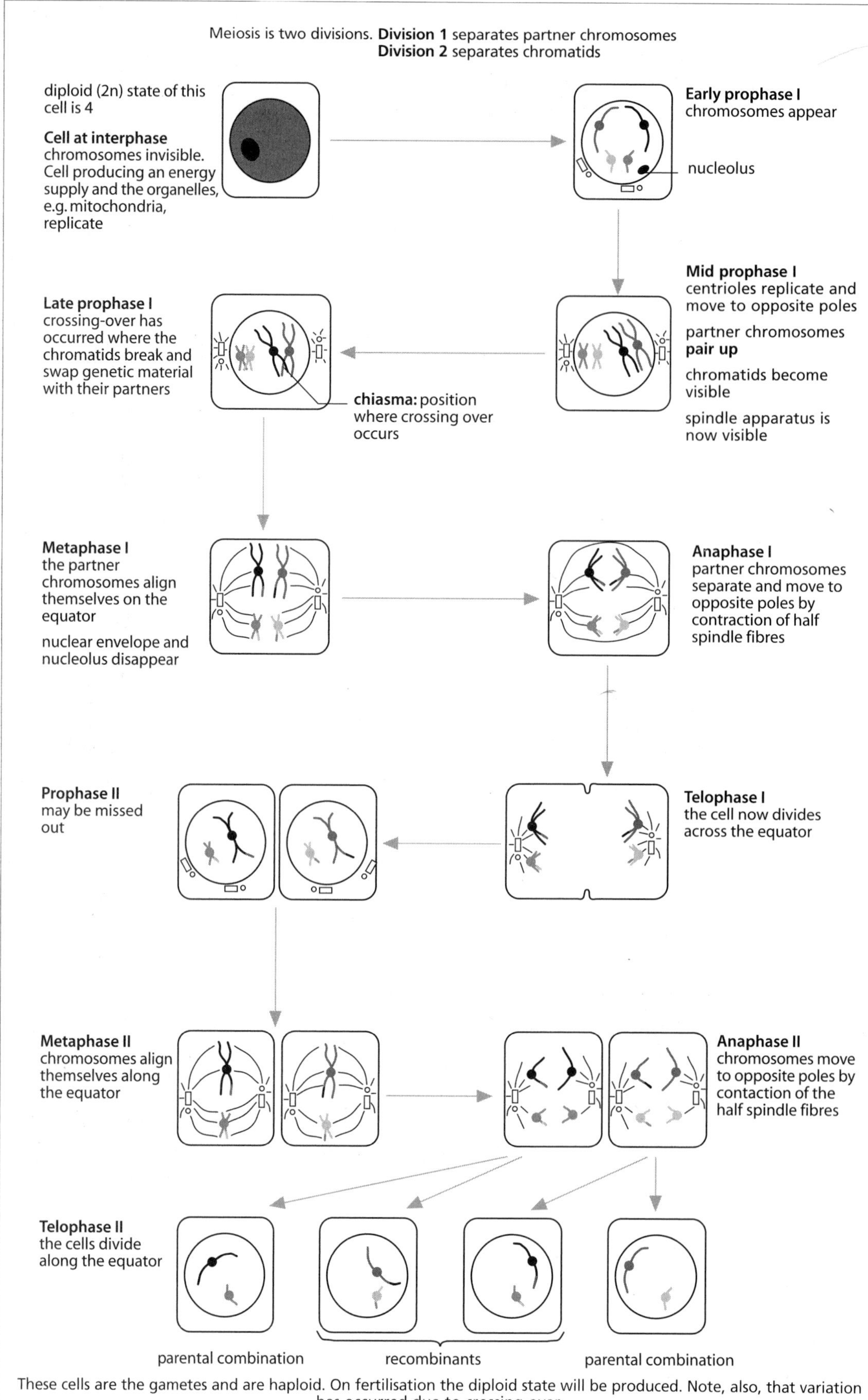

Figure 19.6
Meiosis.

Meiosis

The cells produced in meiosis contain only one copy of each pair of chromosomes present in the parent cell (Figure 19.6). Meiosis actually involves two divisions of the nucleus and cytoplasm of the parent cell:

- **first division** (meiosis I) – separates the members of each pair of chromosomes (homologous chromosomes)
- **second division** (meiosis II) – separates the two copies of each individual chromosome (chromatids).

Q5: How many cells will be produced if a single cell divides by meiosis?

Q6: Which cells in the human body are haploid?

Q7: Where, in the human body, does meiosis take place?

Crossing over

An important event that can occur during meiosis is the ability of the partner (homologous) chromosomes to switch small parts of **DNA** from one to another. This is called **crossing over** and is an important source of genetic variation (see Chapter 21). Figure 19.7 shows the result of this process in a single pair of homologous chromosomes.

Q8: For crossing over to occur the DNA must be cut and then rejoined. Use the information in Chapter 20 to name the enzyme that: (a) cuts the DNA; (b) rejoins the cut ends of DNA.

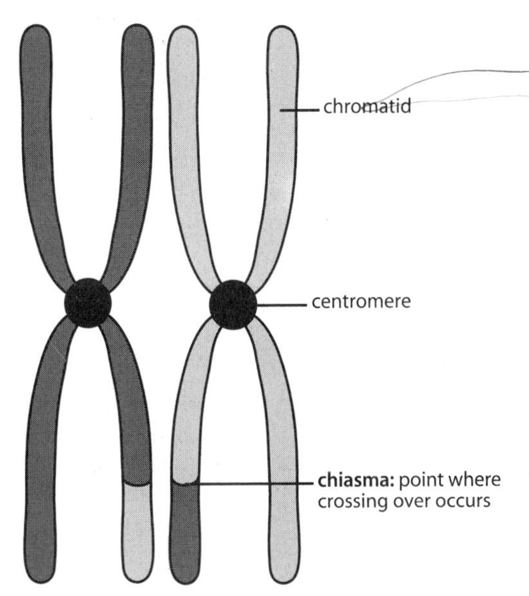

Figure 19.7 Crossing over.

Table 19.1 Comparison between mitosis and meiosis (using human cells as an example)

	Mitosis	Meiosis
Number of cells produced	2	4
Chromosome number in daughter cells of humans	46 (23 pairs)	23
Genetic differences between daughter cells	None – all cells are identical	All cells are genetically different, depending on the combination of individual members of each chromosome pair they contain. Variation is increased further by crossing over. For further details see Chapter 21

Genetic terms

The following glossary should help you as you attempt genetic problems. Do not worry if you need to keep referring back to this glossary.

Allele – one of two or more alternative messages carried by a single gene. For example, the gene controlling ear lobe shape has one allele for fixed lobes and another allele for free lobes.

Chromosome – thin, thread-like structure which carries the genetic information.

Dominant – if an allele is dominant it will always express itself in the phenotype.

Gene – a length of DNA that carries the genetic code for a single protein. It is the basic unit of inheritance, e.g. one gene controls the ABO blood group; another gene controls hair colour, etc.

Genotype – describes an individual's genetic make-up for one characteristic.

Heterozygous – refers to an individual in whom a single characteristic is controlled by two non-identical alleles of the same gene, e.g. **Aa**.

Homozygous (pure-breeding) – refers to an individual in whom a single characteristic is controlled by two identical alleles of the same gene, e.g. **AA**.

Locus – the fixed position on a chromosome where a particular gene is always found.

Phenotype – describes an individual's appearance, e.g. brown-eyed, or chemical make-up, e.g. blood group A.

Recessive – if an allele is recessive it will not express itself if its dominant allele is also present.

Q9: Using symbol **A** to represent the allele for free ear lobes (ear lobes free from the head) and the symbol **a** to represent the allele for fixed ear lobes (ear lobes fixed to the head), answer the following questions:

(a) What is the allele of **A**?

(b) Give the genotype of a homozygous person with free ear lobes.

(c) Give the genotype of a homozygous person with fixed ear lobes.

(d) Give the genotype of a heterozygous person with free ear lobes.

(e) What would be the phenotype of a person whose genotype was: (i) **Aa**; (ii) **aa**?

(f) Why must people with fixed ear lobes always be homozygous?

(g) Why is the genotype of humans always written as pairs of symbols, e.g. **AA**, **Aa** or **aa**?

(h) What is the meant by the term locus?

(i) What genotypes exist for humans with free ear lobes?

Monohybrid inheritance

This is the inheritance of a single characteristic, e.g. shape of ear lobes, height in pea plants, albinism. The basic 'laws' of genetics were first developed by an Austrian monk, called Gregor Mendel, who studied genetics using pea plants. Although he worked with plants, the 'laws' of genetics that he discovered apply equally in humans.

Mendel crossed a homozygous tall pea plant with a homozygous dwarf pea plant and collected their seeds. When he planted these seeds, he found that the plants that grew from them [known as the first offspring generation – offspring (1) – or sometimes as the F_1 generation] were all tall. He then self-fertilised these tall plants (this is possible in plants but occurs very rarely in animals) and found that in the second offspring generation [offspring (2) – or F_2 generation] he obtained both tall and dwarf plants in an approximate 3:1 ratio:

Parental phenotypes	tall	x	dwarf		
		↓			
Offspring (1) phenotypes		tall	x	tall	(self-fertilised)
Offspring (2) phenotypes	tall		dwarf		
		3:1			

This pattern of inheritance can be explained quite easily. Looking at the offspring (1) generation we can deduce that tallness is due to a dominant allele of the gene for plant height. The allele which causes dwarfness is recessive. We represent these alleles as: **T** = allele for tallness; **t** = allele for dwarfness. Using these symbols and a standard format for laying out genetics crosses, we can represent the first stages of our genetics cross as:

Parental phenotypes	Homozygous tall	Homozygous dwarf
Parental genotypes	**TT**	**tt**

NB: Each parent is diploid therefore must have two symbols.

> **Q10**: Why must the tall parent plants have been **TT** and not **Tt**?

Now we can now continue our flow chart as shown in Figure 19.8.

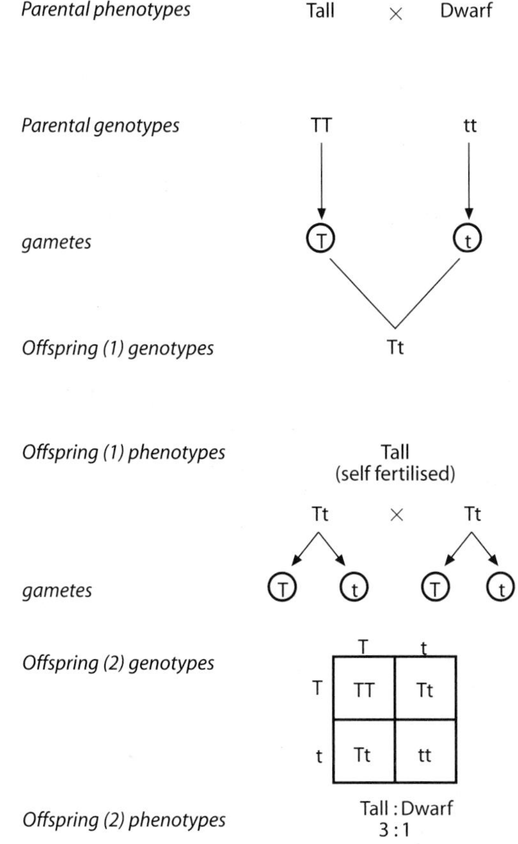

Figure 19.8 Diagrammatic representation showing the results of a cross between tall and dwarf plants.

NB:

1 We have represented the types of gamete not the number of gametes.

2 We have used a method for laying out this cross (in italics) that will be used in your examinations and that you must always use

3 To represent the offspring (2) generation, we have used a device called a **Punnett square**. This is often easier to use.

As can be seen in Figure 19.8, we have a three tall : one dwarf ratio, which is what Mendel found. It must be realised that these ratios are never exact. This is due to what is called the **sampling error**.

To become familiar with genetics you need to practise answering problems. There are several at the end of this book but, to give more help, we will attempt one involving tongue-rolling (Figure 19.9). Tongue-rolling is another characteristic that is thought to be a case of monohybrid inheritance in which the allele for ability to roll the tongue (**R**) is thought to be dominant over an allele causing an inability to roll the tongue (**r**). **N.B.** It has recently been shown that tongue rolling is a condition that can be learnt.

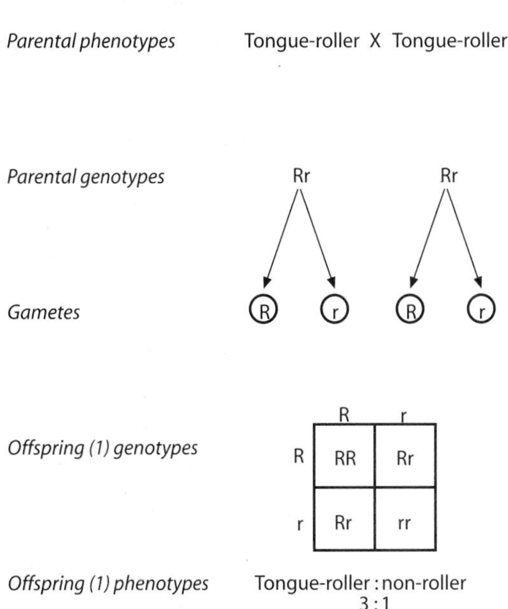

Figure 19.9 Example of monohybrid inheritance (tongue-rolling).

Q11: From Figure 19.9, what are the chances of a non-roller child being produced?

Supposing two people who can roll their tongues have a daughter who cannot roll her tongue. As both parents can roll their tongues then both must have one **R** allele. However, their child has the genotype **rr**. She must have inherited one **r** allele from each parent.

Q12: What would the possible genotypes be of: (a) someone who can roll their tongue; (b) someone who cannot roll their tongue?

Another example of a condition governed by a recessive allele is cystic fibrosis (see page 165). Huntington's disease is a condition governed by a dominant allele (see page 180).

Codominance and multiple alleles

In the previous examples, we have stated that an allele is either dominant or recessive. However this need not be the case; sometimes neither is recessive, in which case the alleles are said to be **codominant**.

We have also assumed that a gene only ever has two alleles. This is also not the case; sometimes there are more than two alleles of a gene controlling a single characteristic. These are referred to as **multiple alleles**. The inheritance of the ABO blood groups is a good example to demonstrate both these concepts.

The ABO blood group is explained on page 30. On the surface membrane of our red blood cells are proteins called antigens:

antigen A – controlled by allele $\mathbf{I^A}$
antigen B – controlled by allele $\mathbf{I^B}$
neither antigen A nor antigen B – controlled by allele $\mathbf{I^o}$

Alleles $\mathbf{I^A}$ and $\mathbf{I^B}$ are codominant; both are dominant over the recessive allele $\mathbf{I^o}$. All possible combinations of these alleles can occur, giving the genotypes and phenotypes shown in Table 19.2. Note the new way of representing alleles: this notation is always used with multiple alleles. In this case, the **I** stands for immunoglobulin (the type of protein in the blood) and the A, B and o refer to the particular immunoglobulin.

Table 19.2 Phenotypes and genotypes of blood groups

Blood group name (Phenotype)	Genotype
Group A	$I^A I^A$ or $I^A I^o$
Group B	$I^B I^B$ or $I^B I^o$
Group AB	$I^A I^B$
Group O	$I^o I^o$

To become familiar with this notation, suppose a woman is heterozygous for group B and her husband is heterozygous for group A. We can represent the inheritance of ABO blood groups among their children using a diagram like the one in Figure 19.10.

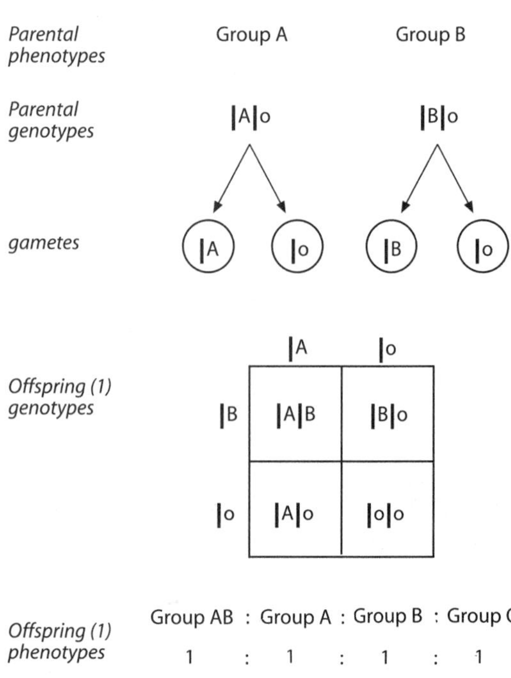

Figure 19.10 Inheritance of ABO blood groups.

Q13: Do you find anything strange about the results in Figure 19.10? If so, what?

Sex determination

Except for gametes and red blood cells (that lack a nucleus), all human cells contain:

- 22 pairs of chromosomes (autosomes)
- 1 pair of sex chromosomes.

Females have twenty two pairs of autosomes and two **X** chromosomes. Males have twenty two pairs of chromosomes, one **X** chromosome and a smaller **Y** chromosome. To represent the female and male genotypes, we must use symbols to show whole chromosomes, not just individual genes. We do not need to show the autosomes, only the sex chromosomes are important. Consequently, we represent a female as **XX** and a male as **XY**.

NB: males are the exception to the rule that homologous chromosomes are identical.

Figure 19.11 shows that, in theory, there should be equal numbers of females and males born. In fact, this is not quite true. Since the **Y** chromosome is much smaller than the **X** chromosome, sperm cells that carry the **Y** are slightly faster than sperm cells that carry the **X** chromosome. Consequently, **XY** fertilisations are slightly more common than **XX** fertilisations.

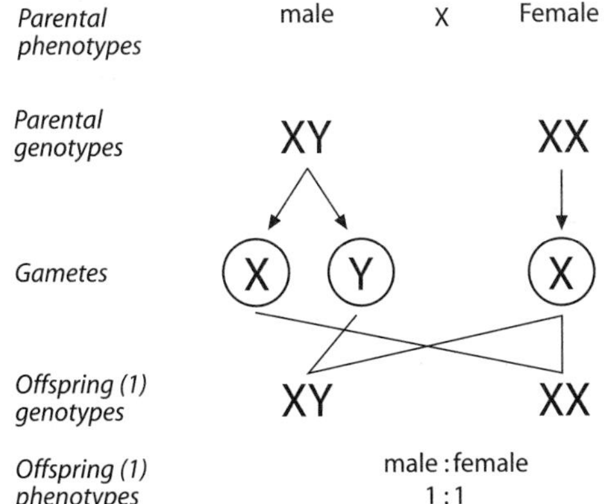

Figure 19.11 Sex determination.

Sex linkage

Some genes that have nothing to do with sex are carried on the sex chromosomes (Figure 19.12). These are most likely to be on the **X** chromosome as the **Y** chromosome is smaller and carries very few genes. Genes carried on the **X** or **Y** chromosome are said to be **sex-linked**.

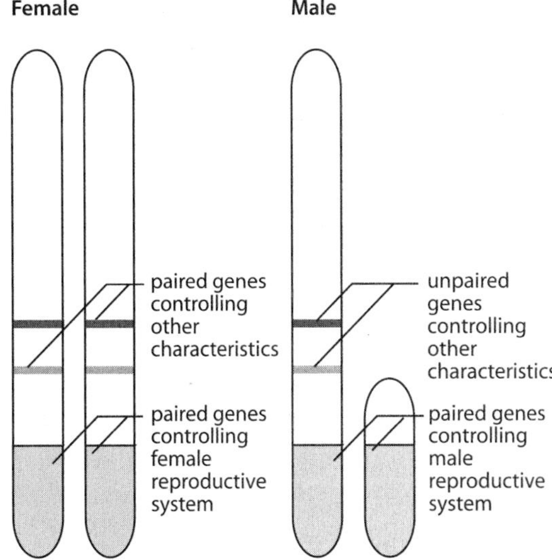

Figure 19.12 Sex linkage.

Examples of characteristics that are controlled by sex-linked genes are red/green colour-blindness and haemophilia (blood fails to clot). Let us construct a diagram to show how two people with normal colour vision can produce a colour-blind child. The gene for colour vision is carried on the **X** chromosome. The allele for normal colour vision is dominant and represented as $\mathbf{X^N}$. The recessive allele for colour-blindness is represented as $\mathbf{X^n}$. (Note that the symbol **C** for colour has not been used since it is difficult to distinguish between the upper case **C** and a lower case **c**.)

- The woman is **XX** and the man is **XY**
- They both have normal vision, so the man is $\mathbf{X^NY}$
- They have a colour-blind child, so the woman must carry a recessive allele. She is, therefore, $\mathbf{X^NX^n}$.
- We can now do the cross as shown in Figure 19.13 on page 160.

There is a 1 in 4 (or 25%) chance of a colour-blind child being born to this couple.

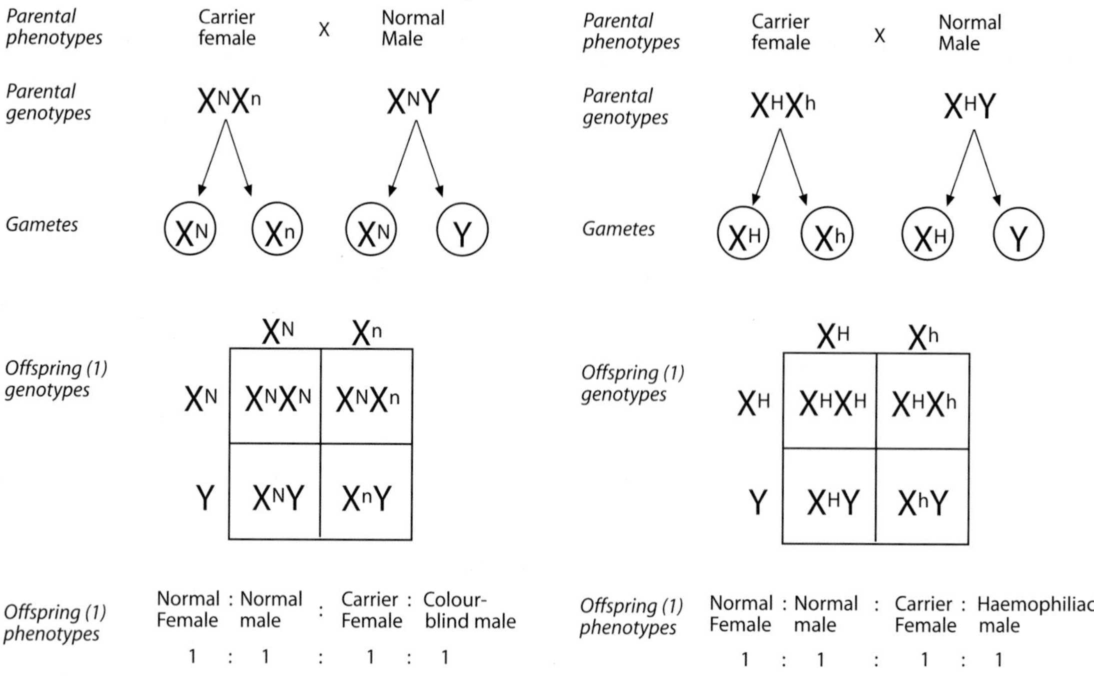

Figure 19.13 Sex linkage and colour-blindness.

Figure 19.14 Sex linkage and haemophilia.

The genetics of haemophilia are exactly the same as in the previous example, i.e. the gene is carried by the **X** chromosome only and the allele for the disease is recessive. Imagine two normal people produce a haemophiliac son. If we use the symbol $\mathbf{X^H}$ to represent an **X** chromosome carrying the allele for normal blood clotting and the symbol $\mathbf{X^h}$ to represent an **X** chromosome carrying the recessive allele for haemophilia, we can construct a diagram to explain what has happened to this couple.

- The woman is **XX** and the man is **XY**.
- Both have blood that clots normally, so the man is $\mathbf{X^HY}$.
- They have a haemophiliac child, so the woman must carry a recessive allele. She is, therefore, $\mathbf{X^HX^h}$.
- We can now do the cross as shown in Figure 19.14.

As with red-green colour-blindness, there is a 1 in 4 (or a 25%) chance that a haemophiliac child will be born to this couple. This is taken into account when genetic counselling is given (page 103).

Males are much more likely to show harmful sex-linked characteristics than are females. This can be explained. If a female has the recessive harmful allele on one of her **X** chromosomes, it will usually be masked by a dominant allele on her other **X** chromosome. However the male only has one **X** chromosome therefore if he inherits the harmful allele, he will suffer from that condition.

Summary

- Variation between individuals of the same species can be either inherited or non-inherited (environmental).
- Chromosomes are long thin structures, made from DNA, that carry genes. Before a cell divides it copies each of its chromosomes, so that each is temporarily made up of two chromatids.
- Genes are parts of a chromosome that control individual characteristics.
- In a diploid cell, chromosomes are found in homologous pairs – one copy from each parent's gamete.
- In a haploid cell only one of each pair of homologous chromosomes is found.
- Mitosis is a type of division which produces two identical cells.
- Meiosis is a type of division which produces haploid cells. It has two divisions: meiosis I separates homologous chromosomes; meiosis II separates chromatids.
- Monohybrid inheritance is the inheritance of a single characteristic.
- An allele is the alternative form of a gene at the same locus on a chromosome.
- Multiple alleles – where more than two alleles exist in the population.
- The locus is the point on a chromosome where a particular gene is always found.
- The genotype describes the alleles of a gene that are present in an organism.
- The phenotype describes an organism's appearance. It is the result of the activity of the genes and of environmental influences.
- Homozygous genotypes have identical alleles of a gene.
- Heterozygous genotypes have different alleles of a gene.
- Genetic sex is determined by a pair of sex chromosomes. Autosomes are chromosomes that do not carry genes determining sex.
- Genetics crosses can be represented using a standard format:

  Parental phenotypes
  Parental genotypes
  Gametes
  Offspring (1) genotypes
  Offspring (1) phenotypes
  Offspring (2) genotypes
  Offspring (2) phenotypes

Self check
See page 249

CHAPTER 20

DNA, biotechnology and genetic engineering

In this chapter you will learn about the structure of DNA and how it controls protein synthesis. You will also look at biotechnology, with particular emphasis on genetic engineering and basic microbiology.

Structure of DNA

The genetic material in the cell is deoxyribonucleic acid (DNA). This controls the structure and activities of cells by controlling the production of its proteins. DNA is made up of three constituents, each of which is obtained from our diet:

- a five-carbon sugar (deoxyribose)
- a phosphate group
- one of four nitrogen bases – adenine, thymine, cytosine, guanine.

Figures 20.1 and 20.2 show the structure of a DNA molecule. Note that:

- it is made of two strands twisted around each other – the so-called double helix
- one strand is upside down compared to the other
- the two strands are held together by weak hydrogen bonds between the nitrogen bases
- the nitrogen bases always pair in a precise way: cytosine always pairs with guanine (C–G) and adenine always pairs with thymine (A–T).

Q1: If one strand of DNA had a base sequence of AAT CCG TTG, what would the corresponding sequence be on the other strand?

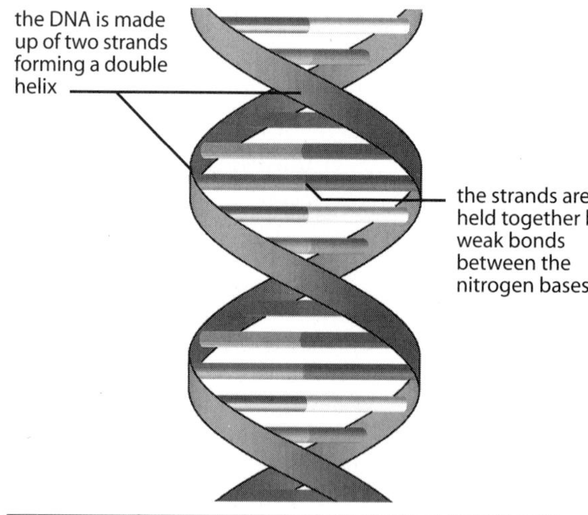

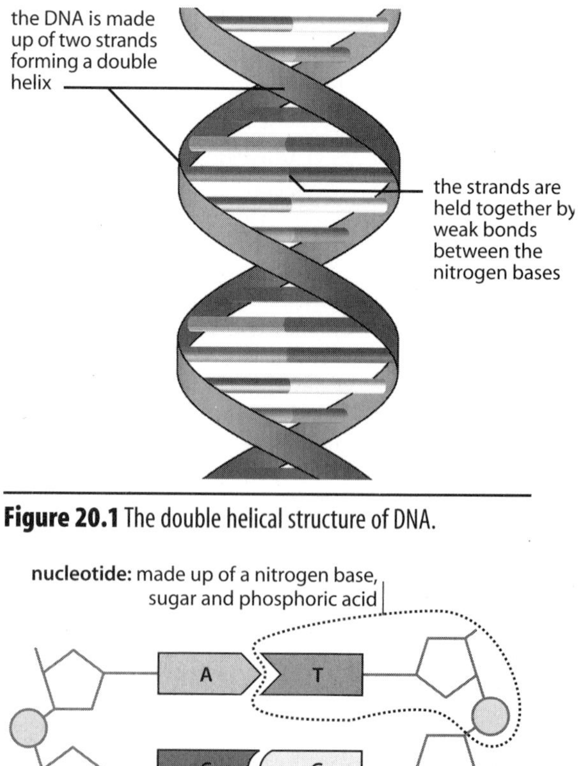

Figure 20.1 The double helical structure of DNA.

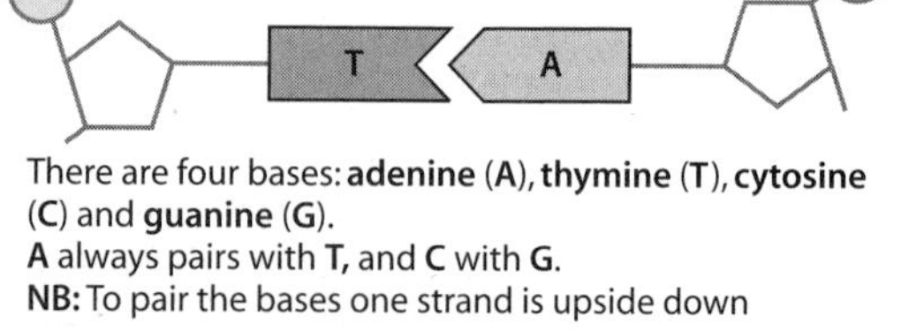

nucleotide: made up of a nitrogen base, sugar and phosphoric acid

A T
C G
T A

There are four bases: **adenine** (A), **thymine** (T), **cytosine** (C) and **guanine** (G).
A always pairs with **T**, and **C** with **G**.
NB: To pair the bases one strand is upside down

Figure 20.2 The structure of DNA.

Protein synthesis

Proteins are made up of amino acids linked together in a certain order. It is the role of DNA to link these amino acids in the correct order. To do this two processes are involved:

- **transcription**
- **translation.**

Figure 20.3 shows these two processes during the formation of proteins. Note that, although ribosomes actually make the proteins, two other nucleic acids have important roles to play. Messenger ribonucleic acid (**mRNA**) carries the genetic code for a single gene, copied from the cell's DNA; transfer RNA (**tRNA**) carries the code for a single amino acid. Note also that in mRNA and tRNA, the nitrogen base thymine is replaced by **uracil**.

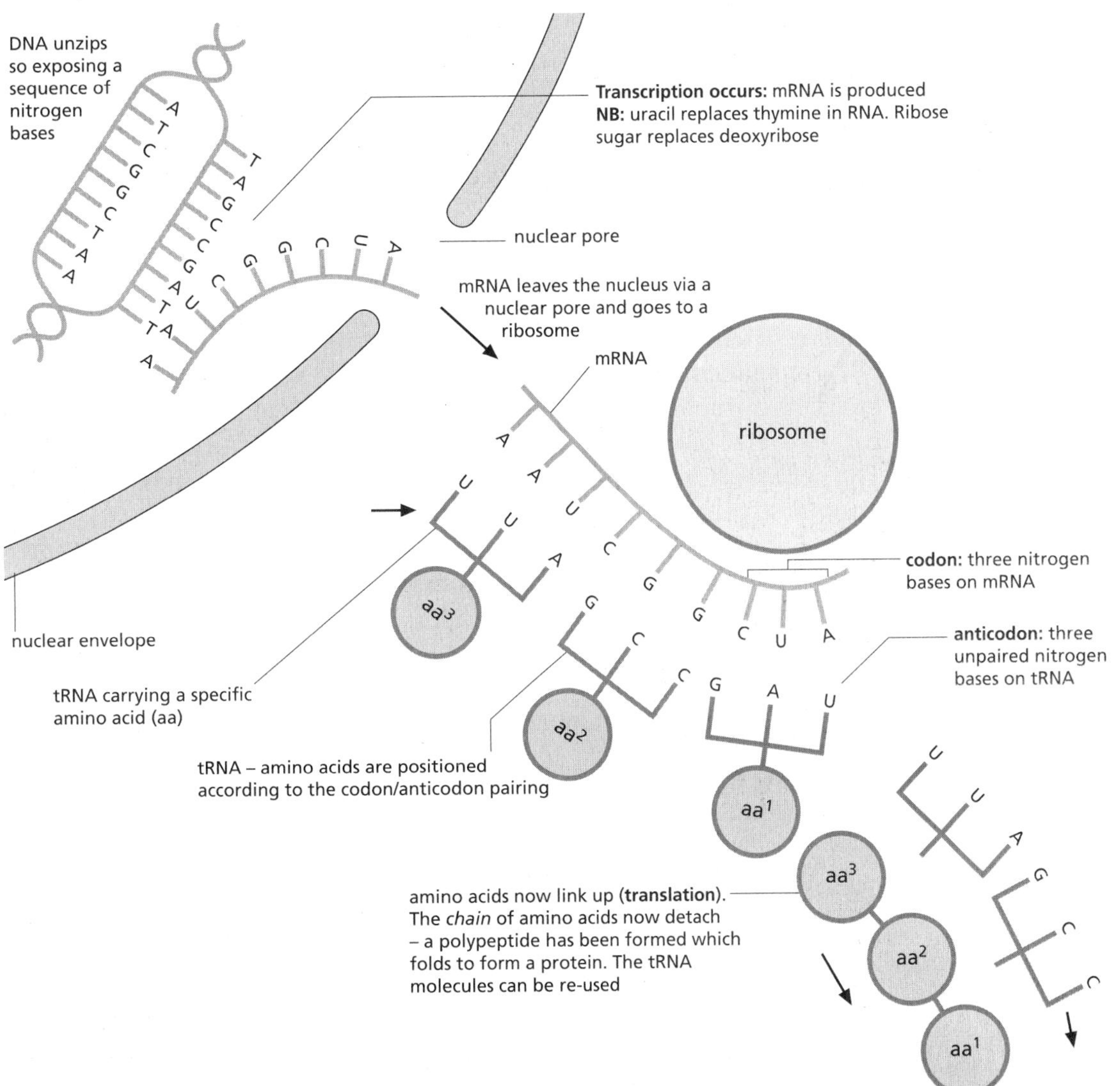

Figure 20.3 Formation of proteins.

Q2: (a) How many nitrogen-containing bases code for a single amino acid? (b) During transcription, an mRNA molecule was made from a DNA section with a nitrogen base sequence of ATC GTC GGA. What would be the nitrogen base sequence of the mRNA? (c) State the anticodon on the tRNA which would complement the codons on this mRNA.

Genetic engineering (recombinant DNA technology)

For many years, humans have changed the genotypes of certain organisms through rearing specific animals and plants. Later, specific breeding programmes were developed (Chapter 21). However, as our knowledge of genetics has increased, it has become possible to take a gene from one organism and transfer it to another. This is known as **recombinant DNA technology** or, more commonly, **genetic engineering** and has allowed us to turn microorganisms into factories capable of producing useful products.

Recombinant DNA technology involves three stages:

- a gene is isolated from a donor
- this gene is inserted into a carrier (vector)
- the gene within its vector is transferred to the host.

Isolation of the gene

- The cell with the desired gene is broken up using enzymes.
- DNA (genetic material) is extracted from the cell. This looks like very long pieces of string. The DNA is cut into shorter lengths using **restriction enzymes**. These cut the DNA at a precise sequence of nitrogen bases. As a result, one long strand will be cut in several places.
- The gene required must now be found from these pieces.
- To do this a **gene probe** may be used which binds to part of the desired gene.
- This probe is a single-stranded piece of DNA (Figure 20.4).
- The probe is slightly radioactive, enabling us to find our gene from amongst the other fragments.

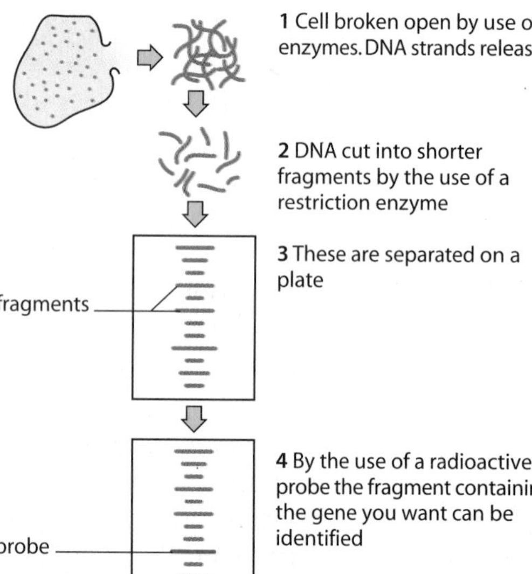

Figure 20.4 Stages in isolating a gene.

Q3: If you know that part of the gene required has a base sequence of ATC GTT TCC, what base sequence might the probe have?

Insertion of the isolated gene into a vector (carrier)

Several vectors are known, e.g. certain viruses and circular strands of DNA (**plasmids**) that are found in some bacteria. The rest of this account will concentrate on the use of viruses.

- A virus operates by attaching to the outside of its host cell and injecting its own nucleic acid into the cell. This provides a way of getting the isolated gene into another cell.
- The isolated gene is placed inside the virus. Generally, viruses are used that attack either bacteria or yeast cells.
- One enzyme, a restriction enzyme, is used to cut the viral DNA and another enzyme, **DNA ligase**, is used to join the desired gene to the DNA of the virus.

Transfer to a new host

- Host cells are now infected with the modified virus. The virus attaches to some of the host cells and injects its own DNA (along with the required gene) into them.
- The host cell will now manufacture the desired product (Figure 20.5).
- In a fermenter, the microorganisms divide repeatedly and produce large amounts of the product.
- The product is harvested and used.

Biotechnology

This area of science brings together engineers, biologists, chemists and physicists. It is a multi-billion pound industry and is beginning to change the world's economy.

Fermenters

The aim of fermenters is to grow microorganisms in an environment where conditions such as temperature, pH and food source can be closely monitored and regulated. As the

Table 20.1 Examples of recombinant DNA technology

Application	Method
Human insulin	This is secreted by the pancreas and controls blood sugar levels. Diabetics must inject themselves with insulin. Originally, this insulin was obtained from slaughtered pigs and cows but this is gradually being replaced by the genetically engineered type (**humulin**)
Human growth hormone	This hormone is secreted by the pituitary gland and regulates our growth rate. The gene controlling its production was the first to be made by a 'gene machine'. It is placed in the bacterium *Escherichia coli* (*E. coli*) which then manufactures the hormone. The manufactured hormone is used in the treatment of a type of dwarfism that affects about ten people per million
Cystic fibrosis	This is a condition where internal membranes, including those of the lungs, produce a very sticky mucus. This allows bacteria to thrive and can be life-threatening unless regular physiotherapy is given to help the patient. The gene for the production of normal mucus has been isolated, inserted into a vector (in this case a virus) and given as an aerosol spray into the lungs. The hope is that the virus will attach to the surface membranes of cells lining the alveoli and inject its DNA (along with the gene) into the cells. As a result, normal mucus will be produced. Early results of the treatment have been encouraging
Toxin (poison) production in plants	A bacterium *Bacillus thuringiensis* produces a toxin that kills the larvae of moths and butterflies. The bacterial gene controlling toxin production has been isolated, inserted into a vector, and transferred into the cells of tobacco and tomato plants. These modified plants now produce the toxin so giving them protection against damage by butterfly larvae. The toxin is harmless to humans

microorganisms flourish, they produce the desired products, e.g. ethanol (alcohol) in brewing (Figure 20.6) or antibiotics. In **batch culture** the cells are grown in a fixed volume of liquid medium in a closed vessel. In **continuous culture** the nutrients are added and the cells harvested at a given steady rate. Figure 20.7 on page 166 illustrates the internal structure of a typical fermenter.

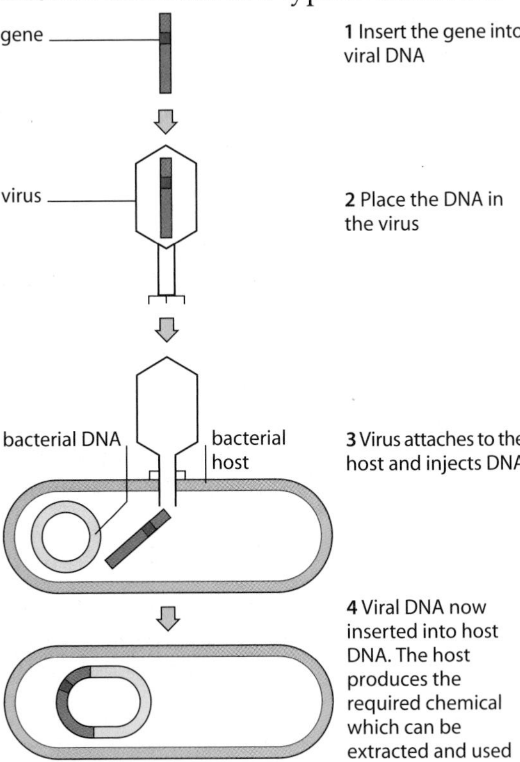

Figure 20.5 Transfer of the gene into a host.

Q4: With reference to cystic fibrosis, what process normally taking place in the lungs will be slowed down by the thick mucus?

Q5: Suggest what might have been used to protect tobacco and tomato plants from attack by larvae before the use of genetic engineering.

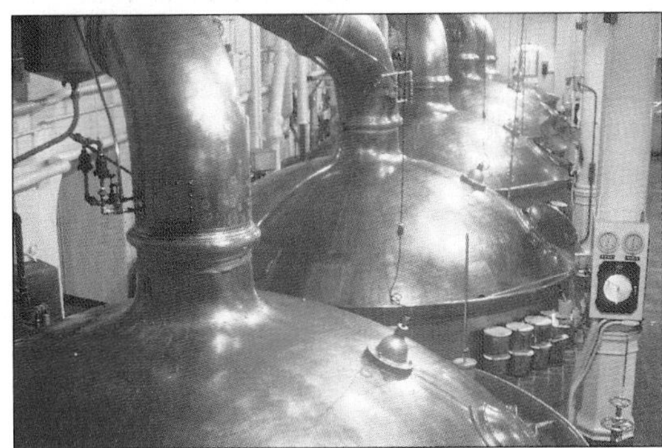

Figure20.6 Fermenters in a brewery.

Waste technology

Both water and sewage must be treated to remove harmful microorganisms and other impurities. Details of these processes are given in Chapter 27. Waste can also be used in the production of **biogas**. This gas is mainly methane and can be produced from the anaerobic digestion of human excreta and the leafy remains of vegetable crops. The process is summarised in Figure 20.8 on page 166.

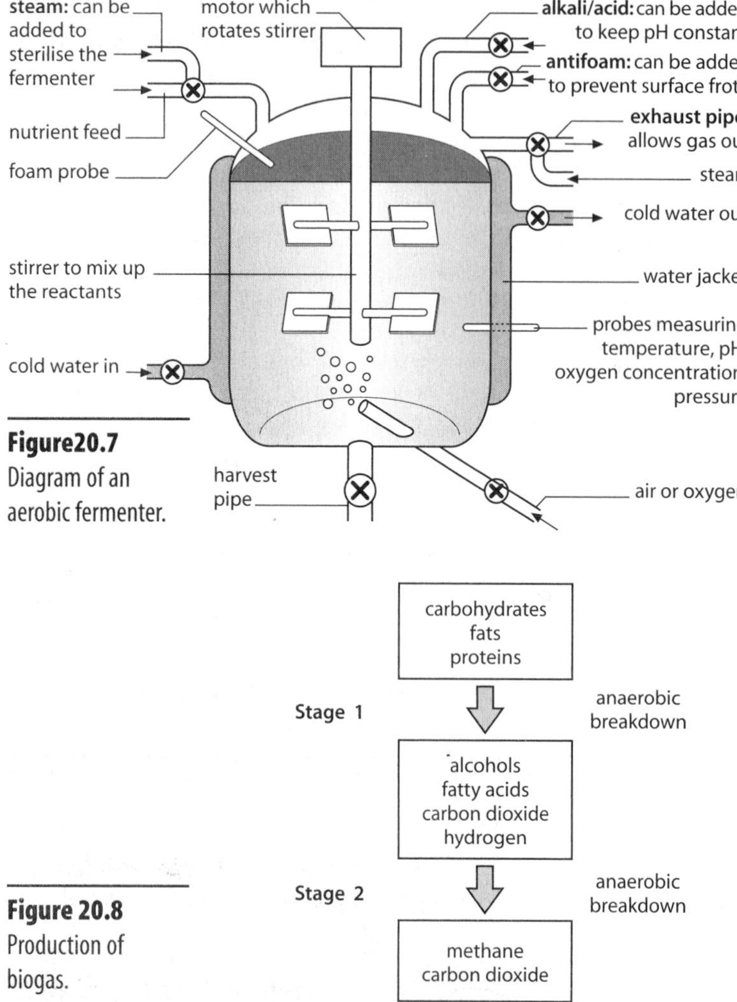

Figure 20.7 Diagram of an aerobic fermenter.

Figure 20.8 Production of biogas.

In some parts of the world, individual homes have their own biogas generators and use household waste to make their own biogas (Figure 20.9).

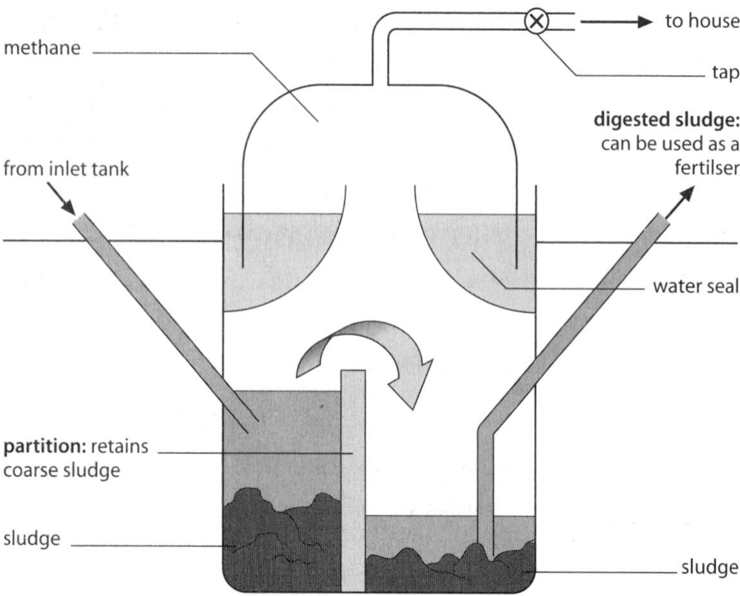

Figure 20.9 A domestic biogas generator.

Ethanol (alcohol) can be mixed with petrol and used as a fuel in combustion engines. It is a particularly valuable fuel in countries that do not have their own oil reserves but do have an abundant source of carbohydrate. In Brazil, alcohol for fuel is produced from the anaerobic fermentation of sugar-cane juice or from maize starch.

Enzyme technology

Enzymes are very important chemicals in the home and industry. Some of their uses are summarised here.

- **Protease and lipase** – found in detergents; digest protein and fat-based stains respectively.
- **Catalase** – can be used to convert latex into foam rubber due to the production of oxygen by catalase when mixed with hydrogen peroxide.
- **Isomerase** – glucose is not as sweet as fructose. Using this enzyme, glucose can be converted into fructose and therefore used in less quantities as a sweetener. This helps in 'slimming' foods.
- **Amylase** – used to convert starch into syrup which is used in the food industry.
- **Protease** – used to get rid of gluten in strong flour in the manufacture of biscuits; to make leather more pliable and in the production of some cheeses.
- **Lactase** – used to convert lactose to simple sugars in the preparation of lactose-free milk. It makes the milk sweeter and allows people to drink it who are lactose-intolerant, i.e. don't produce their own lactase.

A great deal of time and trouble is involved in isolating and purifying enzymes which are needed to catalyse chemical reactions in industry. This costs money and the enzymes, once used, are wasted. However, a technique of immobilising enzymes has now been developed in which the enzyme is attached to a support medium, e.g. beads. Attached to its beads, the enzyme can now be re-isolated and re-used (Figure 20.10).

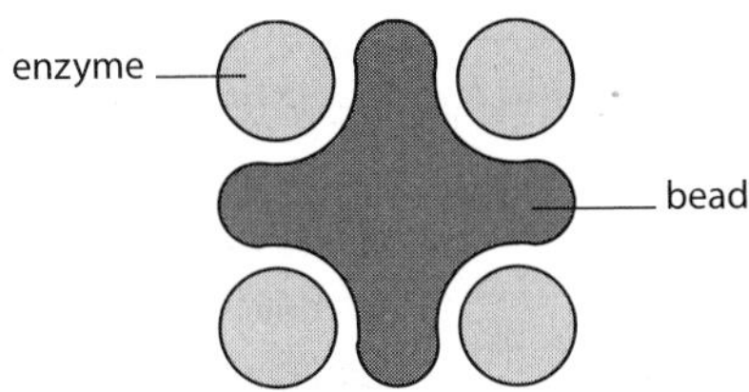

Q6: What effect will enzyme immobilisation have on the cost of the process?

Figure 20.10 Enzymes attached to a bead.

Practical 20.1 To investigate the effect of pectinase in fruit juice production

Pectins are components of plant cell walls. Because they act as a 'cement' which holds the cells together, they cause fruits to retain their juice. Hence, they limit the extraction of juice from fruit.

Requirements

- Range of fruits, including apple
- Blender
- Small beakers
- Filter funnels
- Filter papers
- Measuring cylinders
- Pectinase solution
- Pipette, to measure 1 cm³
- Tablespoon
- Stop clock
- Balance

1 Blend an apple to produce apple sauce. Place 10 g of this apple sauce into each of two labelled beakers.

2 To one beaker, add 1 cm^3 of H_2O. To the other beaker, add 1 cm^3 of pectinase solution.

3 Stir each mixture carefully and leave for 15 minutes at 30°C.

4 After this time filter each mixture.

5 Record the volume of juice that comes through the filter after 5 minutes.

6 Repeat instructions 1 to 5 with other fruit.

Practical 20.2 To demonstrate the use of immobilised enzymes

In industry, the immobilised enzyme glucose isomerase is used to catalyse the conversion of glucose to fructose:

$$\text{glucose} \xrightarrow{\text{glucose isomerase}} \text{fructose}$$

In this experiment, the principle of using immobilised enzymes will be demonstrated using the reverse of this process, i.e. converting fructose to glucose. This allows us to measure glucose easily using clinistix.

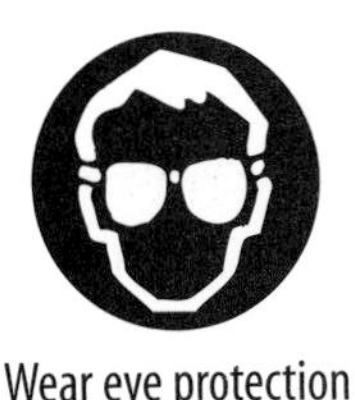

Wear eye protection

Requirements

- Fructose solution
- De-ionised water
- Measuring cylinders
- Test tubes
- Clinistix
- Glucose isomerase immobilised on beads
- Pasteur pipettes
- Water baths at 40°C and 65°C.
- Filter funnels
- Filter paper
- Small beakers
- Stop clocks
- Chinagraph pencil
- Balance

To find the optimum temperature for the reaction:

1 Dissolve 1.5 g fructose in 25 cm^3 de-ionised water.

2 Pipette 5 cm^3 of this into a clean test tube.

3 Dip a clinistix into the solution, remove and record the colour (check against the standard).

4 Add 0.1 g glucose isomerase to the tube and incubate at 20°C, shaking occasionally.

5 Every 30 minutes, remove a small sample using a Pasteur pipette. Allow the sample to cool if necessary, and test with a clinistix.

6 Record the colour of the clinistix and repeat instructions 1 to 5 until a maximum intensity of colour has been obtained.

7 Repeat instructions 1 to 6 at 40°C and 65°C. Wear eye protection when heating the mixture.

8 Can you obtain the enzyme from the reaction mixture? Work out a method for doing this and then carry it out.

9 Estimate your percentage yield (remember that you initially added 0.1 g of immobilised enzyme).

10 Does the enzyme still work? If so, does it work as well as before?

11 Repeat instructions 1 to 6.

12 Write up your account of the experiment.

13 What conclusions can you draw about immobilised enzymes?

Medicine

- **Antibiotics** are produced by some fungi and bacteria. Examples are penicillin produced by the fungus *Penicillium* and streptomycin produced by the bacterium *Streptomyces*. Antibiotics attack pathogens and help a person overcome infection. In penicillin production a species of the fungus, *Penicillium*, is grown in a fermenter containing an aerated liquid culture medium. After rapid growth, when there is adequate sugar, the fungus begins to produce penicillin. The optimum yield of penicillin is achieved after six to eight days when the antibiotic is extracted from the culture medium by filtration (Figure 20.11).

Figure 20.11 Penicillin production.

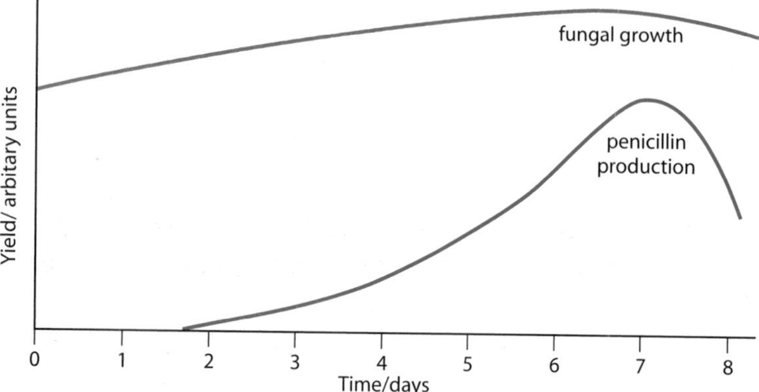

- **Vaccines** are normally made from dead or weakened pathogens. When they are injected, the recipient responds by producing antibodies against the active pathogen.
- **Gene therapy** involves placing genes inside humans in an attempt to correct serious conditions, e.g. cystic fibrosis (pages 101, 165).
- **Monoclonal antibodies** – antibodies are proteins produced by certain lymphocytes (page 29). They are very specific and will 'attack' only cells with a particular protein (antigen) on their surface membranes. If one type of antibody can be produced that is specific to the surface antigen of only one type of cell in the body, diseases of those cells could be targeted. This method has been used successfully in cancer treatment by attaching an anti-cancer drug to an antibody that is specific to one type of cell. In this way, the drug attacks only those cells, leading to fewer of the side-effects commonly associated with cancer treatment.

Forensic science

Genetic fingerprinting is now a common tool in forensic science. To make a genetic fingerprint, DNA can be extracted from human fluid, such as a blood sample.

Using enzymes, these strands of DNA can be chopped up into smaller fragments.

Q7: Why would human red blood cells not be suitable to obtain a sample of DNA?

Q8: What name is given to these enzymes?

These fragments are then separated to form a bar code (**genetic fingerprint**) which is unique to that person (Figure 20.12). These can be used in rape cases or disputed paternity suits (Figure 20.13).

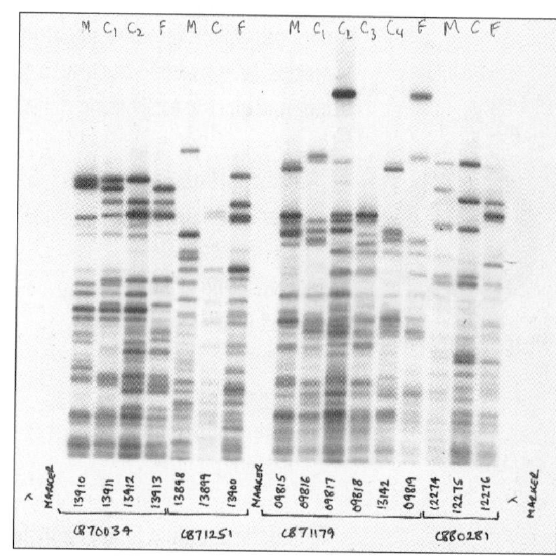

Figure 20.12 A DNA fingerprint – note bar code arrangement.

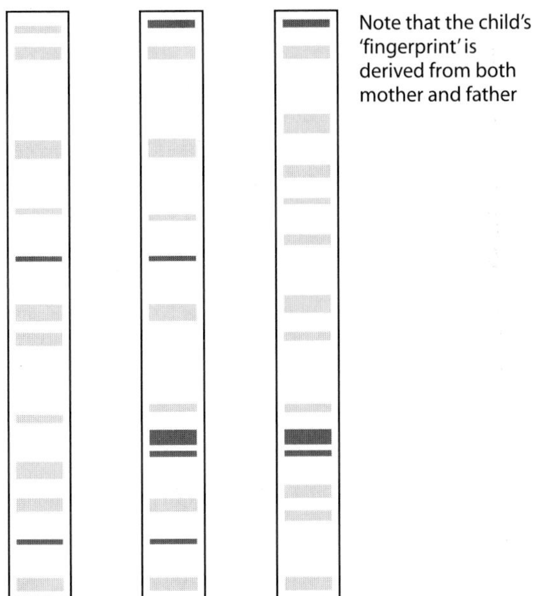

Figure 20.13 Hypothetical situation of a child and its parents.

Agriculture

Examples of biotechnology used in agriculture are given in Table 20.2.

Table 20.2 Uses of biotechnology in agriculture

Example	Use
Disease resistance	Toxin production by genetically engineered plants is described on page 165
Cuttings	About 20 cm of stem is cut from a healthy plant. This cutting is trimmed at the base and put into a growth medium, such as soil or a nutrient jelly. The cutting produces roots and begins to grow into a healthy plant. Plant growth substances, such as auxins, may be used to stimulate root formation
Plant tissue culture (micropropagation)	In the past, plants have been produced by various methods, e.g. growing seed, taking of cuttings (see above) and grafting. However tissue culture is now replacing many of these. The main stages involved in tissue culture are shown in Figure 20.14. Its advantages over other methods include the fact that it takes up little space, can be carried out all year round and its production rate is very high. It has been used to produce genetically modified tomato plants, the fruits of which are now on sale in British supermarkets

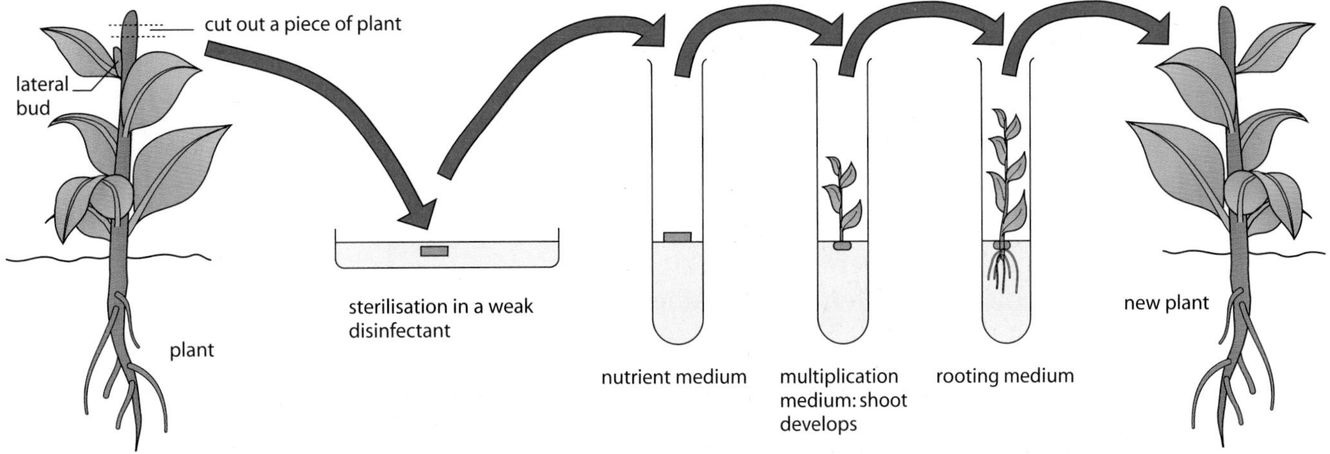

Figure 20.14 Stages in plant tissue culture – shoots and roots can be formed by varying the concentration of plant growth substances, e.g. auxin.

Food and drink industry

Bread production

Humans are known to have made a bread-like food for thousands of years.

The following flow chart summarises the process by which bread is made:

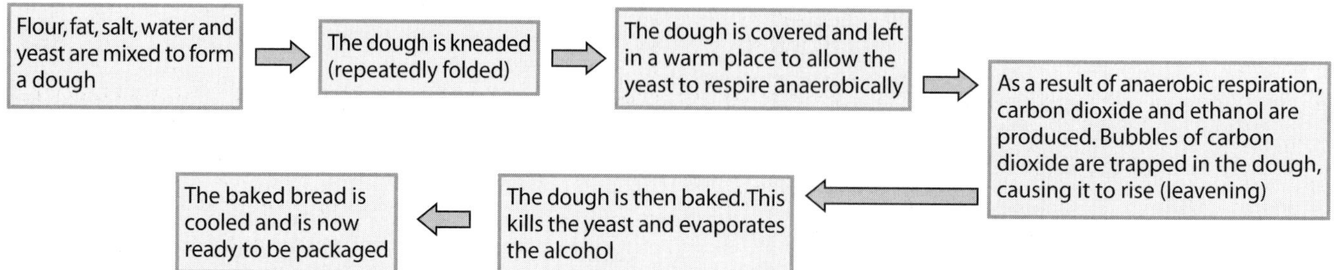

Beer production

Like bread, beer is a product of fermentation by yeast and has been made by humans for thousands of years. Different beers are made using different strains of yeast and slightly different ingredients but the brewing process relies on the stages shown in the flow chart opposite.

Nowadays, special genetically designed yeasts are available. Some of these produce low-carbohydrate ('lite') beer whereas others have high tolerance to alcohol and make a stronger beer.

Malting – barley seeds (grains) are soaked in water and allowed to germinate. Enzymes produced during germination convert stored starch to sugar and stored proteins to amino acids. Germination is stopped by heating to 80°C, producing malted barley

Milling – the malted barley is broken up

Mashing – hot water is added to the grains which softens them and extracts a nutrient-rich liquid (wort)

Boiling – female flowers from hop plants (hops) are mixed with the wort to give flavour. The mixture is heated to a high temperature and allowed to cool

Fermentation – yeast is added and converts sugar to ethanol (alcohol) and carbon dioxide

Filtration – the alcoholic liquid (beer) is extracted

Finishing – the beer is now packaged for sale

Wine production

Wines are made in a similar way to beer except that barley seeds are not the source of sugar for the fermentation process. Traditionally, wines are made from grapes but they can also be produced from other sugar-rich fruits or root crops, e.g. parsnips.

Vinegar production

A continuous culture system is used in what is called a **tower process**. The starting material is wine, beer or a liquid from the fermentation of fruit juices. This is trickled over wood shavings on which the bacteria live. These shavings are held in a vertical tower (fermenter), rather like that in Figure 20.7, and provide a large surface area for the growth of aerobic bacteria. Air is blown through the mixture and the vinegar produced from the alcohol is drawn off from the base of the tower.

Single cell protein (SCP) production

This product is made up of the dried cells of bacteria, fungi or algae. It is very rich in protein. SCP is mainly used as animal feed.

Yoghurt production

Yoghurt is a Turkish word and yoghurt was probably first made by the nomadic tribes of the Middle East who kept cows, sheep, goats and camels. The great advantage of yoghurt over the milk from which it is made is that yoghurt lasts longer before going off. The way to succeed when making yoghurt is to provide the right conditions for the growth of the desired lactate bacteria, while keeping the number of other microorganisms to a minimum.

Practical 20.3 To investigate the effect of temperature on the fermentation of baker's yeast in dough

Requirements

Freshly made dough (made from plain flour, glucose, fresh yeast and warm water)
Water baths at 20°C, 30°C, 40°C and 70°C
Ice and beaker for ice bath
100 cm³ measuring cylinders × 5
Stop clock
Ruler

1 Take five pieces of the dough which was made just before the start of the experiment using the ingredients listed above.

2 Carefully drop each piece of dough into a 100 cm³ measuring cylinder, having first smeared the inside with a small amount of cooking oil.

3 Place the measuring cylinders in a water bath at each of five temperatures – 5°C, 20°C, 30°C, 40°C and 70°C, and allow the dough so settle for five minutes. Then note the volumes of the dough pieces and start the stopclock.

4 Read the volumes of each piece of dough every five minutes until the skin of the dough shows signs of collapse.

5 Record your results.

6 At which temperature did the dough rise by the greatest amount?

7 What does this tell you about the optimum temperature for yeast growth?

Practical 20.4 To make yoghurt

Biohazard

Requirements

UHT (ultra high temperature) milk
Plain live yoghurt, one teaspoonful
Thermometer
Domestic cooker or Bunsen burner, tripod and gauze
Insulated ('thermos'-type) flask
Refrigerator (if possible)

1 Warm 500 cm³ of UHT milk to 48°C exactly.

2 Add a small teaspoon of plain live yoghurt and stir. Pour the mixture into an insulated flask; put the lid on, but do not screw it down.

3 After 8 to 12 hours, pour the mixture from the flask, whisk it and refrigerate for two hours. You now should have yoghurt.

SAFETY: Do not taste the yoghurt you have made unless you have carried out this practical under hygienic conditions at home or in a domestic science laboratory. Under no circumstances taste the yoghurt if you have carried out the work in a science laboratory.

Mycoprotein – food from fungi

A fungus called *Fusarium* has been used in the biotechnology industry to make food for human consumption. The fungus is grown on waste products generated during the manufacture of flour. The resulting mycelium is harvested and a material extracted called **mycoprotein**. Mycoprotein is high in protein and fibre, but contains no cholesterol. It can be made to look attractive and taste like chicken or beef. It is sold under the brand name 'Quorn' and is becoming increasingly popular because:

- its consumption is acceptable to vegetarians and others who prefer not to eat meat
- it is less expensive than most meats
- the absence of cholesterol may be good for some people's health.

Growth and culture of bacteria

Most bacteria are heterotrophic, i.e. they cannot manufacture their own food but have to obtain food from their surroundings. This food should contain sources of energy, e.g. fats, carbohydrates or proteins, together with mineral ions and vitamins for making special enzymes or part of the cell structure. In order to grow bacteria in the laboratory,

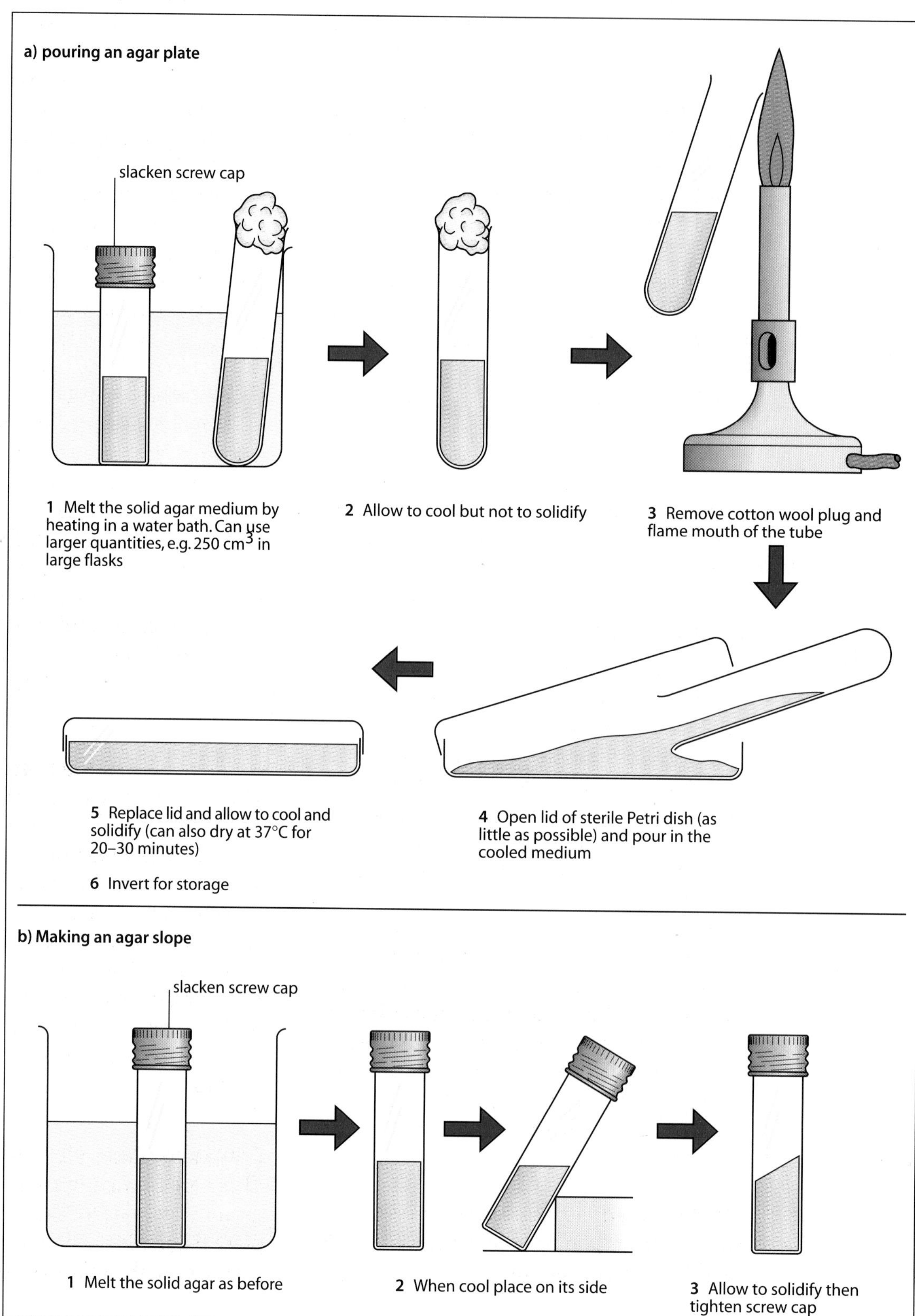

Figure 20.15 Pouring of **a)** an agar plate and **b)** an agar slope.

it is necessary to provide the bacteria with these substances. Bacteria are normally grown on either nutrient broth or nutrient agar.

- **Nutrient broth** is a liquid containing sugar, some amino acids, vitamins and minerals. Bacteria grow in the broth and turn it cloudy, usually at a neutral pH (pH 7).
- **Nutrient agar** has a similar composition to nutrient broth but has agar added to it. Agar is liquid at high temperatures but at room temperature it will cause the broth to set into a firm jelly. Agar is poured into a Petri dish to produce an **agar plate** or poured into a test tube or McCartney bottle and cooled at an angle to make an **agar slope** (Figure 20.15). When bacteria are placed on the surface of the agar (inoculated), they grow and reproduce to form visible colonies. Bacteria grow best within a certain temperature range – often about 40°C – so broths and plates are incubated at this temperature for 1–7 days to produce optimum growth.

Aseptic technique

When bacteria are grown, it is essential that only the required bacteria from a certain source, e.g. milk samples, develop. The sample must not become contaminated with bacteria from other sources. Great care has to be taken with the way in which the practical work is carried out.

- All the equipment and media used must be sterilised *before* and *after* use.
- The procedure is conducted in such a way that contamination by introducing microorganisms from the environment (including the student) into the cultures is not possible. Neither must the release of microorganisms from the cultures into the environment be allowed. This procedure is described as **aseptic technique**.

Sterilisation of equipment or media

Some of the common sterilisation methods used in laboratories are:

- **dry heat** – placed in a hot-air oven; suitable for glassware
  – heated in a Bunsen flame to red heat; suitable for inoculating loops
- **wet heat** – boiled in water; suitable for glassware
  – boiled; suitable for sterilising heat-stable media
- **steam heat** – using an autoclave, material can be heated under a pressure of 100 kPa for 15 minutes. This treatment will even kill resistant bacterial spores and is suitable for glassware, heat-stable media and for sterilising any material before its disposal.

Any item which comes into contact with sterilised equipment or media must itself be sterilised. Remember:

- disinfect the bench
- on opening any jar, test tube, flask or bottle, flame the neck by passing it through a Bunsen flame
- wire loops or mounted needles which are being used to transfer bacteria to, or from, the broth or agar must be sterilised before and after use by heating them in a Bunsen flame until they are red hot
- all growth media must be kept covered when not in use and before placing in an incubator.

Isolation of a single species of bacterium

This can be done by producing a streak plate (Figure 20.16 on page 174). The bacteria in a mixed sample are dragged across the surface of an agar plate. The bacteria become separated into individual cells and, when incubated, multiply and appear as a single colony on the plate. Each single colony represents millions of bacterial cells, all produced from the one individual, so they will all be of the same species.

Confluent plates ('lawns')

These are formed when bacteria grow to uniformly cover the surface of an agar plate (Figure 20.17 on page 174). They are used to test the effectiveness of antibiotics.

1 Sterilise inoculating loop

2 Holding loop in hand, remove stopper from culture tube containing broth culture

3 Flame neck of the tube

4 With cooled loop pick up some of the broth containing bacteria

5 Remove loop, flame tube and replace stopper (or cotton wool)

6 Streak heavily over first 1/3 of the plate after lifting top of Petri dish as little as possible. Replace lid

7 Sterilise loop (*see* 1). Using the cooled loop drag some of the inoculum from the first sector into the second one

8 Sterilise loop (*see* 1). Using the cooled loop drag some of the inoculum from the second sector into the third one

9 Invert plate and incubate

This technique is often used for separating mixed cultures into pure ones because the individual colonies which become separated can be used to inoculate fresh plates or tubes

Expected results

Heavy continuous growth

Individual colonies

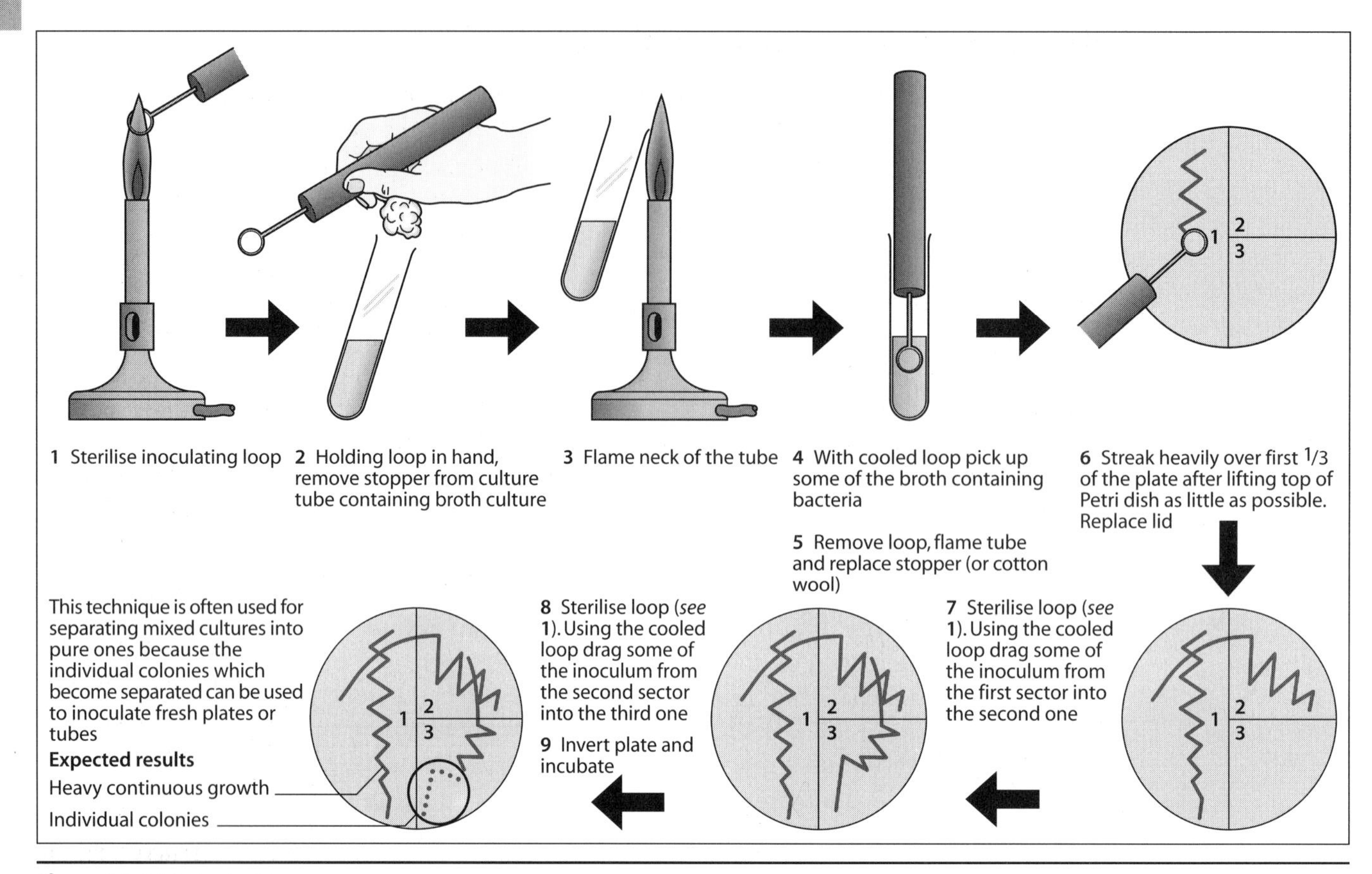

Figure 20.16 A streak plate.

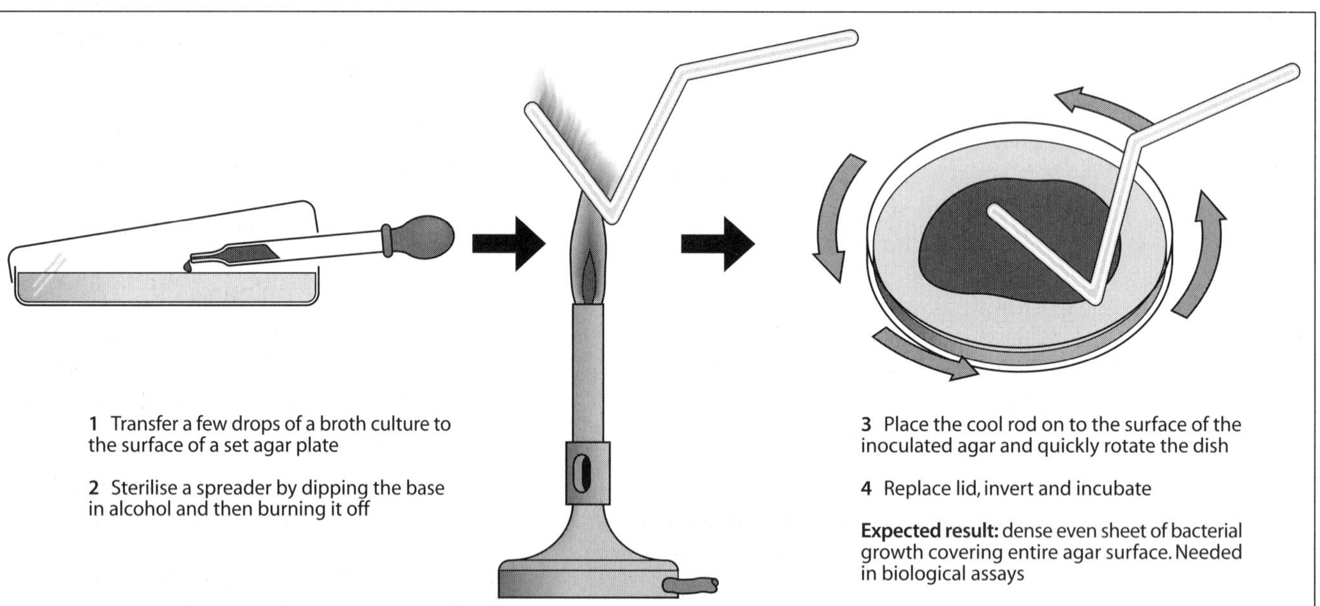

Figure 20.17 A confluent plate (lawn).

Culturing of viruses

Although microorganisms such as bacteria and fungi can be easily grown on nutrient agar or nutrient broth, viruses pose more of a problem. This is because they cannot multiply outside a living host cell. They have been successfully grown in fertilised hen's eggs. Today this method has been widely replaced by growing the required virus in animal cell cultures.

Safety precautions in microbiology

In order to study microorganisms, they must be grown and handled. It must always be remembered that all microorganisms should be treated as pathogens, i.e. to assume that careless behaviour can result in infections and disease. Therefore it is most important to follow a few important rules.

In order to infect you, pathogens must come into contact with you. They can enter your bodies in a number of ways:

- through the nose and mouth carried in the air
- through the mouth by contact with contaminated hands or equipment
- through the lining of the mouth or intestine in contaminated food
- through cuts in the skin after contact with contaminated equipment.

Observing the rules listed below should prevent contamination.

1 *Make sure that any cuts or grazes on exposed parts of the body are covered by waterproof dressings.*

2 *Before and after experiments involving microorganisms, wipe down your workbench top with a disinfectant solution.*

3 *All hand-to-mouth operations, such as eating or licking labels, are forbidden.*

4 *Never pipette by mouth. Do not squirt liquids which might contain microorganisms quickly into a container as this might form an aerosol and cause the dispersal of spores.*

5 *If a culture (i.e. solution containing microorganisms) or any medium is spilled or dropped, report this immediately to your teacher/lecturer.*

6 *When transferring microorganisms from one medium to another, ensure that the inoculating instrument (i.e. the loop, pipette or needle) is heat-sterilised before and after use.*

7 *Only open containers of cultures when told to do so. Never sniff them or remove them from the laboratory. It is usual to observe cultures in the unopened containers in which they have been grown.*

8 *After use, dispose of all glassware, Petri dishes, etc. by the method instructed, ready for sterile disposal.*

9 *Wash and dry your hands thoroughly before leaving the laboratory. Use warm water, soap and paper towels.*

Practical 20.5 To investigate the effect of different sterilisation methods

The aim of the experiment is to investigate the effect of various sterilisation procedures on the growth of bacteria in a sample of nutrient broth. The effect of autoclaving the culture medium, oven-sterilising test tubes and using cotton wool stoppers will be investigated both independently and in combination. You should read the section *Safety precautions in microbiology* before proceeding.

BIOHAZARD

Requirements

4 sterilised test tubes with cotton wool stoppers
4 unsterilised test tubes with cotton wool stoppers
Chinagraph pencil
Test tube rack
Bunsen burner
Matches
Protective mat
10 cm^3 of autoclaved nutrient broth
10 cm^3 of nutrient broth that has not been autoclaved
Incubator at 25°C

1 Label four unsterilised, stoppered test tubes 1–4.

2 Label four sterilised, stoppered test tubes 5–8.

3 To tubes 1, 3, 5 and 7 add 2 cm^3 of autoclaved broth (remembering to flame the necks of both the flask and the test tubes before and after pouring the broth and replacing the stoppers).

4 To tubes 2, 4, 6 and 8 add 2 cm^3 of non-autoclaved broth (taking the same precautions as in 3 above).

5 Remove the cotton-wool stoppers from tubes 1, 2, 5 and 6 only and incubate all tubes at 25°C for 48 hours.

6 After this time, record the growth in each of the test tubes.

7 Before disposing of your test tubes, replace their stoppers and hand them in to your lecturer or teacher to be autoclaved.

Summary

- DNA is made up of deoxyribose sugar, phosphate and nitrogen bases.
- There are four nitrogen bases in DNA. Cytosine always joins with guanine and adenine with thymine.
- DNA is a double helix where the two strands are held together by weak hydrogen bonds between the base pairs. One strand is upside down compared with its partner.
- RNA differs from DNA in that it is single-stranded, contains ribose not deoxyribose sugar and has the base uracil instead of thymine.
- Proteins are chains of amino acids arranged in a certain order.
- Each amino acid is coded for by a triplet of nitrogen bases.
- In the formation of proteins, transcription occurs first, followed by translation.
  - Transcription is the formation of mRNA from part of the nitrogen base sequence of DNA.
  - Translation is attaching the amino acids in a certain order through the nitrogen base pairing between codons on the mRNA and anticodons on the tRNA.
- The three stages in recombinant DNA technology (genetic engineering) are: isolation of the gene from a donor; insertion of the isolated gene into a carrier; transfer of the gene into a host.
- Examples of genetic engineering are the production of useful chemicals, e.g. human insulin, the treatment of genetic conditions, e.g. cystic fibrosis, and toxin production, e.g. protection of edible plants against butterfly larvae.
- Examples of biotechnology are fermenters, waste technology, enzyme technology, medicine, forensic science and agriculture.
- Immobilised enzymes are enzymes attached to a support, e.g. beads.
- Sterilisation of equipment and growth media is either by dry heat, wet heat or steam heat under pressure (autoclave).
- Aseptic techniques are used in microbiology to avoid contamination by microorganisms.
- Nutrient broth and nutrient agar can be used to grow bacteria and fungi.
- Viruses need living cells in order to multiply.

Self check
See page 251

CHAPTER 21

Evolution

In this chapter you will learn about Darwin's theory of evolution through natural selection. To understand this, you will study the causes of variation, natural selection in action and, finally, how humans artificially select the plants and animals they use to produce food.

Darwin's theory of natural selection

Darwin published his theory in 1859. Since then, research has led to its modification, so that a modern summary includes the following key ideas.

- **Variation:** In any population of organisms that reproduce sexually, there is variation between individuals. Some of this variation results from environmental differences. However, some is inherited (Chapter 19). It is this inherited variation that is important in evolution.
- **Competition:** Organisms generally produce more offspring than the environment can support. Therefore, there is competition (page 188) for such resources as space, food or a mate. Darwin called this a *'struggle for existence'*.
- **Natural Selection:** Darwin argued that those organisms that were best able to compete or escape predation would be more likely to survive. As a result, they would reproduce and be the parents of the next generation. If their favourable characteristics were inherited, this would result in organisms in the next generation inheriting those favourable genes, i.e. the next generation would be genetically better able to survive. Darwin called this *'survival of the fittest'*.

We now know that poorly adapted organisms need not die for their genes to be lost from the population. Organisms that are not successful in competition might survive but they produce fewer offspring than those that are successful in competition. For example, an animal that is unable to find sufficient food, or a plant that is unable to produce as much chlorophyll as other plants, lacks the energy needed to produce large numbers of offspring.

Evolution of the giraffe

Darwin might have explained the evolution of the present-day giraffe as follows:

- He would have assumed that the ancestral giraffes had shorter necks and legs than present-day giraffes.
- He would then suggest that, in the

ancestral population, there were some animals with longer necks and longer legs, i.e. there was variation. These characteristics were inherited.

- Finding enough food was probably a major problem for the giraffe, i.e. there would have been competition for food. (Darwin would have said there was a struggle for existence.)
- Those animals best able to get food would survive. In this case, having longer legs and necks would be an advantage, enabling animals to reach leaves at the tops of trees. These animals would survive and produce more offspring, i.e. survival of the fittest.
- Nature has, therefore, selected those best suited at that time, i.e. natural selection has occurred.
- If this continued generation after generation, the present-day giraffe would eventually evolve (Figure 21.1).

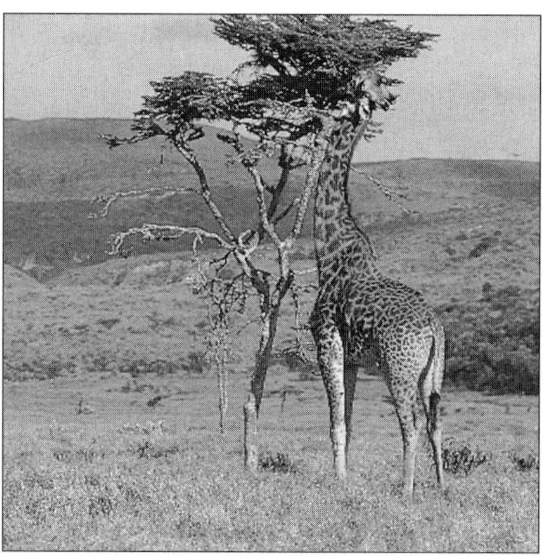

Figure 21.1 Giraffe reaching up for leaves.

Q1: Would animals with shorter legs or necks have to die in order for natural selection to change the giraffe population?

Inherited variation

In Chapter 19 we looked briefly at inherited and non-inherited variation. We will now look more closely at inherited variation.

If you look at a group of people, you will see variation in a number of human features.

Continuous variation

A feature such as human height follows the pattern shown in Figure 21.2. This pattern is called a **normal distribution**. Although the graph in Figure 21.2 is symmetrical, this need not always be the case and the graph may be skewed as in Figure 21.3. Where the differences in a feature show a smooth gradation, we call this **continuous variation**.

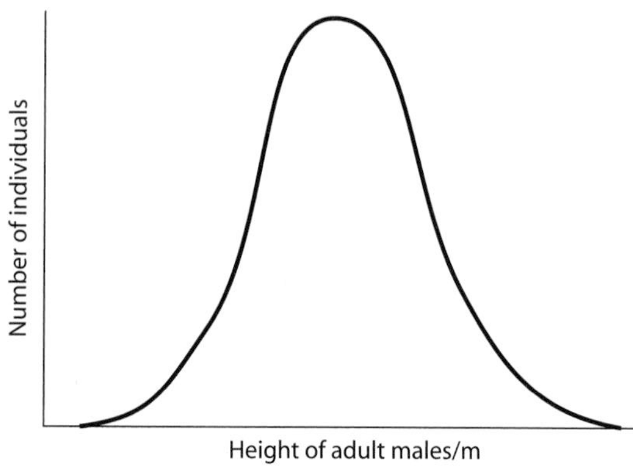

Figure 21.2 Normal distribution curve.

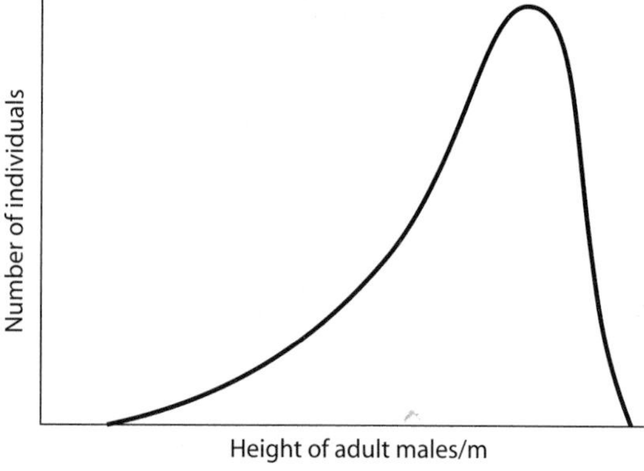

Figure 21.3 Skewed distribution curve.

Continuous variation usually occurs when an individual feature is controlled by a number of genes, i.e. it is **polygenic**. A simple way of looking at this is to imagine a characteristic such as seed mass in a cereal crop being controlled by five pairs of alleles **Aa**, **Bb**, **Cc**, **Dd** and **Ee**. If we assume that an allele represented by a large letter contributes a mass of 1 mg to the phenotype and an allele represented by a small letter contributes a mass of 0.5 mg to the phenotype:

- the heaviest seed will be 10 mg with a genotype of **AA BB CC DD EE**
- the lightest seed will be 5 mg with a

genotype of **aa bb cc dd ee**.
Other genotypes will result in seeds with masses between these two values. Although this is not a human example, it illustrates how polygenic inheritance works.

Q2: What would be the possible genotypes of seeds weighing 7.5 mg?

Discontinuous variation

A feature such as the human ABO blood group shows a small number of discrete phenotypes: group A, group B, group AB and group O. There is no smooth gradation between blood groups. Where the differences in a feature result in a small number of distinct types, we call this **discontinuous variation**.

Discontinuous variation usually occurs when an individual feature is controlled by a single gene. This pattern of inheritance is described in Chapter 19.

Examples of continuous and discontinuous variation in humans are shown in Table 21.1.

Table 21.1 Examples of continuous and discontinuous variation in humans

Continuous variation	Discontinuous variation
Height	Fixed ear lobes or free ear lobes
Weight	ABO blood group
Skin colour	Rhesus blood group
Hair colour	Genetic sex

Q3: Which of the following features show discontinuous variation: haemophilia; intelligence; eye colour; cystic fibrosis; lung capacity?

Causes of genetic variation

Natural selection works on genetic differences between the organisms in a population. Such genetic differences arise through:

- **random assortment** of chromosomes during meiosis I (Figure 21.4)
- **random fertilisation**, i.e. pure chance determines which gamete fuses with another (e.g. Figure 19.11)
- **crossing over** during meiosis (Figure 19.7) which separates genes that were linked together on a single chromosome
- **mutation**, i.e. a change in either a single gene (**gene mutation**) or in a whole chromosome (**chromosome mutation**).

Q4: Which is the only source of genetic variation in organisms that only reproduce asexually? Explain your answer.

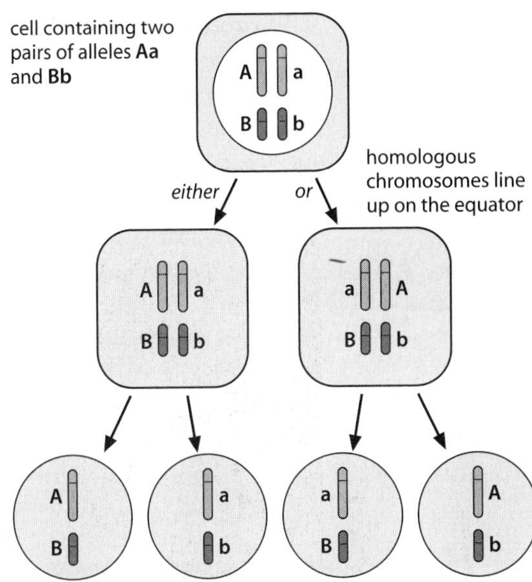

Figure 21.4 Random assortment of chromosomes.

Gene mutations

A gene is a length of DNA that codes for the production of a single protein (page 163). A spontaneous change in the base sequence of this DNA is called a **gene mutation**. All genes mutate at a very low rate but this rate is increased if organisms are exposed to mutagens, such as radiation and certain chemicals. Most mutations are harmful, but some give the organism an advantage over others, e.g. a mutation giving a rat resistance to warfarin, a commonly used rat poison, gives its possessor an advantage over susceptible rats.

Q5: Define the term 'mutagen'.

The majority of mutations result in recessive alleles, e.g. the alleles causing cystic fibrosis. However some mutant alleles are dominant, e.g. the allele causing Huntington's disease which is a condition involving a gradual deterioration of the nervous system.

Sickle cell anaemia is a condition that is thought to have resulted from a gene mutation. Red blood cells contain the oxygen-carrying pigment haemoglobin. The production of normal haemoglobin is controlled by a gene (**H**) with two alleles. The allele $\mathbf{H^N}$ controls the production of normal haemoglobin. However at some stage in human ancestry, a gene mutation led to a new allele, $\mathbf{H^S}$. This allele controls the production of a haemoglobin molecule with a different amino acid at one point along its length. This simple difference reduces the ability of the haemoglobin molecule to carry oxygen. At low oxygen concentrations, cells with abnormal haemoglobin collapse into a sickle shape (Figure 21.5), hence the name of the disorder.

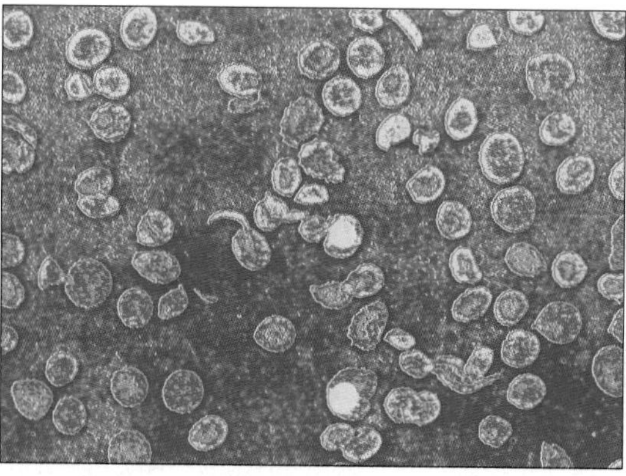

Figure 21.5 Photomicrograph of normal red blood cells and those showing the sickle cell condition.

People can have one of three genotypes: $\mathbf{H^NH^N}$; $\mathbf{H^NH^S}$; $\mathbf{H^SH^S}$. Those with the genotype $\mathbf{H^NH^N}$ only produce red blood cells with normal haemoglobin. Those with the genotype $\mathbf{H^SH^S}$ only produce red blood cells with the abnormal haemoglobin. This is called **sickle cell anaemia** and, without constant medical treatment, people with this condition are likely to be very ill and often die when they are young. The blood shown in Figure 21.5 is from such a person. People with the genotype $\mathbf{H^NH^S}$ produce red blood cells with some normal haemoglobin and some abnormal haemoglobin. This condition is known as the **sickle cell trait.**

Q6: As sickle cell anaemia is usually fatal, what might you expect to happen to the $\mathbf{H^S}$ allele controlling its production?

People with the sickle cell trait only suffer a reduced ability to transport oxygen at abnormally low oxygen concentrations, so they survive normally. In fact, in some parts of the world this condition is advantageous. This strange event occurs because the sickle cell trait gives resistance to malaria. It appears that *Plasmodium*, the parasite causing malaria (page 147), finds it much more difficult to infect red blood cells that contain the abnormal haemoglobin.

Q7: In which parts of the world would the sickle cell trait be advantageous?

Gene mutations are frequent in the influenza virus. Because this virus mutates so often, it is very difficult to get a vaccine against 'flu'.

Chromosome mutations

This is a spontaneous change in:

- the structure of one (or more) chromosome(s) *or*
- the number of chromosomes in a cell.

In mammals, such mutations are usually lethal, but plants seem to be able to withstand them better and, in some cases, flourish as a result of them.

Human cells are sometimes found in which the chromosome number is greater than the expected 46. This occurs from the fusion of an egg cell or a sperm cell that was produced after a pair of homologous chromosomes failed to separate during meiosis (Figure 21.6). It is called **chromosome non-disjunction.**

Probably the most common example of chromosome non-disjunction in humans is **Down's syndrome**. People with this syndrome have an extra copy of chromosome 21 in each of their cells. Children with this syndrome have a characteristic appearance with a roundish face and almond-shaped eyes. In addition, they suffer varying degrees of mental retardation, stunted physical growth, heart abnormalities and reduced resistance to disease. The presence of Down's syndrome in a fetus can be detected by an amniocentesis (page 103).

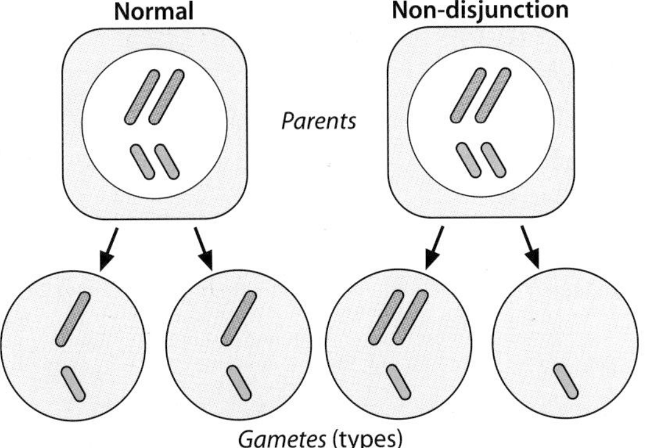

Figure 21.6 Chromosome non-disjunction.

Q8: (a) How many chromosomes will there be in the body cells of someone with Down's syndrome? (b) Suggest why people with Down's syndrome are usually sterile.

Natural selection in action

In this chapter, we have already looked at examples of natural selection, including the effect of a long neck in giraffes and the effect of the sickle cell trait in countries where malaria is endemic. Many other examples of natural selection involve the development of resistance to chemical pesticides, e.g. bacterial resistance to antibiotics, resistance of some mosquitos to DDT, resistance of rats to warfarin. A further example is of historical interest because it was the first example of natural selection to be studied and because it was published exactly one hundred years after Darwin had proposed his theory of natural selection. It involves populations of the peppered moth, *Biston betularia,* a normally light-coloured moth. Figure 21. 7 shows the two colour forms of *B. betularia* – speckled white and black (melanic).

In the 1850s it was found that in industrial parts of the country, e.g. Birmingham and Manchester, the black form was becoming more common than the speckled form. By 1895 the black form had increased to 98% of the population.

Since the 1970s, the speckled form has once more become the more common form in Birmingham and Manchester.

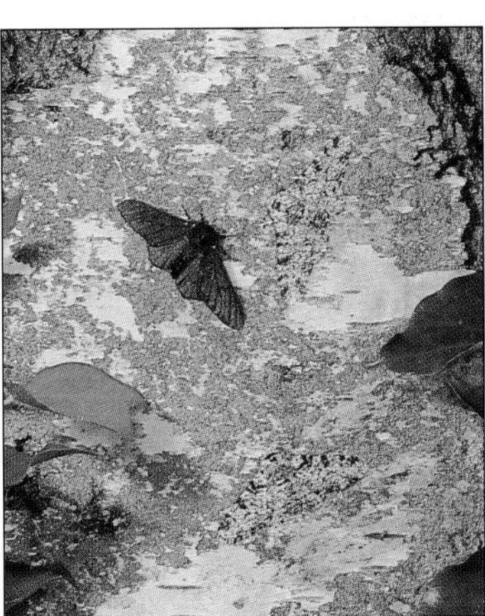

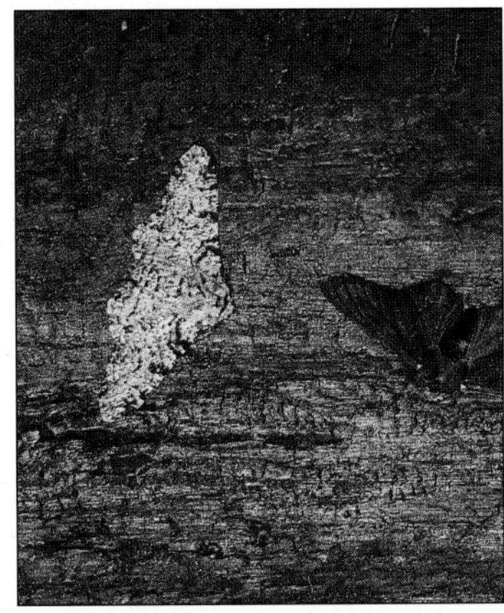

Figure 21.7 Speckled and black forms of the peppered moth, *Biston betularia*, on tree bark in **left:** rural and **right:** industrial areas.

Q9: Which of Darwin's points is illustrated by this statement – About two hundred years ago, most of the moths in Britain were speckled?

Q10: Use your knowledge of natural selection and the information in Figure 21.7 to suggest why most moths were speckled at this time.

Q11: How might the black form have arisen?

Q12: Use your own knowledge and the information in Figure 21.7 to suggest why the black form became dominant in industrial areas in the 1850s.

Q13: Use your own knowledge to suggest why the speckled form has once again become the more common form in Birmingham and Manchester.

Artificial selection

In the examples described so far, the success or failure of organisms to reproduce has been an entirely natural phenomenon. However, if animals or plants are of value to humans, we can decide which we will allow to reproduce. This is called **artificial selection** and involves breeders choosing organisms with the qualities they require and breeding from them. Table 21.2 shows some of the qualities that are useful to the breeders of a number of commercially exploited organisms.

Table 21.2 Qualities selected in breeding different animals and plants

Organism	Quality selected
Cattle	Early maturation; lean meat; high milk yield
Chickens	Rapid growth; high rate of egg laying
Maize (corn)	High yield; resistance to disease
Potatoes	Suitability for different cooking methods; resistance to disease

Breeding animals

At its simplest, the breeder might only need to choose a male and female animal with the required qualities, put them in a pen together and let them mate. This technique has been used with several animals, e.g. pigs and sheep. Artificial insemination and embryo transplantation are modern refinements used by animal breeders.

Embryo transplantation

- A female with many desired qualities can be made to produce more eggs than normal by treatment with hormones.
- These eggs can be fertilised by artificial insemination (see above right).
- The embryos can be recovered and placed inside other females which will allow them to develop normally inside them.
- Recent developments even allow the embryos to be tested for their genetic sex before implantation so that the desired sex of offspring can be obtained.

Artificial insemination

This technique allows the sperm from one male with many desired qualities to be used to fertilise a large number of different females.

- Semen (containing the sperm) is taken by a vet, tested for motility (ability of the sperm to swim) and stored at low temperatures.
- When required, the semen can be placed into the vagina or uterus of the recipient female using a long syringe.
- Since the semen can be diluted, the semen from one male can be used to inseminate large numbers of females.

This method has been used extensively with cattle, reducing the need for dairy farmers to keep their own bulls.

Breeding plants

The most common technique is to remove pollen from the anthers of a particular flower and transfer it to the stigmas of another plant of the same species. The pollinated flower is then covered using a small plastic bag to prevent other pollen getting in. Several methods can be used to prevent pollination before this treatment, e.g. covering the flowers with small plastic bags or removing the anthers.

Inbreeding and outbreeding

Inbreeding involves sexual reproduction between closely related organisms, e.g. between offspring of the same parents. This is commonly used in breeding 'show' animals, such as dogs. However, used over several generations, this can lead to a decrease in fitness. For example, the offspring may become smaller, less resistant to disease or more prone to physical abnormalities such as weak hips.

Outbreeding involves sexual reproduction between individuals who are members of different varieties or strains of a species. The offspring are known as **hybrids** and are usually strong and healthy: they are said to show **hybrid vigour**. Figure 21.8 shows how F1 hybrids are produced in maize plants (corn).

Marquis wheat

Wheat is grown around the world. Its flour is used for making such foods as bread, pasta and roti. A type of wheat known as **Marquis** was developed using selective breeding.

- In the early 1900s, most of the wheat grown in Canada was a type known as Red Fife.
- The advantages of Red Fife were that it produced a lot of grain and it produced flour that was good for bread-making.
- However, Red Fife plants suffered the disadvantage of susceptibility to damage by late autumn frosts.
- Scientists decided to breed a type of wheat that was faster growing so that the frosts would not affect it. They did this by cross-breeding Red Fife wheat with a type from India that ripened earlier.
- The result was the Marquis type of wheat which ripened earlier so that frost damage was minimal.

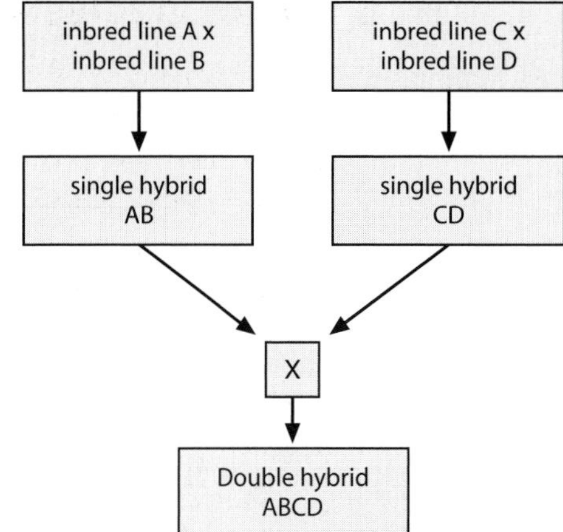

Figure 21.8 F1 hybrids in maize.

Summary

- Darwin's theory of natural selection rests on three concepts: inherited variation; a struggle for existence (competition); survival of the fittest.
- Variation can be inherited (genetic) or non-inherited (environmental). Natural selection can act only on inherited variation.
- Inherited variation is either continuous (e.g. human height) or discontinuous (e.g. human blood groups).
- Genetic variation results from crossing over of chromosomes during meiosis, random assortment of chromosomes during meiosis, random fertilisation of genetically different gametes and mutations.
- Mutations might involve a change in the structure of a gene or in the structure or number of chromosomes in a cell. Although mutations occur naturally, their rate is increased by mutagens.
- Examples of natural selection include the evolution of resistance to antibiotics among bacteria, the maintenance of the sickle cell trait among human populations in parts of the world where malaria is endemic and the balance of different body forms in populations of the moth *Biston betularia*.
- Artificial selection occurs when breeders select organisms with the qualities they require and breed from them. Among the methods used are artificial insemination and embryo transplantation.
- Inbreeding is selective reproduction between closely related organisms. Outbreeding is selective reproduction between organisms that are not closely related. At its extreme, two closely related species can be interbred so forming a hybrid.

Self check

See page 253

CHAPTER 22

Habitats and ecosystems

In this chapter you will learn how, in nature, organisms are grouped into ecosystems. We shall examine two natural and one artificial ecosystem and see how the organisms found in a place may change over time.

The variety of ecosystems

Think of the names you could use to describe different areas in the wild. You might use words like woodland, stream, estuary, desert or coral reef. Different organisms are found in these different places. Now think of a small wood. A small wood is an example of an **ecosystem**. An ecosystem consists of all the interacting organisms in a relatively self-contained area together with the non-living components of their environment.

Think again of a small wood such as that in Figure 22.1. We used the word 'small' because a really big wood – a forest – doesn't consist of only one ecosystem since many of the organisms in it are too far apart to 'interact'. On the other hand, a single tree isn't really big enough to be an ecosystem: it is too small to be 'relatively self-contained'. An ecosystem is self-contained if most of the organisms found in it can spend their entire life cycles in it. Look again at Figure 22.1. Some of the largest animals, such as birds and mammals, may move from this wood to another one, but the majority of woodland organisms will spend their entire lives in just that wood.

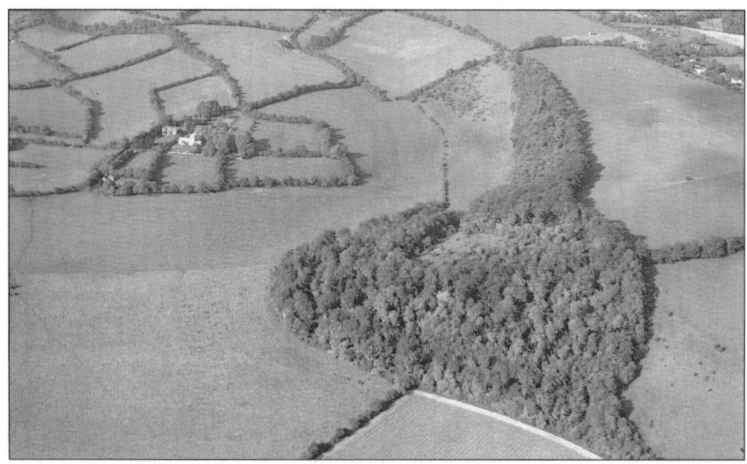

Figure 22.1 A small wood is an example of an ecosystem because it is relatively self-contained.

Q1: Which of the following would probably be the right size to be considered a single ecosystem: an ocean, a lake, a puddle?

An ecosystem has one further characteristic. It tends to be relatively stable in the sense that it exists in the same place for a long period of time. This is because the organisms in an ecosystem reproduce with the result that the same ecosystem persists for generations, even though the individual organisms within it age and die. If this wasn't the case, think how difficult maps would be to produce. It would, for instance, be impossible to show woods on them.

Oak woodland

One example of an ecosystem is oak woodland. Oak woodland is the most common natural woodland vegetation type found throughout much of England and Wales. A diagram of oak woodland is shown in Figure 22.2. Notice the following components of oak woodland.

- **Producers** – these are the plants. They are called producers because they produce the food on which the other organisms in the ecosystem depend. Another name for a producer is an **autotroph**. Autotroph means 'self feeder'. Plants are autotrophs because they make their own food as a result of photosynthesis (see Chapter 23). In an oak woodland some of the plants are trees, such as oak, ash and hornbeam. Other plants are bushes, such as holly, hazel and woodland hawthorn; while others are herbs, such as bluebells, oxlips and anemones.
- **Primary consumers** – these are the animals that feed on the plants. For example, squirrels and dormice are primary consumers, as are butterflies – both as adults (when they feed on nectar) and as larvae (when they are caterpillars and feed on leaves). Another name for a primary consumer is a **herbivore**.
- **Secondary consumers** – these are the animals that feed on the primary consumers. For example, titmice are secondary consumers. Another name for a secondary consumer is a **carnivore**. In fact, although titmice are carnivores, because they eat insects they can also be called **insectivores**.
- **Top carnivores** – these are carnivores which are themselves not preyed upon. Examples in Figure 22.2 are sparrowhawks and weasels. Sparrowhawks eat mainly small birds; weasels eat small mammals.
- **Decomposers** – these are organisms which break down dead organisms and the urine and faeces of animals. Many fungi and bacteria are decomposers.
- **Omnivores** – these are animals which eat both plants and animals. An example is the woodmouse which eats both insects and herbs.

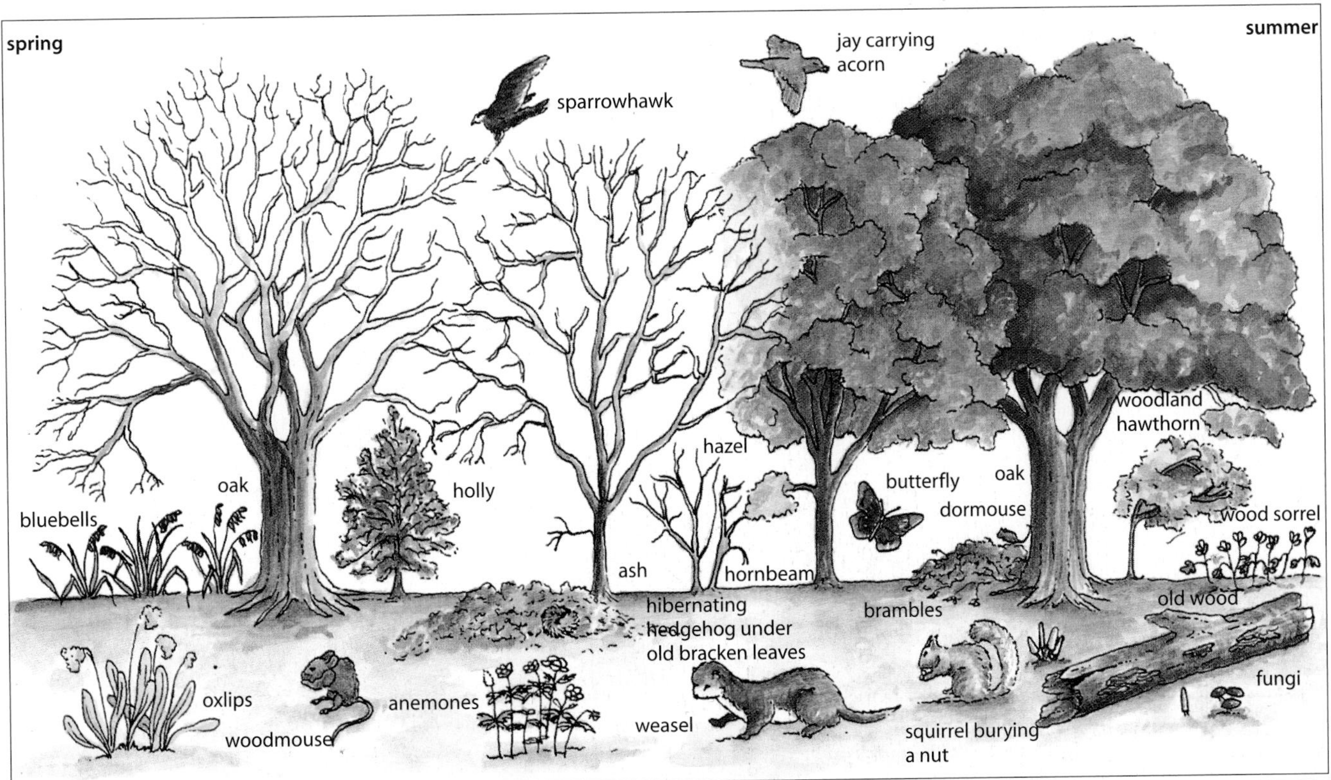

Figure 22.2 Oak woodland in spring (on the left) and in late summer (on the right).

Freshwater ponds

A cross-section through a pond, showing some of the animals and plants that might live there, is shown in Figure 22.3.

Q2: Identify (a) three producers, (b) two herbivores, (c) an omnivore and (d) three carnivores in Figure 22.3.

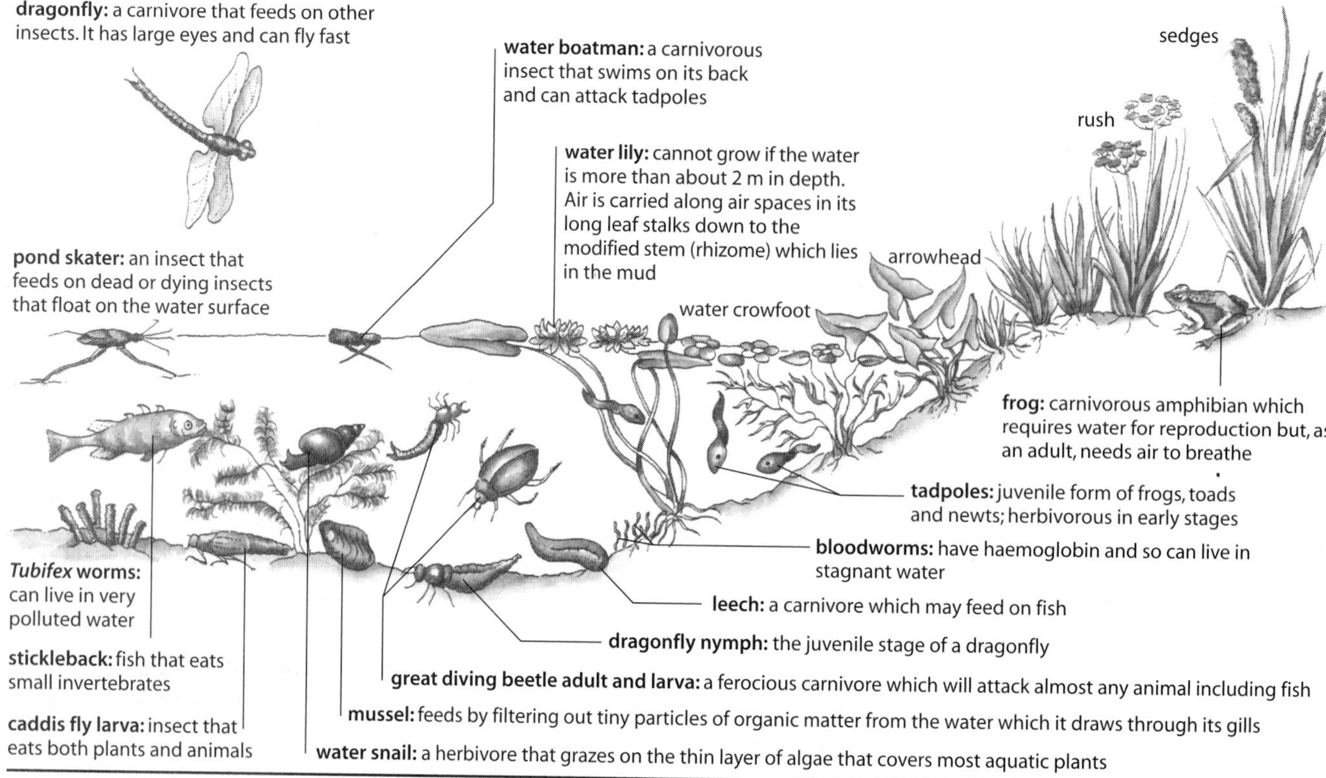

Figure 22.3 Cross-section through a typical pond showing some of the organisms that may be found there.

A greenhouse

Woods and ponds are examples of natural ecosystems. However, ecosystems can be artificial, like that in a greenhouse. Imagine a greenhouse, such as that in Figure 22.4, used to grow tomatoes. Like natural ecosystems, a greenhouse will have:

- producers (tomatoes)
- herbivores (both people who harvest the tomatoes and pests that live on the tomatoes)
- decomposers (these break down plant roots and other organic matter in the soil).

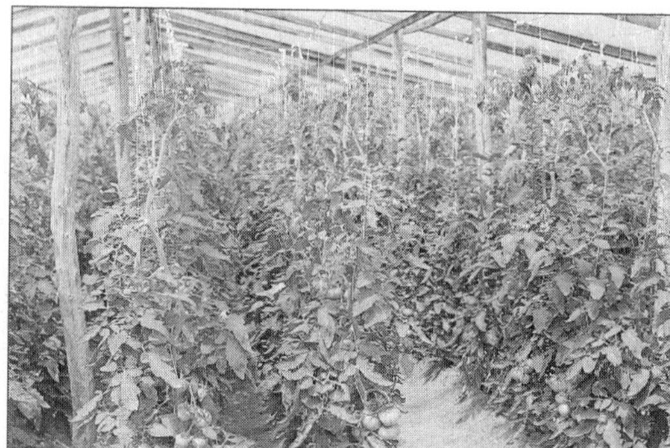

Figure 22.4 A greenhouse ecosystem.

In addition, there might be carnivorous insects introduced to eat any herbivorous insect pests as a form of **biological control**. For example, the parasitic wasp *Encarsia* can be used to control whitefly.

However, a greenhouse ecosystem will differ from a natural ecosystem in a number of important respects:

- there are few species, i.e. **species diversity** is low
- there is little recycling of nutrients
- the ecosystem is not very self-contained – young tomato plants and fertiliser are brought into the green-house and tomato fruits are taken from it
- the ecosystem is not very stable – if left to itself for a few years it would not continue to produce tomatoes.

Habitats and communities

The place where an organism is found is its **habitat**. Table 22.1 gives the habitats of some familiar organisms. The different organisms that are found in a habitat make up a **community**. So one can identify rock pool communities, sand dune communities and grassland communities, for example.

Table 22.1 The habitats of some familiar organisms

Organism	Habitat
Oak tree	Woodland
Rush	Wet grassland, fens
Dandelion	Wasteland
Red squirrel	Woodland with conifer trees
Grey squirrel	Woodland with broad-leaved (deciduous) trees
Mallard	River, freshwater lake
Frog	Pond
Earthworm	Alkaline or neutral soil
Edible wild mushrooms	Grassland

Abiotic components of an ecosystem

The non-living aspects of an ecosystem are called the **abiotic** (or **physical**) components. These include such things as the:

- temperature
- water content (of air or soil)
- pH (of soil or water)
- oxygen levels (of soil or water)
- light levels
- nutrient levels (of soil or water)
- topography (altitude, slope and direction, e.g. south-facing)
- currents (of air or water).

The abiotic components of an ecosystem affect the organisms that can live there. For example, many of the organisms that live in woods in northern Scotland are different from the organisms that live in woods in southern England.

Q3: Suggest two differences in the abiotic factors found in woods in northern Scotland and southern England.

Abiotic factors can also vary within an ecosystem. Figure 22.5 shows some of these differences between the surface water and the mud at the bottom of a pond.

Q4: Near the surface of a pond the pH levels usually rise during the day, especially if it is sunny, and then fall at night. Why is this?

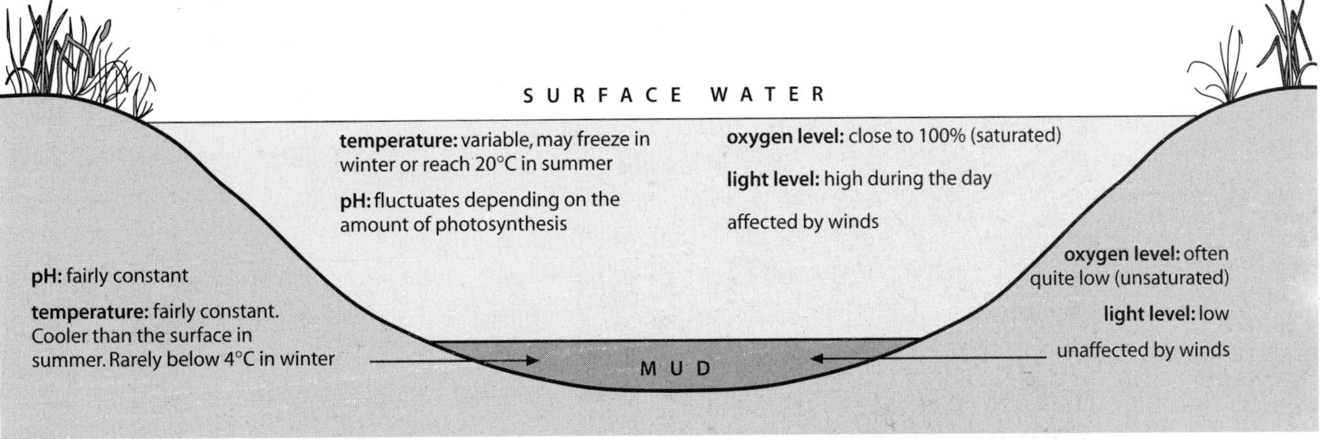

Figure 22.5 Differences between the surface water and mud at the bottom of a pond with respect to various abiotic factors.

Practical 22.1 To compare the water content of two different soils

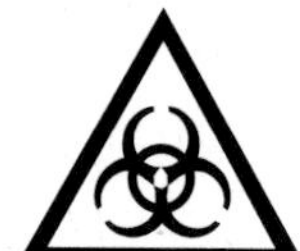

Requirements

Two soil samples, fresh, each 60–100 g
Heat-proof container, e.g. aluminium dish
Balance, accurate to at least 0.1 g
Oven
Tongs
Desiccator, if available

1 Obtain samples from two different soils just before you carry out the practical if possible. This will ensure that their water contents when measured will be close to actual values.

2 Carry out steps 3 to 10 below for each soil, separately.

3 Weigh a small heat-proof container, such as an aluminium dish ($W_{container}$).

4 Spread the soil sample evenly in the container. Weigh it again ($W_{soil + container}$).

5 Calculate the mass of the soil ($W_{soil} = W_{soil + container} - W_{container}$).

6 Place the container with the soil in an oven at 110°C for at least three hours.

7 Remove the container with the soil from the oven and allow to cool, ideally in a desiccator (to prevent the absorption of water from air).

8 Weigh the container with the oven-dried soil. Find the mass of the soil by subtracting the original mass of the container from the mass of the container with the oven-dried soil.

9 Repeat steps 6 to 8 until you obtain the same mass for the oven-dried soil. This means that all the soil water has been driven off and you have the mass of the dry soil ($W_{dry\ soil}$).

10 The % of the water content in the original soil is given by:

$$\frac{W_{soil} - W_{dry\ soil}}{W_{soil}} \times 100\%$$

11 Compare the water content of the two different soils. If they differ, propose a hypothesis to explain why this is the case. How could you test this hypothesis?

SAFETY: Always wash your hands after handling soil.
SAFETY: Take care not to burn yourself on removing the container from the oven.

Biotic components of an ecosystem

The living components of an ecosystem are called the **biotic** components. The main biotic factors that affect a rabbit are shown in Figure 22.6. Note that these fall into two categories:

- **intraspecific** factors – these operate within a species; the intraspecific factors for a rabbit are therefore other rabbits, including those it competes with for food, any rabbits with which it mates and any baby rabbits it has
- **interspecific** factors – these operate between species; interspecific factors

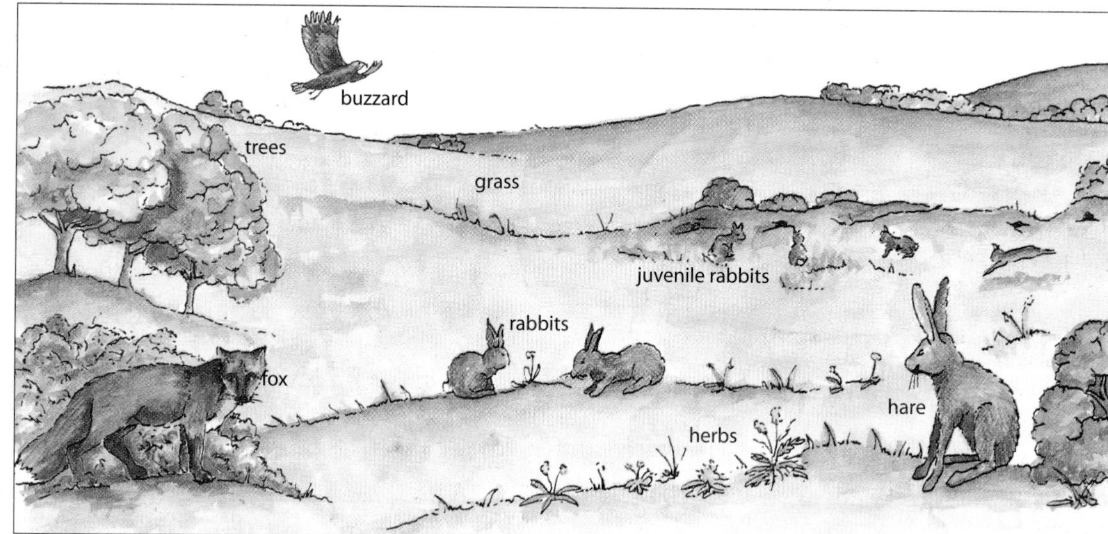

Figure 22.6 The main biotic factors that affect a wild rabbit.

for a rabbit include the food it eats (plants such as grass and herbs), other species with which it competes for food (e.g. hares), parasites (e.g. rabbit fleas) and predators (such as foxes and buzzards).

Q5: Identify three of the biotic factors that affect a woodmouse in an oak wood such as that shown in Figure 22.2.

Succession

In most parts of the UK, if a pond such as that shown in Figure 22.3 is left alone for long enough it eventually turns into woodland (Figure 22.7). The woodland is known as the **climax community**. The development of a wood from a pond occurs as follows:

- plants growing in the pond or at its edges die
- some of this plant matter decomposes but some of it accumulates at the bottom of the pond
- gradually the pond fills up with mud and partly decomposed plant matter
- the pond becomes shallower and shallower
- once the pond has dried out, terrestrial grasses, herbs and small bushes invade
- eventually trees invade and a mature woodland results.

This entire process may take hundreds of years. The development of woodland from open water is an example of **succession**. Succession is simply a change over time in the vegetation and associated animals and other organisms found in an area.

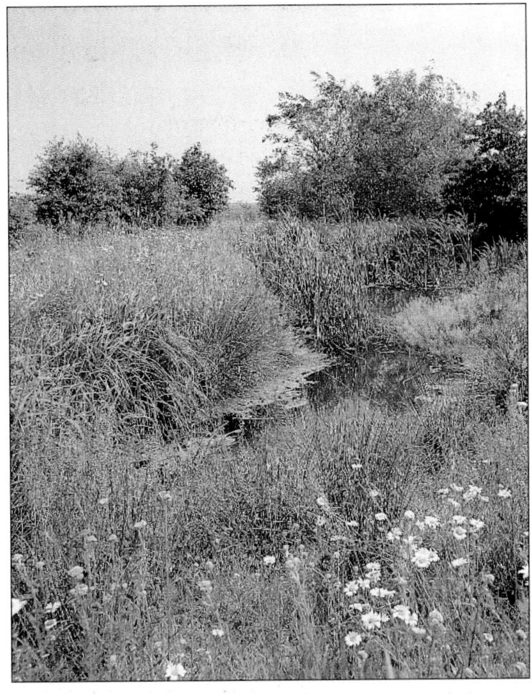

Figure 22.7 Unless it is regularly cleared out, a pond eventually becomes filled in as vegetation invades. This is an example of succession.

Two types of natural succession occur:

- **Primary succession** – here the succession starts in an area where there is no soil. The main examples are succession from open water or from bare rock (Figure 22.8).
- **Secondary succession** – here the succession starts in an area where there is soil. For example, it might occur on an area where the vegetation has recently been destroyed by fire.

Q6: Would you expect primary succession to take place more quickly or more slowly than secondary succession? Explain your answer.

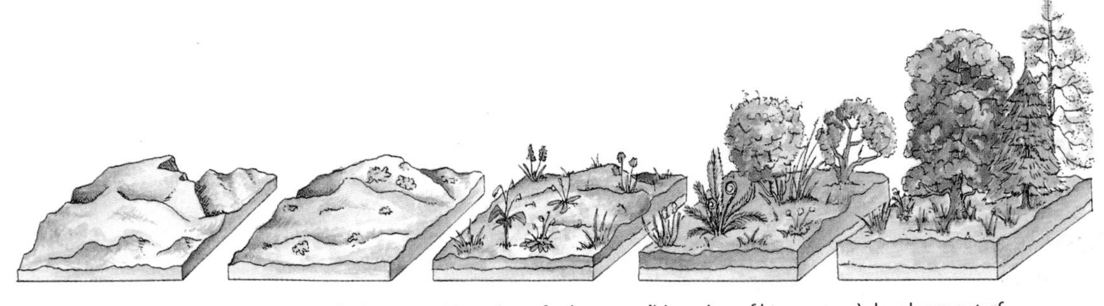

Figure 22.8 Primary succession on bare rock usually ends up with woodland. In nature, bare rock is found when a glacier retreats or when larva is produced by a volcano.

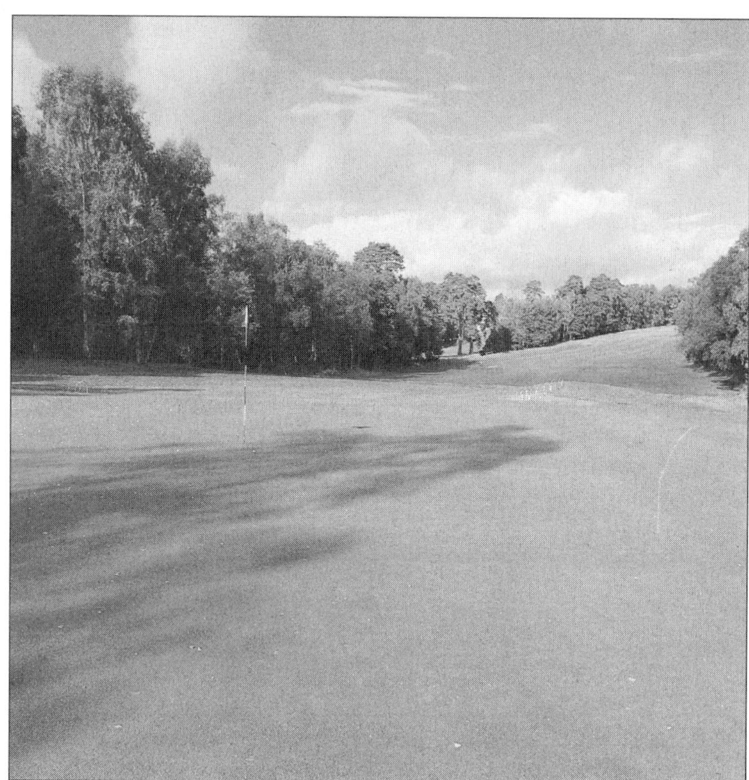

Deflected succession

If left to itself, succession results in the climax community. However, it is possible to prevent this from happening. For example, grassland can be maintained by:

- grazing
- burning
- cutting (Figure 22.9).

Grassland is an example of a **deflected succession**. The succession is said to be 'deflected' from its natural path.

Q7: Explain what would happen to the vegetation if the greens and fairways on a golf course, such as that in Figure 22.9, were abandoned.

Figure 22.9 Grassland, such as that found on a golf course, is an example of a deflected succession.

Summary

- An ecosystem consists of all the interacting organisms in a relatively self-contained area together with the non-living components of their environment.
- Ecosystems tend to be relatively stable over time.
- Plants are known as producers or autotrophs.
- Animals that feed on plants are known as primary consumers or herbivores.
- Animals that feed on herbivores are known as secondary consumers or carnivores.
- Top carnivores are not preyed upon.
- Decomposers break down dead organisms and the urine and faeces of animals.
- Omnivores are animals that eat both plants and animals.
- The place where an organism is found is its habitat.
- The different organisms that are found in a habitat make up a community.
- The non-living components of an ecosystem are called the abiotic or physical components.
- The abiotic components of an ecosystem include such things as the temperature, pH and light levels.
- The living components of an ecosystem are called the biotic components.
- Succession is the change over time in the vegetation and associated animals and other organisms found in an area.
- The natural endpoint of a succession is the climax community.
- Primary succession starts where there is neither vegetation nor soil.
- Secondary succession starts where there is soil but no vegetation.
- A deflected succession results when something prevents a succession from continuing through to the climax community.

Self check

See page 253

CHAPTER 23

Photosynthesis and food chains

In this chapter you will learn how plants make organic chemicals by the process of photosynthesis and how feeding relationships can be described by means of food chains and food webs. We shall also examine some of the ways in which different species interact with each other.

The process of photosynthesis

Plants make their own food by **photosynthesis**, turning the energy from light into chemical energy stored in starch and other organic molecules (Figure 23.1). The word literally means 'making by light'. For photosynthesis to take place the following are needed:

- **chloroplasts** with **chlorophyll** and a number of **enzymes**
- **light energy** – either from the Sun or from artificial sources (e.g. lamps)
- **carbon dioxide**
- **water.**

Photosynthesis results in the formation of:

- **glucose**
- **oxygen.**

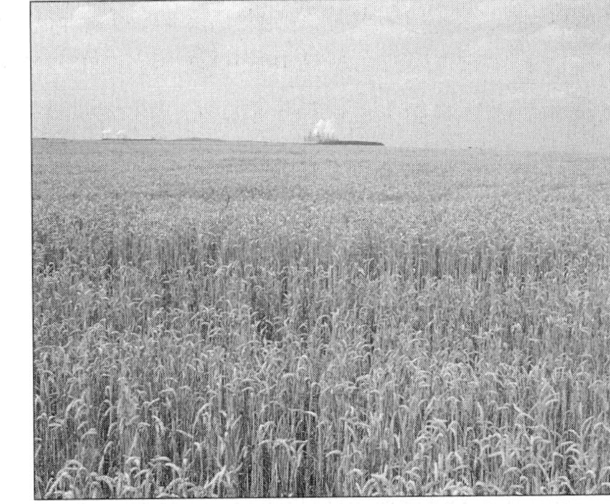

Figure 23.1 The wheat in this field has grown as a result of photosynthesis. In less than a year it has developed from individual grains into whole plants.

Overall, we can write a word equation for photosynthesis as follows:

$$\text{carbon dioxide} + \text{water} \xrightarrow[\text{chloroplasts}]{\text{light energy}} \text{glucose} + \text{oxygen}$$

A simplified chemical equation for photosynthesis is:

$$6CO_2 + 6H_2O \rightarrow C_6H_{12}O_6 + 6O_2$$

Q1: How many molecules of carbon dioxide does it take to make one molecule of glucose?

Q2: For each molecule of water that a plant uses in photosynthesis, how many molecules of oxygen does it produce?

Q3: Does photosynthesis require an input of energy or result in the release of energy?

Glucose is an example of a **monosaccharide sugar** (see page 14). Plants use the glucose made in photosynthesis for several things.

- Much of the glucose is converted into **starch** and then stored. Starch, like glucose, is a **carbohydrate**. However starch, unlike glucose, is an extremely large molecule known as a **poly-saccharide** (see page 15). Starch is a convenient storage molecule for plants because it neither dissolves in water nor attracts lots of water molecules (i.e. it has little osmotic effect).

- Some of the glucose is converted into the **disaccharide, sucrose** (see page 14). This is the chemical form in which organic compounds are moved from one part of a plant to another, for example from leaves to growing roots or shoots.
- Some of the glucose is converted into other carbohydrates, such as **cellulose** which is an important component of plant cell walls.
- Some of the glucose is combined with nitrogen and phosphorus to make nucleic acids.
- Some of the glucose is combined with nitrogen, sulphur and other elements to make proteins.
- Some of the glucose is respired to release energy that may be needed for the plant to grow.
- Some of the glucose is converted into lipids, such as oils found in many seeds (Figure 23.2).

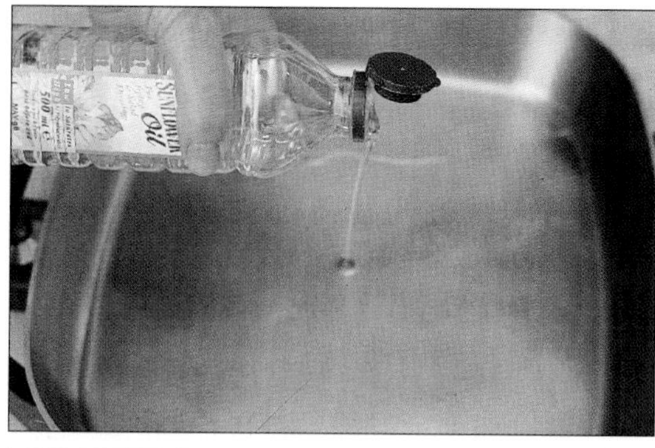

Figure 23.2 Most of the oils we use in cooking come from plant seeds.

Practical 23.1 To demonstrate the evolution of oxygen by a photosynthesising plant

An aquatic plant, such as Canadian pondweed, can be used to investigate the rate of photosynthesis. As the plant photosynthesises, small bubbles of gas are released and can be counted. These bubbles contain oxygen, one of the products of photosynthesis.

Requirements

Test tube
Glass beaker, 250 cm^3
Glass funnel
Funnel supports, 2
Water, 20–25°C
Thermometer
Lamp
Stopclock
Pondweed, fresh
Sodium hydrogencarbonate (not essential)
Scissors
Splint
Matches

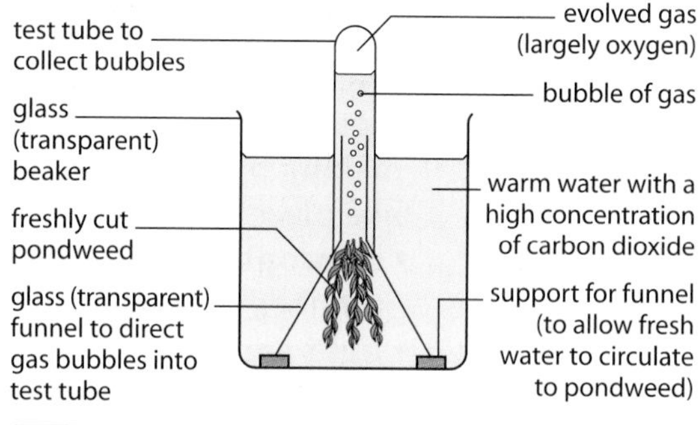

Figure 23.3 Apparatus for Practical 23.1.

1 Assemble the apparatus as shown in Figure 23.3. Use water with a temperature of 20–25°C and increase the carbon dioxide concentration either by blowing through it or by adding some sodium hydrogencarbonate. Cut a short length of pondweed with scissors under water.

2 Check that the pondweed is producing bubbles.

3 Record the number of bubbles produced over 60 seconds.

4 Increase the light intensity by shining a lamp onto the apparatus. Wait three to five minutes to acclimatise the plant to the new environmental conditions.

5 Record the number of bubbles produced over 60 seconds.

6 Remove the lamp so that the conditions are the same as when you counted the bubbles in step 3. Again, wait three to five minutes.

7 Count the number of bubbles produced over 60 seconds.

8 What effect did increasing the light intensity have on the rate of photosynthesis?

9 Why was it a good idea to carry out steps 6 and 7?

10 Explain the advantages of using warm water with a high concentration of carbon dioxide for this investigation.

Note to students: You may wish, after you have completed your investigation, to test the composition of the evolved gas collected in the test tube. Place a thumb over the end of the test tube while it is still underwater. Slowly remove the test tube from the beaker. Remove your thumb and immediately insert a glowing splint. It may ignite, showing that the evolved gas is largely oxygen. However, don't be surprised if it doesn't! A lot of nitrogen will also be present and this may prevent the glowing splint from igniting.

Practical 23.2 To test a leaf for the presence of starch

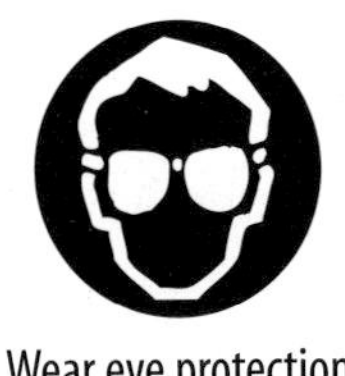

Wear eye protection

FLAMMABLE
Ethanol

Requirements

- Beaker, 250 cm^3
- Test tube
- Tweezers
- Ethanol
- Bunsen burner
- Matches
- Water bath at 85°C
- Thermometer
- White tile
- Dilute iodine solution
- Eye protection

The biochemical test for starch simply involves seeing if iodine solution, which is brown, turns blue-black. The complications when testing for the presence of starch in leaves come from the fact that:

- the chlorophyll in leaves makes any colour change more difficult to see
- leaves are not very permeable to iodine solution.

For these reasons the following procedure is used.

1 Remove the leaf to be tested from the plant.

2 Place it in boiling water for 20 seconds. This makes the leaf more permeable to iodine solution.

SAFETY: Wear eye protection and take care not to burn yourself.

3 Ensure all Bunsen burners are turned off.

SAFETY: Ethanol is flammable. All Bunsen burners must be extinguished before the lid of the bottle in which ethanol is kept is removed.

4 Place the leaf in a test tube of ethanol. Place the test tube with the ethanol and the leaf in a water bath of water at about 85°C as shown in Figure 23.4. The ethanol will boil and decolourise the leaf.

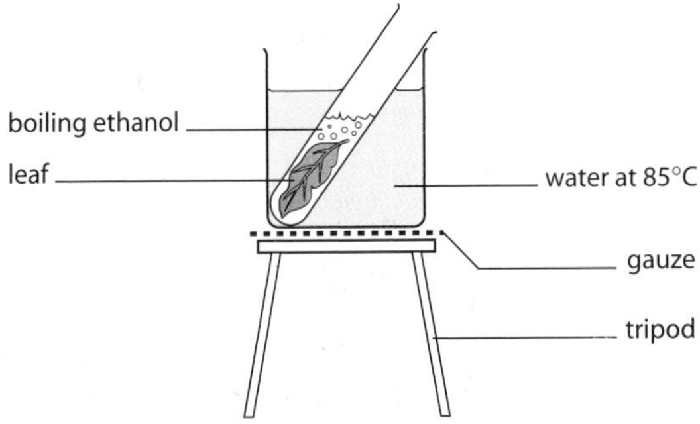

Figure 23.4 Apparatus for Practical 23.2.

5 After ten minutes, remove the leaf from the ethanol and wash it in the water bath for 20 seconds.

6 Spread the leaf out on a white tile and test with dilute iodine solution.

Practical 23.3 To investigate the factors needed for photosynthesis in a terrestrial plant

The arrangement in Practical 23.1 can be used to investigate how (a) light intensity, (b) the wavelength of light, (c) temperature and (d) carbon dioxide concentration affect the rate of photosynthesis. A different procedure can be used to demonstrate that a terrestrial plant, such as a geranium, needs light and carbon dioxide to photosynthesise. This procedure relies on the fact that in most plants much of the glucose made in photosynthesis is converted into starch.

Requirements

- Potted plants (e.g. geranium), 2
- Polythene bags, 2
- Elastic bands, 2
- Dish of dampened soda lime
- Dish of saturated sodium hydrogencarbonate solution
- Requirements for Practical 23.2

The experimental set up to demonstrate that carbon dioxide is needed for photosynthesis is shown in Figure 23.5.

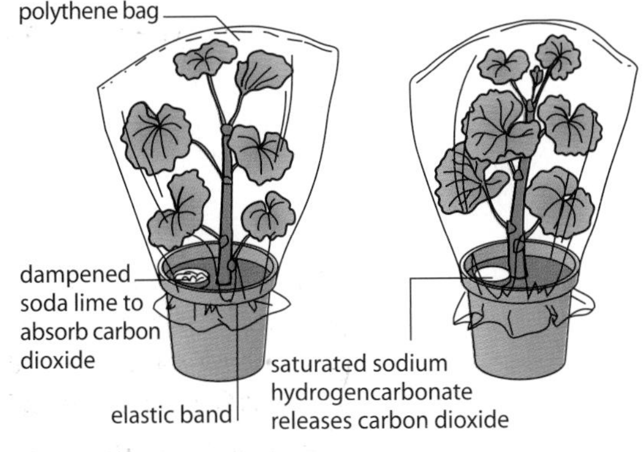

Figure 23.5 Apparatus for Practical 23.3.

Proceed as follows.

1 Put two similar potted plants into the dark for 24 hours. This 'destarches' the plants.

IRRITANT
Soda lime

2 Remove both plants from the dark. In one of them place a dish of dampened soda lime by the plant. (This absorbs carbon dioxide.) In the other put a dish of saturated sodium hydrogencarbonate solution. (This releases carbon dioxide.)

SAFETY: Take care. Soda lime is an irritant.

3 Cover each plant with a polythene bag and hold in place using an elastic band.

4 Place both plants in a warm, well-lit place for 24–48 hours.

5 Remove a leaf from each plant – taking great care not to muddle them up – and test for starch as described in Practical 23.2.

6 Explain your results.

7 Suggest how you could use the same two plants to test the hypothesis that light is required for photosynthesis.

8 Explain how a variegated leaf (part of which is white, part of which is green) could be used to demonstrate that chlorophyll is needed for photosynthesis.

Factors that affect the rate of photosynthesis

If a terrestrial plant is warm, well lit and well watered, the effect of changing the carbon dioxide concentration around the plant is shown in Figure 23.6.

Q4: Describe the relationship between carbon dioxide concentration and the rate of photosynthesis as seen in Figure 23.6.

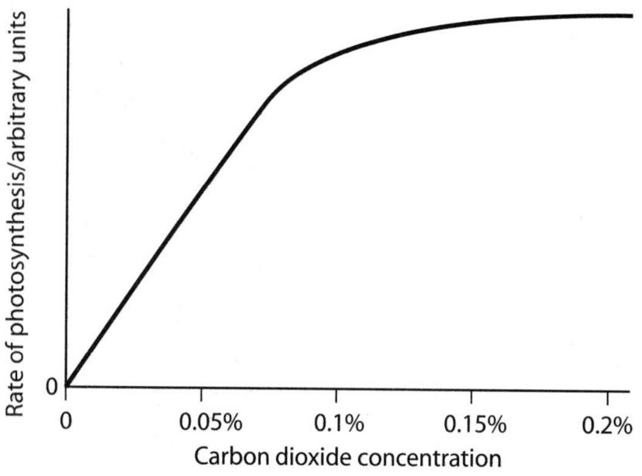

Figure 23.6 The effect of carbon dioxide concentration on the rate of photosynthesis of a warm, well lit and well watered plant.

Q5: Given that the concentration of carbon dioxide in the atmosphere is approximately 0.035% (350 parts per million), suggest why people sometimes burn paraffin in greenhouses that are used to raise commercial crops.

If a plant is well watered, well lit and has plenty of carbon dioxide, the effect of changing the temperature is shown in Figure 23.7.

Q6: Describe the relationship between temperature and the rate of photosynthesis as seen in Figure 23.7.

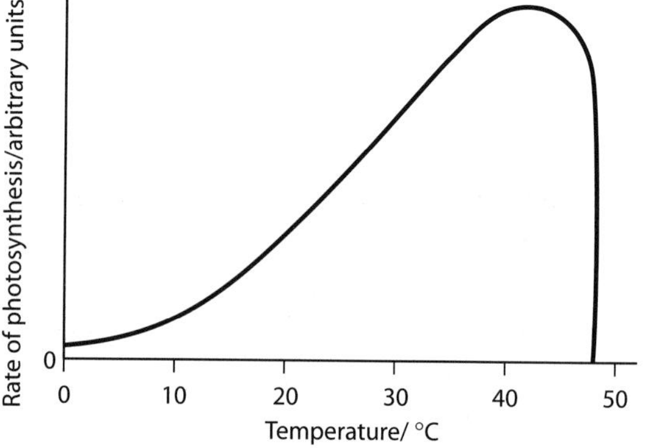

Figure 23.7 The effect of temperature on the rate of photosynthesis of a well watered, well lit plant supplied with plenty of carbon dioxide.

Q7: Why, initially, does increasing the temperature increase the rate of photosynthesis?

Q8: Why does the rate of photosynthesis fall off at high temperatures?

If a plant is warm, well watered and has plenty of carbon dioxide, the effect of changing the light intensity is shown in Figure 23.8.

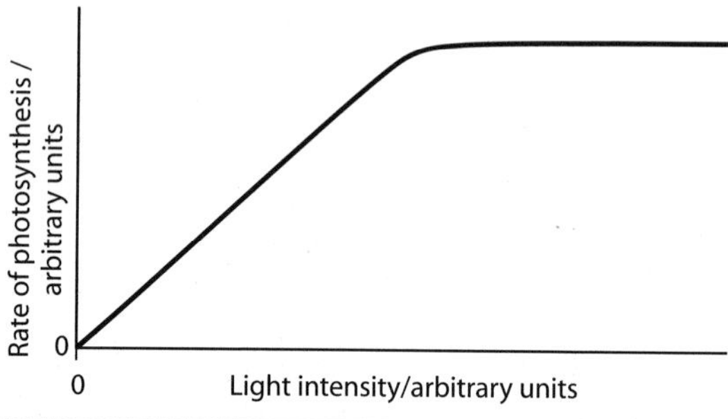

Figure 23.8 The effect of light intensity on the rate of photosynthesis of a warm, well-watered plant supplied with plenty of carbon dioxide.

Q9: Describe the relationship between light intensity and the rate of photosynthesis as seen in Figure 23.8.

It isn't just light *intensity* that is important, the *wavelength* of light is also important as shown in Figure 23.9. Plants have several different photosynthetic pigments, each with a different optimal wavelength for photosynthesis. This allows plants to trap and use a high proportion of the visible light spectrum.

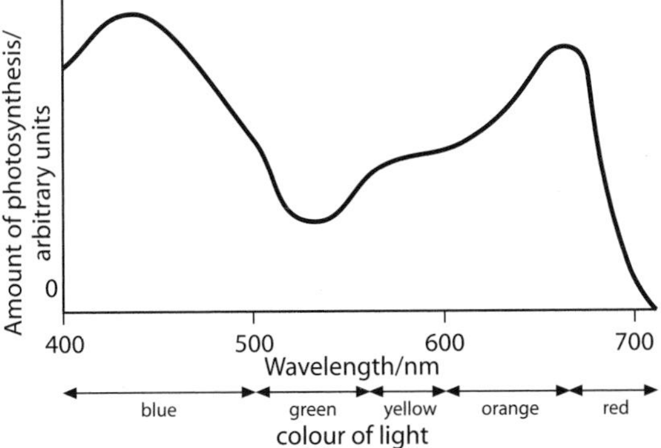

Figure 23.9 The rate at which a plant can photosynthesise is greatly affected by the wavelength of the light it receives.

Q10: (a) Which colour of light is best for photosynthesis? (b) Which is worst?

As well as being affected by carbon dioxide concentration, temperature, light intensity and the wavelength of light, the rate of photosynthesis is also affected by:

- water – a shortage of water results in a decrease in the rate of photosynthesis
- nutrient availability – a shortage of certain nutrients, including magnesium ions, results in a decrease in the rate of photosynthesis
- the internal structure of the plant – in particular the number and arrangement of chloroplasts.

At any one time, there is usually only one **limiting factor** for photosynthesis. For example, if it is warm and sunny, increasing the temperature or light intensity will probably have little if any effect on the rate of photosynthesis. However, increasing the carbon dioxide concentration might greatly increase the rate of photosynthesis. Similarly, if it is warm but quite dark, increasing the temperature or carbon dioxide concentration will probably have little if any effect on the rate of photosynthesis. However, increasing the light intensity will probably have a big effect.

Photosynthesis and plant structure

Photosynthesis takes place in small green structures within the cell (cell organelles) called **chloroplasts**. Chloroplasts are green because they contain the green pigment **chlorophyll**. Chlorophyll can trap some of the light that strikes it, and use the energy that light contains to break water molecules apart. This is a vital step in photosynthesis.

Chloroplasts are found in certain plant cells, especially **palisade cells** and **spongy mesophyll cells** in leaves. The arrangement of these cells in leaves is shown in Figure 23.10. Figure 23.10 also shows the structure of a single palisade cell.

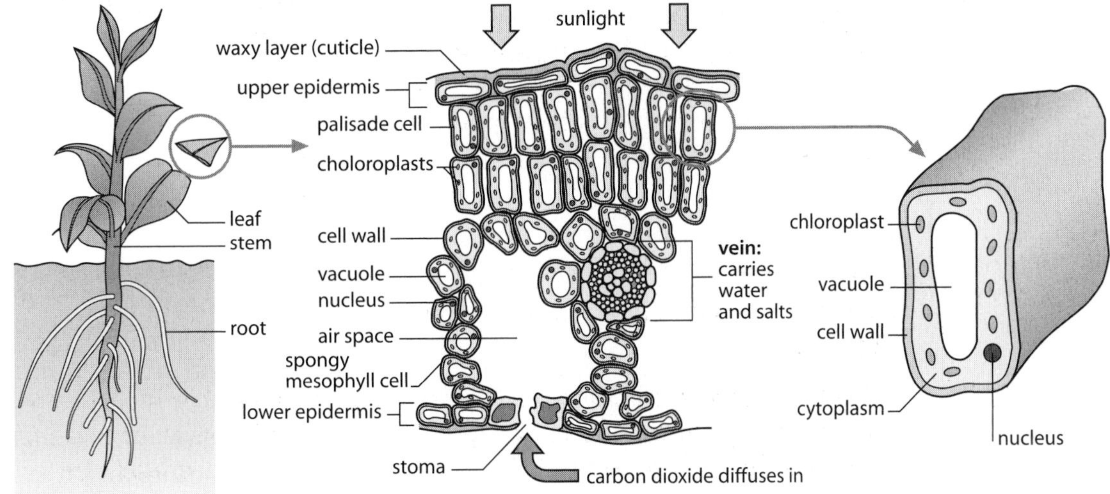

Figure 23.10 The arrangement of cells in a plant enables it to photosynthesise efficiently. Photosynthesis takes place inside chloroplasts which are found in some plant cells.

When it is dark or when a plant is short of water the pores (**stomata**) found on the underside of the leaves shut. This results from a fall in the concentration of potassium ions, K^+, in the **guard cells** on either side of the stoma (singular of stomata). Closure of stomata has the following consequences:

- carbon dioxide required for photosynthesis can no longer diffuse in
- photosynthesis almost ceases
- water can no longer diffuse out through the stomata.

Q11: Plants that are naturally found in deserts, like cacti, generally have fewer stomata than plants found in other habitats. (a) Why is this? (b) What effect would you expect this to have on their maximum rate of photosynthesis, and why?

Photosynthesis and respiration

All living organisms respire and plants are no exception. However, during the day the rate of photosynthesis of most plants is greater than their rate of respiration. This means that there is a *net* uptake of carbon dioxide and a *net* release of oxygen. However, at night the opposite is the case: there is a *net* uptake of oxygen and a *net* release of carbon dioxide.

Q12: Do plants respire during the day while they are carrying out photosynthesis?

Food chains and food webs

As we saw in Chapter 22, plants (also known as **producers** or **autotrophs**) are eaten by **herbivores** (also known as **primary consumers**) which in turn are eaten by **first level carnivores** (also known as **secondary consumers**). Some secondary consumers may be eaten by **second level carnivores** (also known as **tertiary consumers**). Some tertiary consumers may, in turn, be eaten by higher level carnivores.

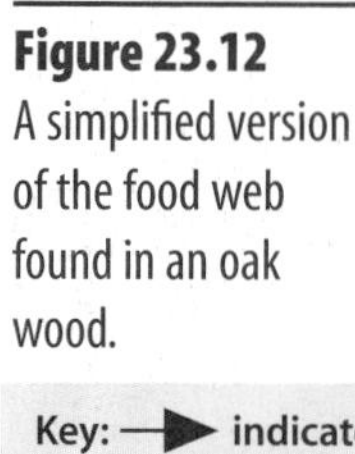

Figure 23.12 A simplified version of the food web found in an oak wood.

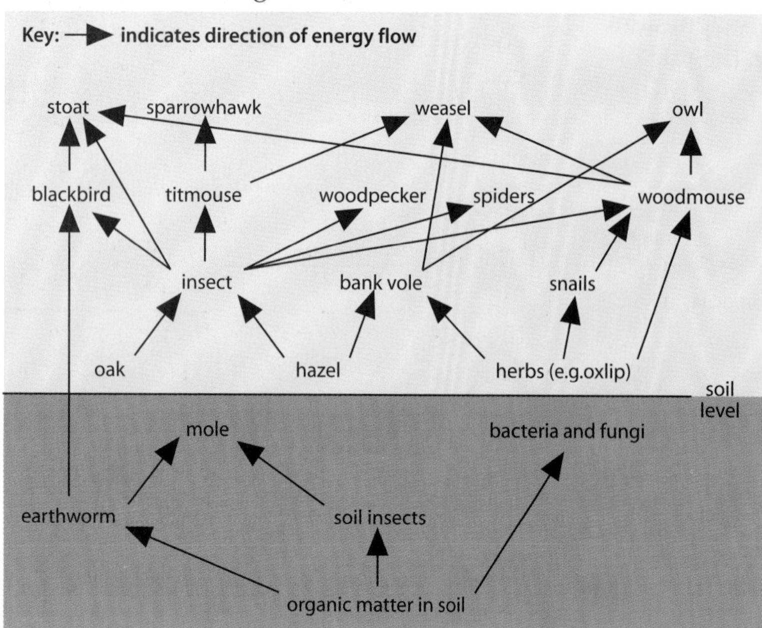

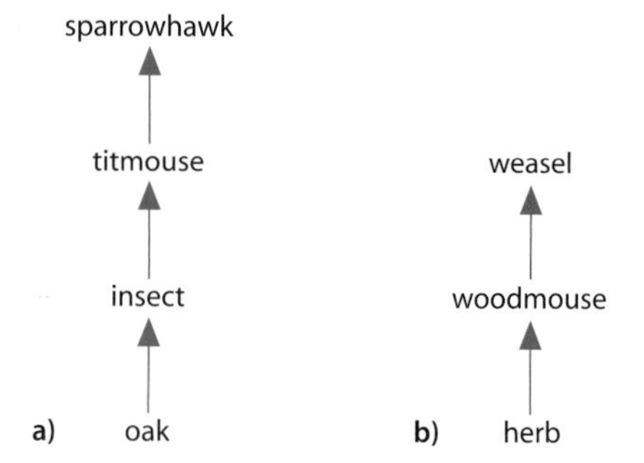

Figure 23.11 Two food chains found in oak woods.

We can show feeding relationships by means of **food chains**. When humans eat food, the food chain ends with us. Figure 23.11 shows two different food chains that are found in oak woods. The arrows show the direction in which the energy goes. Notice how a food chain only has one organism at each feeding level. In reality, though, food chains are an incomplete way of showing the feeding relationships in a community. A better way is to draw a **food web**. Figure 23.12 shows a simplified version of the food web that occurs in an oak woodland. We can see that plants are at the base of all these food chains and food webs.

Figure 23.12 also shows some of what goes on below ground. **Decomposers** (such as fungi and bacteria) break down organic matter in the soil to dark-coloured **humus**. This organic matter also supports earthworms and soil insects. As the decomposers break down soil organic matter, mineral nutrients such as nitrate ions, phosphate ions and magnesium ions are released. These become available for plants which absorb them along with water through the root hairs on their roots (Figure 23.13).

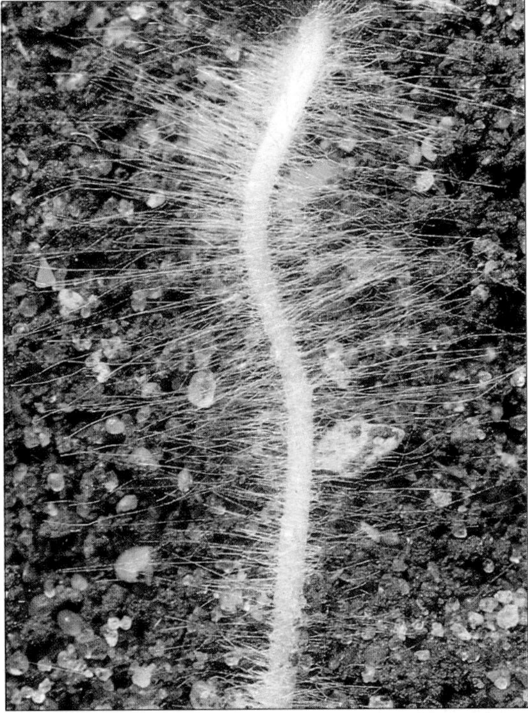

Figure 23.13 Plant roots have very large numbers of tiny root hairs. These greatly increase the surface area available to plants for the absorption of water and minerals.

Symbiosis

The name given to an intimate association between two different species is a **symbiosis**. Examples of symbiosis include:

- **parasitism**, when one organism, the **parasite**, benefits by feeding off another larger organism, the **host**, usually without killing it, but at the host's expense (Figure 23.14)
- **mutualism**, when both organisms benefit (Figure 23.15).

Note, however, that some people only use the term 'symbiosis' when both species in the association benefit.

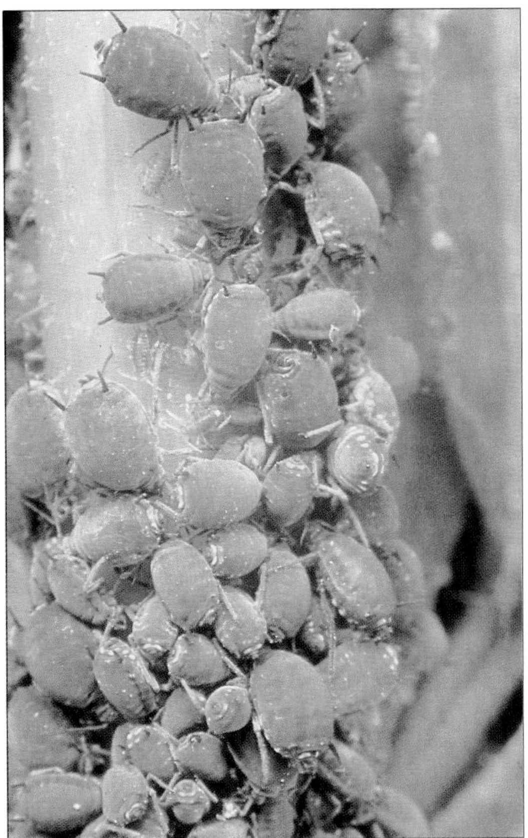

Figure 23.14 Aphids are parasites of many plants. They weaken the plant by taking nutrients from it.

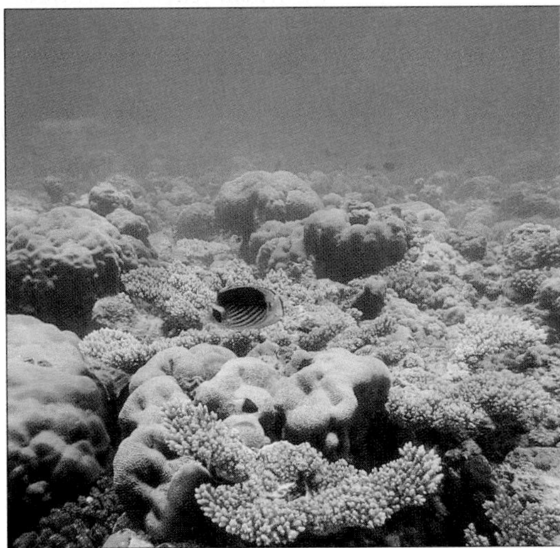

Figure 23.15 Corals, which are found in warm, shallow seas, contain large numbers of one-celled symbiotic organisms. These organisms can photosynthesise. The relationship between the coral and the one-celled organisms is one of mutualism. The one-celled organisms provide the coral with sugars they make by their photosynthesis. The coral provides the tiny organisms with a protected environment, and perhaps also with some of the carbon dioxide they use in photosynthesis.

Q13: Is the relationship between an insect-pollinated plant, e.g. honeysuckle, and the insect that pollinates it, e.g. hawk moth, an example of parasitism or mutualism?

Plant–herbivore relationships

Plants have evolved various ways to make it more difficult for herbivores to eat them. These include:

- physical barriers such as tough leaves or silica in their stems
- chemical defences such as poisons.

In turn, herbivores have evolved ways to help overcome these plant defences. These include:

- strong mouthparts to cut through tough leaves and stems
- the ability to detoxify poisons. For example, the caterpillars of the cabbage white butterfly can safely eat the leaves of cabbages and other brassicas, even though these are poisonous to many other insects.

Predator–prey relationships

A **predator** is a carnivore that kills its **prey** before eating it. Examples of predators catching and eating prey include:

- a fox catching a rabbit
- a pike catching a smaller fish
- a kestrel catching a bank vole.

If the numbers of a predator build up to high levels, the numbers of the prey on which it feeds may decrease. Equally, if the numbers of a prey animal decrease, for whatever reason, fewer predators will be supported.

Q14: Look again at Figure 23.12. Suppose that a disease kills off all the bank voles in a wood. What effects might you expect this to have on the numbers of (a) herbs; (b) owls; (c) woodmice; (d) moles? Give a reason in each case.

Summary

- Photosynthesis requires light, carbon dioxide, water, warmth and a plant with chloroplasts.
- The requirements for photosynthesis can be shown by simple experiments.
- Photosynthesis results in the formation of glucose and oxygen.
- The glucose made in photosynthesis is often converted into starch. It may also be converted into sucrose, cellulose, lipids, combined with various elements to make other organic molecules or respired.
- The formation of starch and oxygen as a result of photosynthesis can be shown by simple experiments.
- The rate of photosynthesis is affected by changes in the temperature, the light intensity, the wavelength of light or the concentration of carbon dioxide.
- At any one time there is usually only one limiting factor for photosynthesis.
- Photosynthesis only takes place in chloroplasts. Large numbers of chloroplasts are found in palisade cells and mesophyll cells in leaves.
- During the day, plants usually photosynthesise at a greater rate than they respire. As a result, they have a net uptake of carbon dioxide and a net loss of oxygen.
- During the night, plants continue to respire. As a result, they take up oxygen and release carbon dioxide.
- Feeding relationships can be shown by means of food chains or, more realistically, by food webs.
- Symbiosis is an intimate association between two different species.

Self check
See page 254

CHAPTER 24

Energy flow and energy loss

In this chapter you will learn how energy flows through ecosystems and how humans rely on both renewable and non-renewable energy sources for industry, for domestic use and for agriculture.

Energy flow through ecosystems

The typical way in which energy flows through an ecosystem, begining with the Sun, is shown in Figure 24.1. Note the following points:

- most of the Sun's energy never reaches producers (plants). Instead it warms up the atmosphere, the soil or the oceans
- some of the Sun's energy that does reach producers is used by them in photosynthesis to make carbohydrates and other organic molecules
- some of the products of photosynthesis are respired, some pass to decomposers and some are eaten by herbivores
- the energy which herbivores get from eating plants may end up being respired by the herbivores, passing to decomposers or passing to carnivores
- energy does not cycle round an ecosystem.

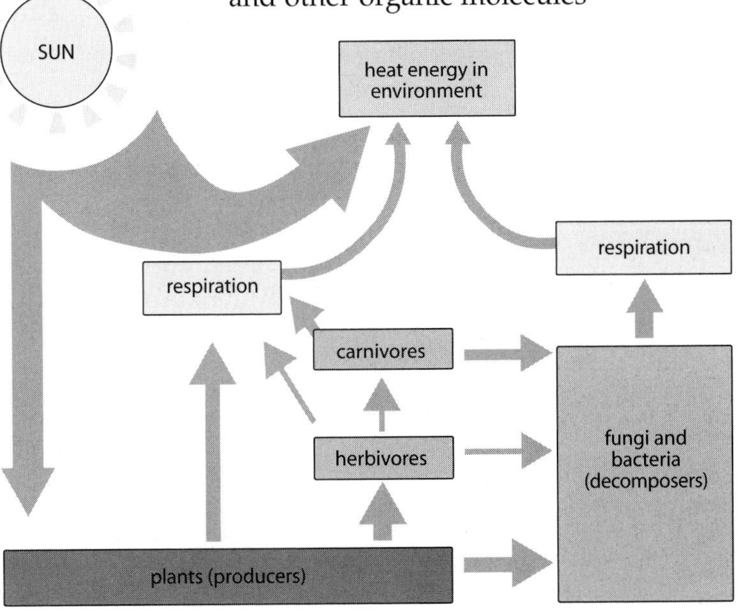

Figure 24.1 The flow of energy through an ecosystem. Note that not all the energy in the producers goes to the consumers: energy is lost as a result of respiration, incomplete consumption, incomplete digestion and excretion.

Q1: Where does all the energy eventually end up in ecosystems such as that shown in Figure 24.1?

Ecological pyramids

A convenient method of showing the way in which energy moves through ecosystems is by diagrams called **ecological pyramids**.

Pyramids of numbers

Imagine a small, self-sustained farm in which sheep are reared and then eaten by the people who live on the farm. The number of plants on the farm will be much greater than the number of sheep. In turn, the number of sheep will be much greater than the number of people. If we draw a diagram to represent the number of producers (plants), the number of herbivores (sheep) and the number of carnivores (people on the farm who live off the sheep) we might get Figure 24.2. Figure 24.2 is an example of a **pyramid of numbers**. It shows the numbers of organisms at each level of the food web in a particular area (in this case the farm). The three feeding levels shown in Figure 24.2 are known as **trophic levels**.

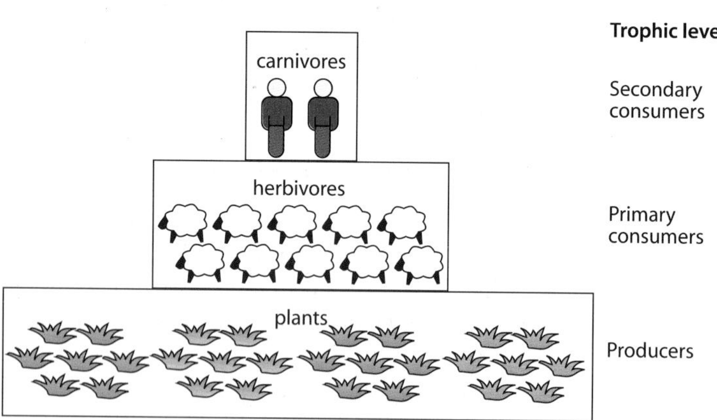

Figure 24.2 A pyramid of numbers.

Figure 24.2 is pyramid-shaped. However, this is not always the case with pyramids of numbers. Figure 24.3 shows a pyramid of numbers for a single oak tree which supports large numbers of herbivores (in this case caterpillars) and a few carnivores (titmice). Note that the producer and herbivore trophic levels form an *inverted* pyramid.

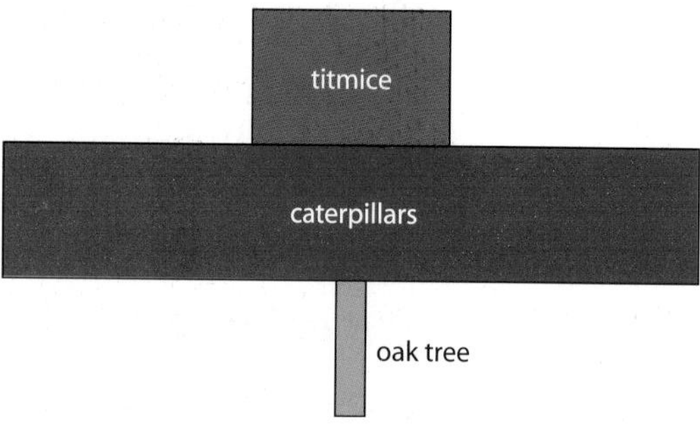

Figure 24.3 An inverted pyramid of numbers.

Q2: Match up the pyramids of numbers shown in Figure 24.4 with (a) a single rose bush supporting large numbers of aphids on which a few ladybirds feed, (b) an area of chalk grassland with very large numbers of individual plants, quite a few rabbits and a single fox, (c) a field with large numbers of plants and a few horses which are heavily infested with parasites such as ticks.

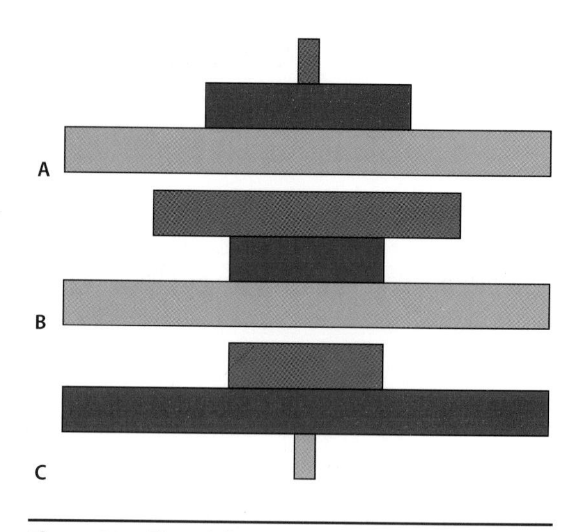

Figure 24.4 Three different types of pyramids of numbers.

Pyramids of biomass

A second sort of ecological pyramid is constructed by showing the biomass (i.e. dry mass of living material) at each trophic level. This is known as a **pyramid of biomass**. This, unlike a pyramid of numbers, takes into account the fact that organisms vary greatly in size. Pyramids of biomass are hardly ever inverted. This is because it takes many kilograms of plants to support 1kg of herbivores, and many kilograms of herbivores to support 1 kg of carnivores.

Q3: Explain why it takes many kilograms of rabbits (herbivores) to support 1 kg of foxes (carnivores).

The typical shape of a pyramid of biomass in a food chain or food web with four trophic levels is shown in Figure 24.5. The units for each level of a pyramid of biomass are mass per unit area (e.g. kg m^{-2}).

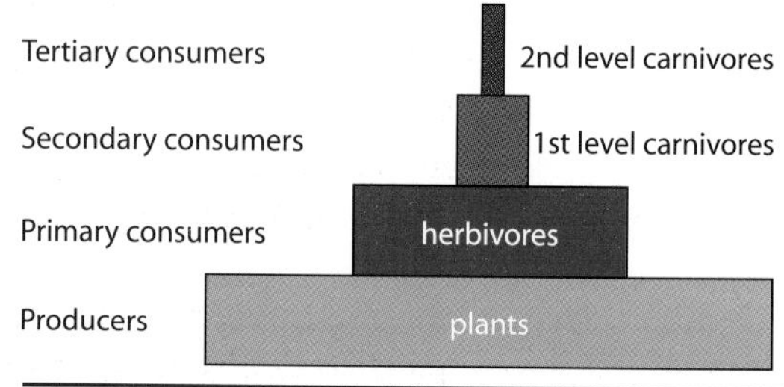

Figure 24.5 A typical pyramid of biomass in an ecosystem with four trophic levels.

Q4: What would be suitable units for each level of a pyramid of numbers?

Pyramids of energy

Pyramids of numbers and pyramids of biomass give a snapshot of an ecosystem *at a moment* in time. A **pyramid of energy**, however, is determined *over a period* of time. This is because it shows the rate (e.g. per day or per year) at which energy flows through a trophic level.

Q5: Explain why kJ m^{-2} $year^{-1}$ would be a suitable unit in which to measure a pyramid of energy.

An example of a pyramid of energy is given in Figure 24.6.

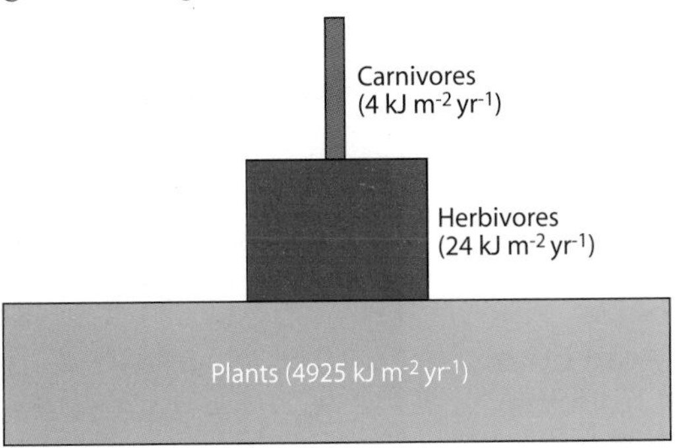

Figure 24.6 A pyramid of energy for Arctic tundra on Devon Island in Canada.

Unlike pyramids of numbers and pyramids of biomass, pyramids of energy can *never* be inverted. To understand why, look again at Figure 24.1. The herbivores get all their energy from the producers. Therefore, the flow of energy through the herbivores cannot exceed that through the producers. Indeed, since producers use some of their organic compounds in respiration while herbivores fail to eat all the producers, the energy flow through the herbivores is significantly less than the energy flow through the producers.

Q6: Explain why the energy flow through the carnivores in an ecosystem must be less than the energy flow through the herbivores.

In most pyramids of energy, 10% or less of the energy that flows through any one trophic level reaches the trophic level above. For example, on a typical farm only about 10% at most of the energy fixed by the grass and other plants in a field ends up in the cows, sheep or other animals that graze that field. Most of the remaining 90% is lost as heat energy, though some also goes to the decomposers in the soil.

Human energy sources

In common with all organisms, humans need energy. In modern, industrial societies our energy consumption is huge (Figure 24.7). Each person in an industrial country like the United Kingdom has an annual energy consumption over twenty times that of a person living in a country with a mainly agricultural economy, such as India.

Q7: List four reasons why *per capita* (per person) energy consumption is so much greater in an industrial than a non-industrial country.

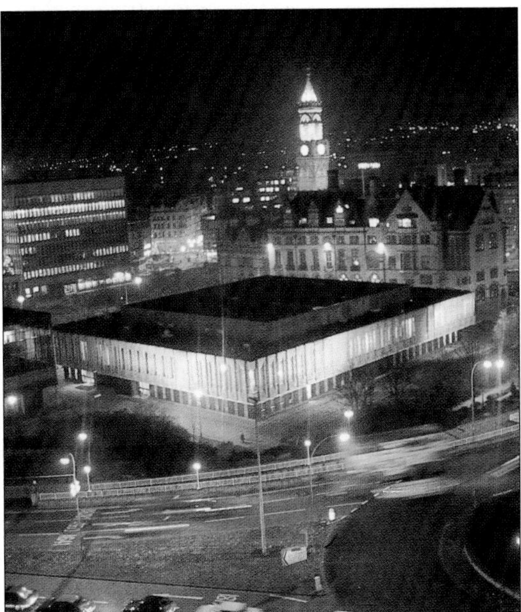

Figure 24.7 The centre of Bradford, a modern industrial city, at night. Modern cities release so much heat energy that their temperature is often 2 to 3°C greater than that of the surrounding countryside.

A useful distinction can be made between two sorts of energy sources:

- **non-renewable energy sources** – these take millions of years to build up and so, in effect, cannot be replaced. They are limited in their abundance
- **renewable energy sources** – these are constantly available and are not used up. In a sense, they are infinitely abundant.

Non-renewable energy sources

Most of our non-renewable energy sources come from **fossil fuels** laid down millions of years ago.

- **Coal** was formed when plants failed to decay, accumulating as **peat** instead. Over millions of years some peat became covered by sands and muds. The pressure and heat caused by these materials on top of the peat gradually converted it into coal. Coal has a very high carbon content. Indeed, some coals are almost pure carbon: anthracite is more than 90% carbon.
- **Natural oil** (also known as crude oil) is a complex mixture of hydrocarbons (chemicals which contain only carbon and hydrogen). It was formed from the organic remains of tiny plants and bacteria found in the sea by the effects of pressure and heat over millions of years. It is a thick liquid-like sludge and is common in certain rocks such as shale.
- **Natural gas** is mainly methane (CH_4). It is often found along with natural oil deposits. It too is formed from the remains of tiny plants and bacteria.

Coal, oil and gas are all burnt to provide heat energy. This energy may be used directly to warm homes and other buildings, or it may be used to generate electricity in power stations. Oil is also an important source of chemicals for the chemical industry, as well as being the raw material for petrol, used to power cars and other vehicles.

Another non-renewable energy source is **nuclear power**. This relies on the splitting (**nuclear fission**) of a heavy atomic nucleus, such as uranium or plutonium, into two smaller atomic nuclei with the release of huge amounts of energy. In a nuclear reactor the energy released in nuclear fission is used to generate electricity (Figure 24.8). In some countries, the contribution of nuclear power to the generation of power is very significant (Table 24.1).

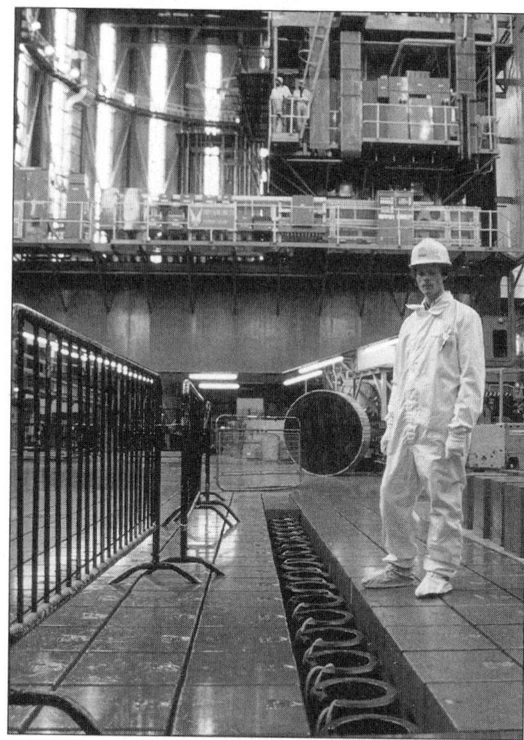

Figure 24.8 Inside a nuclear power station. The fuels used are uranium 235, uranium 238 or plutonium 239. Nuclear power stations have proved more expensive than originally thought, largely because of the tremendous cost of safety precautions.

Table 24.1 The contribution of nuclear power to energy production in selected countries (1990)

Country	Percentage of energy production due to nuclear power
France	75
Belgium	60
Hungary	48
Sweden	46
UK	20
USA	20

Q8: Which non-renewable energy sources directly or indirectly derive their energy from the Sun?

Non-renewable energy sources have been of tremendous importance to humans over the last two hundred years. However, there are two main problems associated with these energy sources:

- they will eventually run out – virtually all the world's major oil and gas reserves will be used up before the year 2050. Coal will last longer – perhaps a few hundred years – and the elements needed for nuclear power longer still
- they can cause serious pollution (see page 219).

Renewable energy sources

Most renewable energy sources derive their energy from the Sun.

- **Solar power** is obtained directly from the heating effect of the Sun's rays. At its simplest, the Sun's rays are used to heat water which can then be used to warm houses. Solar cells are devices that convert the energy from sunlight directly into electricity. Unfortunately the efficiency of solar cells is rather low, and sunlight is not available at night or when it is cloudy.
- **Wind power** has long been used to turn the sails of windmills to grind grain or pump water. Wind is due to the movement of air masses, caused by the heating effect of the Sun. Modern wind farms can generate significant amounts of electricity (Figure 24.9). Unfortunately they take up a lot of space, produce a certain amount of noise and only work when it is windy. Also, some people think they are unattractive.
- **Hydroelectric power** is derived from the gravitational potential energy that is stored in water at a height. A dam can be used to prevent water from flowing down a river or over a waterfall. Water accumulates behind the dam and is then allowed to pass through turbines at the base of the dam, generating electricity as it does so (Figure 24.10). Unfortunately, dams may eventually silt up. They may also involve flooding huge areas of land, which kills many organisms and may force some people to move home.

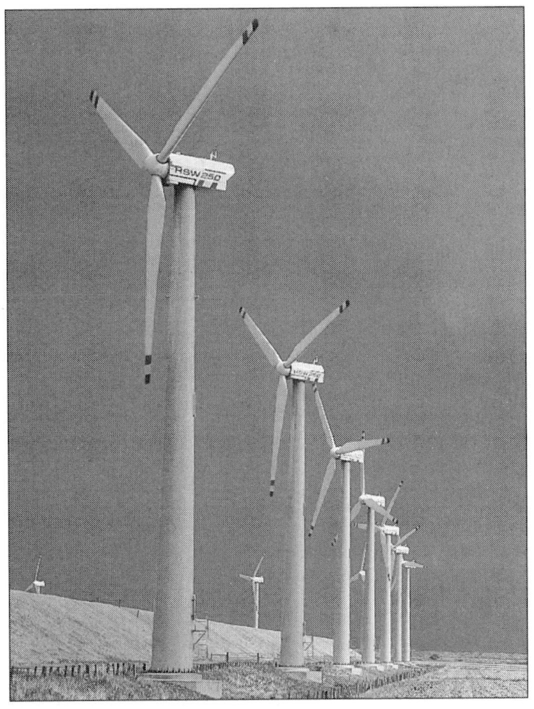

Figure 24.9 Modern wind farms are usually situated in exposed areas where it is windy and where not too many people live. Although unlikely ever to produce a high proportion of an industrial country's energy needs, wind farms can generate significant amounts of electricity.

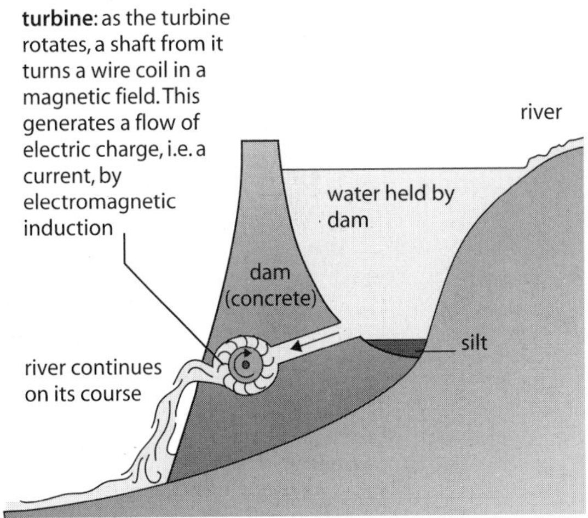

Figure 24.10 The generation of hydroelectric power by a dam.

- **Geothermal power** makes use of the fact that the further down you go through the Earth's surface (crust), the hotter the rocks get. Cold water is poured hundreds of metres or more down bore holes and then pumped back, hotter, to the surface. The hot water can be used for heating or to generate electricity. Strictly speaking, geothermal power isn't renewable since the Earth's interior will eventually cool down, but this won't happen for millions of years.
- **Tidal power** makes use of the tides which result from the gravitational attraction between the Earth and the Moon. As the tide flows, it passes through turbines, generating electricity.
- **Wave power** is still at a research stage. Waves result mainly from the action of wind on water. The hope is that the movement of waves will allow electricity to be generated at a commercially acceptable cost.
- **Wood** has long been used by humans as a source of fuel for burning, as well as for making everything from matches to ships. Wood *can* be a renewable energy source, if the amount taken each year from a wood or farm does not exceed the amount produced by photosynthesis. Fast-growing trees such as willows are now being grown as **biomass for fuels**. This is an example of sustainable development. However, wood can also be used as a non-renewable fuel.

Q9: (a) Which of these renewable energy sources derive their energy from the Sun? (b) When can wood be regarded as a non-renewable energy source?

Energy inputs into agriculture

The major energy inputs into agriculture are indirect. Energy is used to drive farm machinery, to produce fertilisers, pesticides and animal feedstuffs and to transport materials. In most agricultural economies energy from humans and animals is used instead of fuel energy to drive machinery.

Direct energy inputs into agriculture are more important for animals than for plants.

- Crops can have their energy input supplemented if they are given artificial light or heat. This is only used for a few expensive plants in the horticultural trade.
- Most animals kept on farms are given feed supplements at certain times of year, especially in the winter (Figure 24.11). This is a form of energy input.

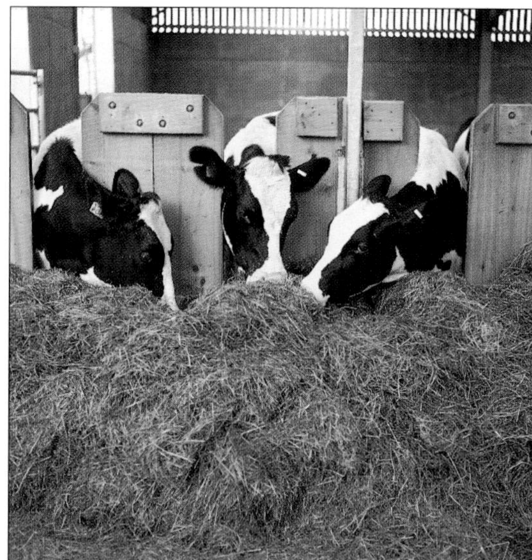

Figure 24.11 Feed supplements are given to farm animals such as cattle and pigs. Such supplements provide protein and energy and result in faster growth rates.

Summary

- Energy flows through ecosystems from the Sun through producers and herbivores to carnivores and decomposers. Eventually it all ends up as heat.
- The way that energy flows through ecosystems can be shown using ecological pyramids.
- Pyramids of numbers show the number of individuals at each trophic level of an ecosystem. They may be inverted.
- Pyramids of biomass show the mass of organisms at each trophic level. They are very rarely inverted.
- Pyramids of energy show the flow of energy through the trophic levels of an ecosystem. They are never inverted.
- Humans obtain energy from both non-renewable and renewable energy sources.
- Non-renewable energy sources include fossil fuels (coal, oil and gas) and nuclear power. Problems with non-renewable energy sources include the fact that they don't last for ever and that they may cause serious pollution.
- Renewable energy sources include solar power, wind power, hydroelectric power, geothermal power, tidal power, wave power and wood. Each of these has advantages and disadvantages.
- Energy inputs into agriculture are used to drive farm machinery, produce fertilisers, pesticides and animal feedstuffs, to transport materials and to provide extra light or heat for certain crops.

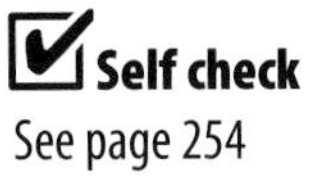

See page 254

CHAPTER 25

Nutrient cycles

In this chapter you will learn how carbon, nitrogen and water are recycled in ecosystems and about the effects that human activity has on these processes.

Carbon cycle

The element carbon (C) is found in all organic molecules. The **carbon cycle** illustrated in Figure 25.1 shows how carbon moves around ecosystems. Note the following:

- carbon dioxide is removed from the atmosphere and from water (e.g. lakes, oceans) by photosynthesis
- carbon dioxide is added to the atmosphere and to water by respiration and by the combustion of fossil fuels and wood
- incomplete decomposition of organic molecules leads to the accumulation of carbon in **sinks** (fossil fuels and certain rocks, e.g. limestones).

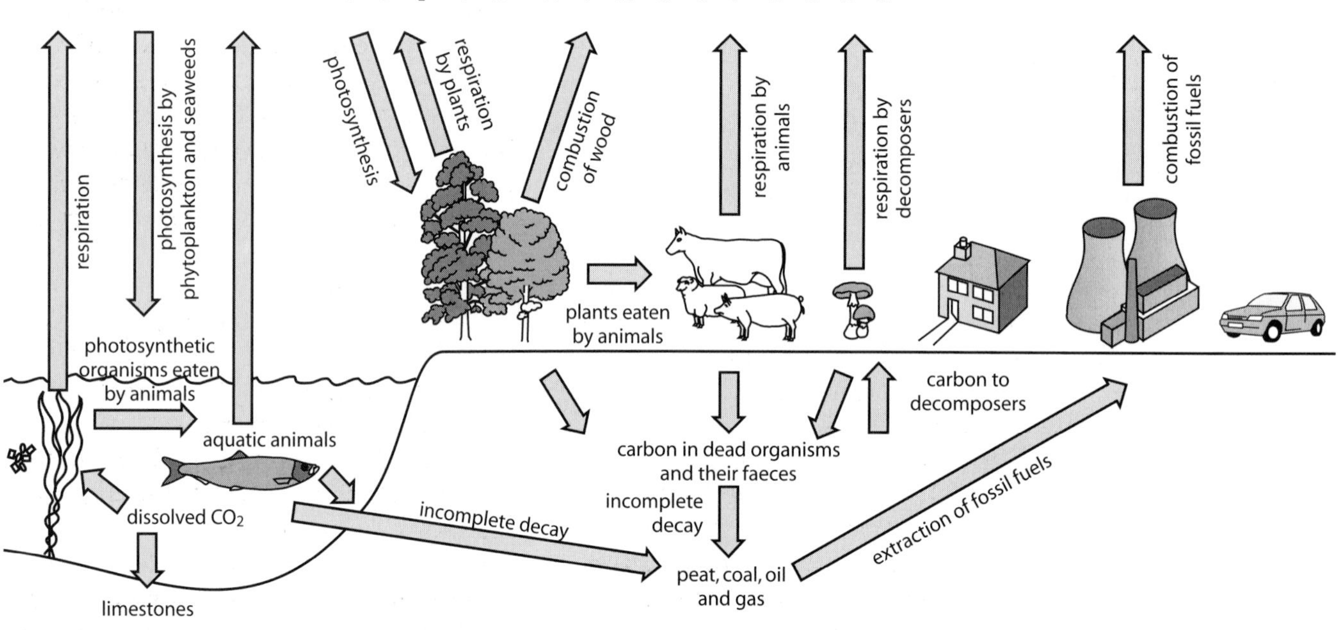

Figure 25.1 The carbon cycle.

Q1: Explain what effect each of the following would be expected to have, *other things being equal*, on atmospheric levels of carbon dioxide: (a) the burning of fossil fuels; (b) an increase in the rate of photosynthesis of plants; (c) a shift from the use of coal to the use of nuclear power in power stations.

The effect of human activity on the carbon cycle

The last hundred years have seen a significant rise in atmospheric carbon dioxide levels (Figure 25.2). This is the result of:

- the burning of fossil fuels, releasing carbon dioxide into the atmosphere
- burning trees both in temperate regions and in the tropics, reducing the amount of carbon locked up in wood.

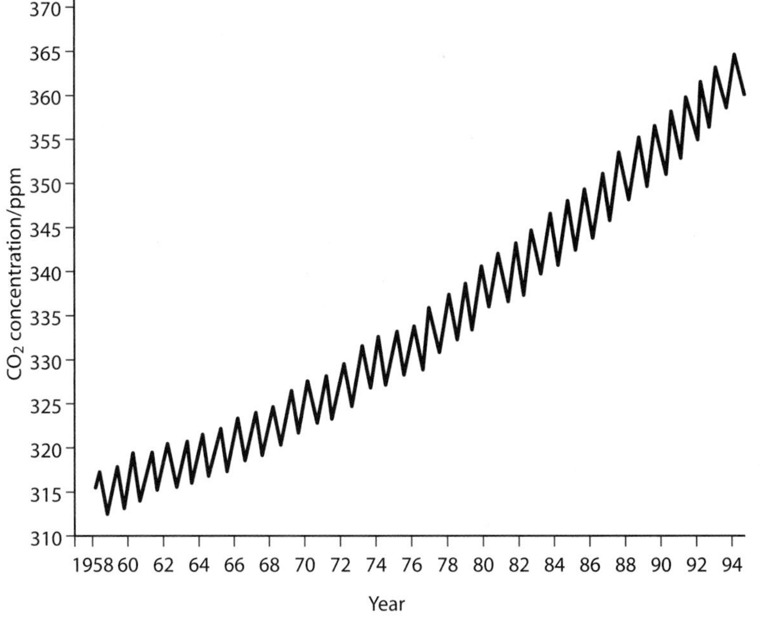

Figure 25.2 Atmospheric levels of carbon dioxide measured in Hawaii over nearly 40 years.

Although it is too early to be certain, this rise in atmospheric carbon dioxide levels is probably contributing to **global warming**. This results from the **greenhouse effect** in which various gases in the Earth's atmosphere, especially carbon dioxide, trap heat energy in much the same way that heat energy is trapped by a greenhouse. Over the last fifty years the Earth's climate has probably become warmer by about 0.5°C. Although this may not sound very much, the following consequences of global warming have already become apparent and may get far worse:

- some of the ice at the Arctic and Antarctic melts
- sea levels rise
- low lying islands (e.g. the Maldives) and coastal land (e.g. large areas of Bangladesh) more likely to flood
- dozens of people killed in floods and thousands made homeless
- less ice at the poles changes the global climate
- rainfall decreases in the tropics, making droughts and famine more likely
- climate becomes windier, increasing the risks of storms and hurricanes
- some species increase in abundance (e.g. in Britain those organisms normally confined to the warmest parts of the county)
- some species become rarer or extinct (e.g. in Britain organisms found on mountain tops).

Q2: Suggest two ways in which global warming might be halted or even reversed.

Nitrogen cycle

The element nitrogen (N) is found in many organic molecules, particularly proteins and nucleic acids. The way that nitrogen moves around ecosystems in shown in the **nitrogen cycle** in Figure 25.3 on page 208. For simplification, the aquatic part of the nitrogen cycle is not shown.

Notice the following:

- N_2 (nitrogen gas) in the atmosphere only becomes available to organisms through **lightning** or the activities of **nitrogen-fixing bacteria**
- nitrogen-fixing bacteria are found in the **root nodules** of certain plants, such as clovers, beans and other legumes (Figure 25.4 on page 208)
- plants that lack nitrogen-fixing bacteria in their roots only take up nitrogen from the soil in the form of nitrate ions (NO_3^-)

- when organisms die (or produce urine and faeces), their remains are broken down to ammonia (NH_3) by bacteria and fungi
- **nitrifying bacteria** can convert ammonia to nitrate
- other bacteria (**denitrifying bacteria**) can convert nitrate to ammonia, nitrate to nitrogen gas, and ammonia to nitrogen gas.

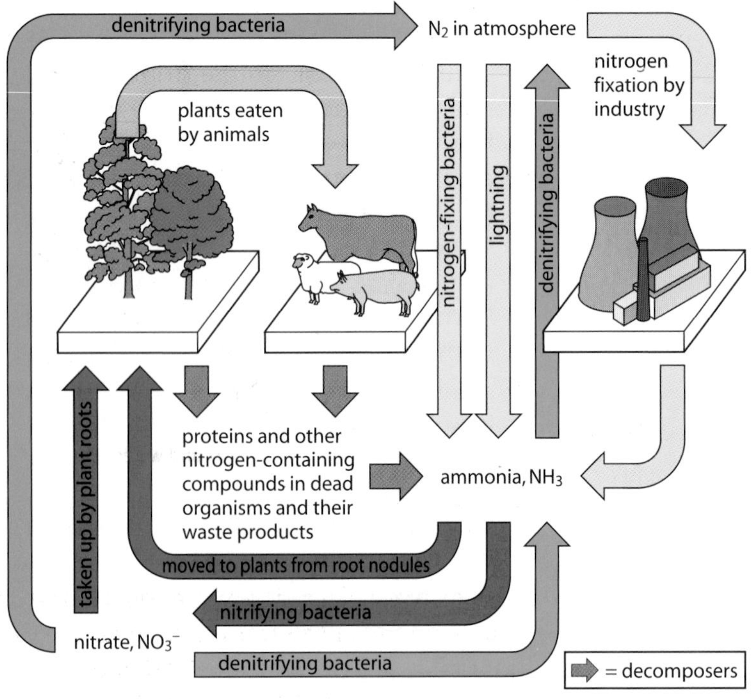

Figure 25.3 The nitrogen cycle on land.

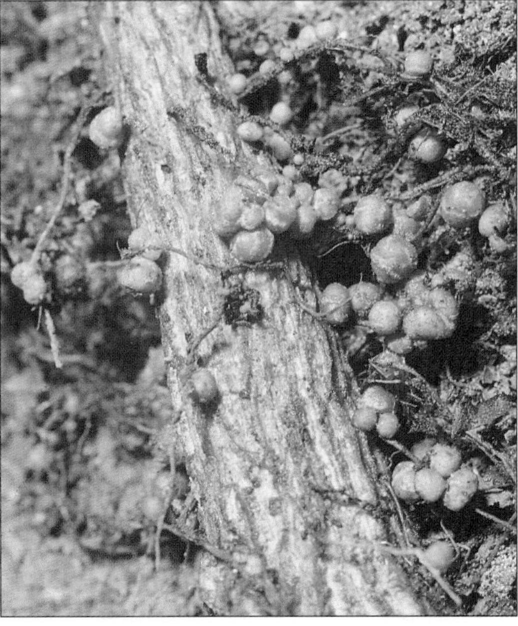

Figure 25.4 A runner bean plant with root nodules visible.

The nitrogen fixed by nitrogen-fixing bacteria in the root nodules of leguminous plants is used by the plants to make proteins. These can be a significant protein source for humans.

The effect of human activity on the nitrogen cycle

Harvesting removes nitrogen from the cycle in the region where the crop is grown. This must be replaced if the soil is to remain fertile. Nitrogen fixation can be carried out by an industrial process called the **Haber process**. This only works at high temperature and pressure. It results in the manufacture of ammonia which is then used to make nitrogen fertilisers for agricultural purposes.

Q3: The natural conversion of ammonia to nitrate requires oxygen. Explain why this conversion takes place less well in waterlogged soils.

Q4: Suggest one reason, connected with the nitrogen cycle, why farmers usually do not want their crops to be waterlogged.

Water cycle

The **water cycle** shows how water (H_2O) moves round ecosystems. It is illustrated in Figure 25.5. Notice the following features:

- **precipitation** – the fall of water as rain, snow, mist or fog
- **drainage** and the **flow of water** in streams and rivers – the descent of liquid water due to the force of gravity
- **evaporation** – the change of state from liquid water to water vapour
- **transpiration** – the loss of water vapour through the open stomata of plants
- **condensation** – the change of state from water vapour to liquid water
- **water table** – the level below which underground water fills all the spaces in the rocks.

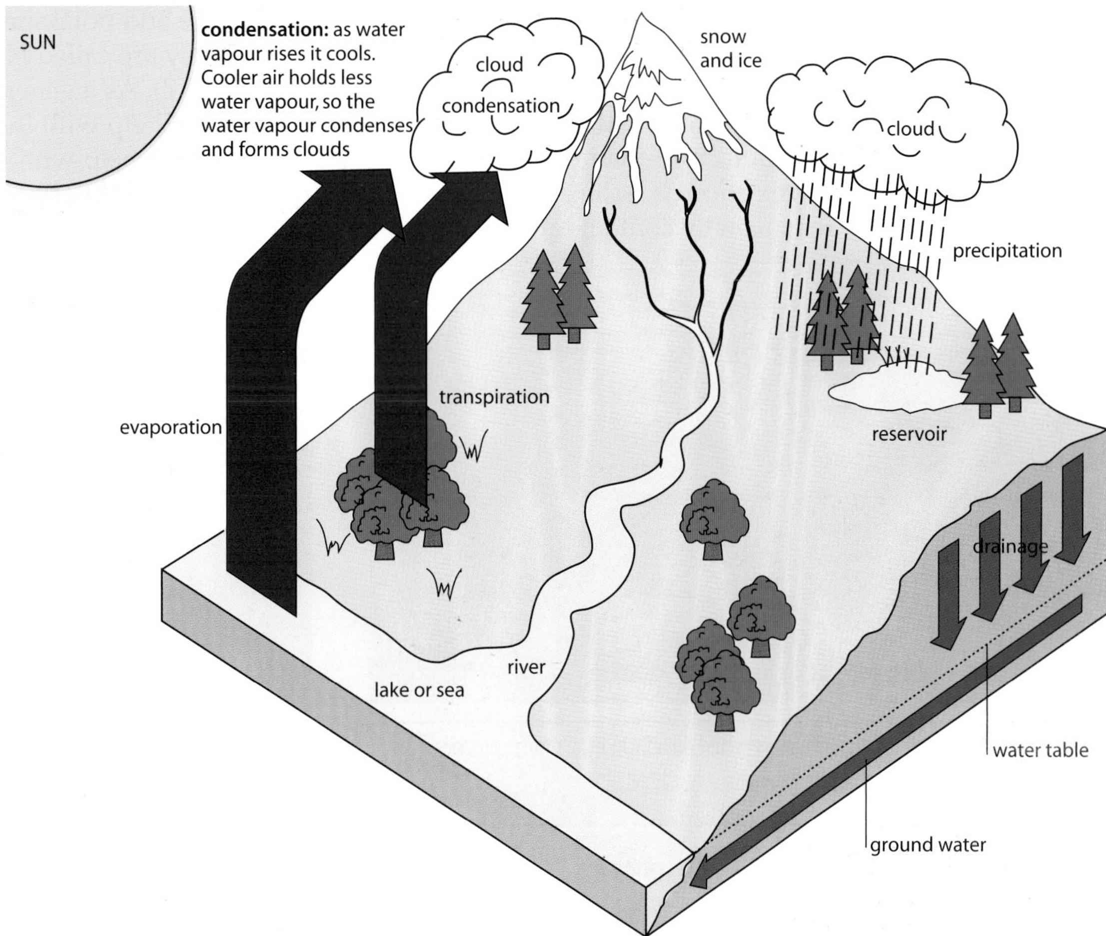

Figure 25.5 The water cycle.

Q5: List those processes which remove water from plants and bare land, and return it to the atmosphere.

The effect of human activity on the water cycle

Humans can affect the water cycle in a number of ways:

- artificial drainage reduces the flow of water into streams and rivers
- extraction of water from wells lowers the water table
- deforestation decreases transpiration and may affect precipitation
- dams affect the flow of water down rivers
- reservoirs store large amounts of water.

Nutrient loss through harvesting

When crops are harvested or animals reared on a farm are taken off to be slaughtered, there is a net **export** (loss) of nutrients from the farm. This tends to be particularly serious for nitrate ions (NO_3^-), phosphate ions (PO_4^{3-}) and potassium ions (K^+) as these ions frequently limit the growth of plants.

Traditional ways of improving soil fertility include:

- planting a crop of legumes every third or fourth year and ploughing it into the soil
- spreading manure from animal faeces (e.g. horse droppings) on a field (known as 'muck spreading')
- leaving a field fallow for a year to allow the soil to build up its nutrient reserves.

Q6: Suggest why deforestation often increases soil erosion by water.

Q7: Explain the benefits of planting a crop of legumes every third or fourth year.

Many farmers still plant legumes or use muck spreaders to improve soil fertility (Figure 25.6). Nowadays, most farmers also use **artificial fertilisers** which are mixtures of factory-made chemicals. Close inspection of fertiliser bags shows that they usually contain nitrate, phosphate and potassium, for which reason they are called NPK fertilisers (Figure 25.7). As a generalisation, nitrate is added to help with leaf growth, phosphate to help with root growth and potassium to aid flower and fruit development.

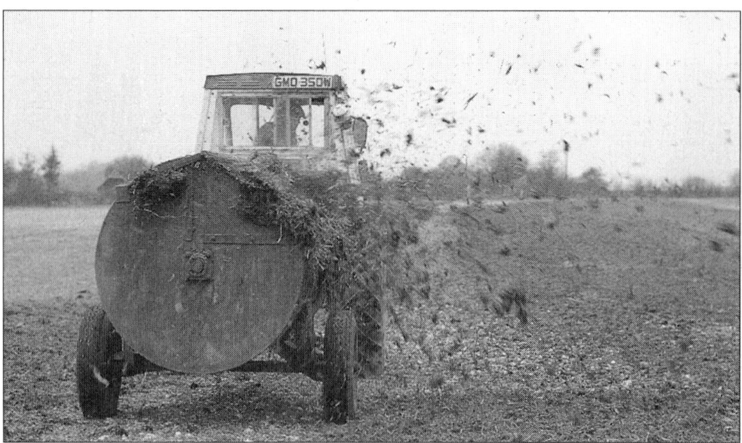

Figure 25.6 Animal droppings can be recycled on a farm by a 'muck spreader'. This helps return nutrients to the soil.

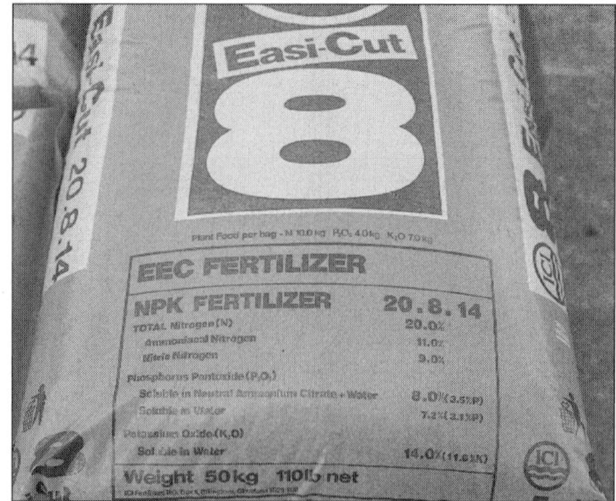

Figure 25.7 This bag of fertiliser contains nitrogen, phosphorus and potassium.

Effects of fertilisers

Fertilisers can significantly increase crop yields. This is their great advantage. However, especially if not properly used, they can have a number of undesirable consequences.

- If applied in excess, they can weaken the stems of crops, causing them to fall over ('lodge').
- If applied when the crop is not growing quickly, they can be carried into streams and ponds (**run-off**) rather than being taken up by the crop. This wastes money. Another problem is that it can cause **eutrophication**. Eutrophication is the enrichment of water with large amounts of nitrate and phosphate. For reasons which are summarised in Figure 25.8, eutrophication can lead to the death of freshwater animals and plants.
- Inevitably, some of the added nitrate ends up in the ground water and thus, eventually, in drinking water. In some parts of the UK, for example East Anglia, nitrate levels in tap water are often 30 to 40 mg dm^{-3}. The upper safety limit for nitrate levels set by the European Union is 50 mg dm^{-3}.

Q8: What effect would pumping air into a eutrophic lake have?

1 Fertiliser run-off from a farm
2 Nitrate and phosphate levels of water rise
3 Algae multiply giving rise to an **algal bloom**
4 Massive increase in aerobic (oxygen-requiring) decomposers (chiefly bacteria)
5 Drop in oxygen levels as these bacteria use up much of the oxygen which is dissolved in the water more quickly than it can be replaced by diffusion from the atmosphere
6 Drop in oxygen leads to death of organisms, such as fish, that require high oxygen level
7 Presence of dead fish leads to even more bacteria

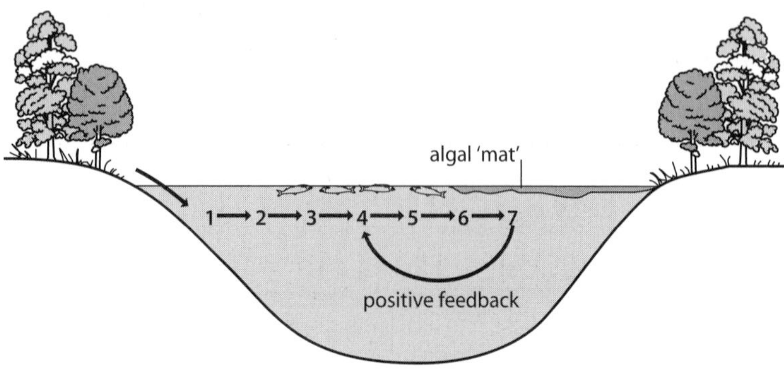

Figure 25.8 The consequences of eutrophication for a small lake.

The effects of nitrates on human health

It is known that high levels of nitrate in drinking water can be dangerous for young babies. This is because nitrate in water can be converted in the stomach to nitrite, and nitrite can combine with fetal haemoglobin (the special sort of haemoglobin which fetuses and young babies have) causing death. This sounds alarming, but the levels of nitrate needed for this to happen are very high and the last case where a baby died in Britain from this was in 1948. Another problem with nitrate, is that there is some evidence, though it is very controversial, that high levels of nitrate consumption can eventually increase the risk of stomach cancer.

Practical 25.1 To test for nitrate and ammonium ion levels in different water sources

BIOHAZARD

DANGER

Requirements
Digital nitrate meter or nitrate testing kit
Access to a variety of water samples/sources

1 Obtain samples of water from a variety of sources, e.g. tap water, rainwater, unpolluted stream or river, ditch by a farm, natural pond, ornamental pond.

SAFETY: If you collect your own samples, do so in pairs, let your parent(s)/guardian(s) and teacher/lecturer know where you are and take care not to fall into any water. Wash your hands after collecting each sample. Under no circumstances drink any of the water you have sampled.

2 Within 24 hours test each water source for the level of ammonium ions and the level of nitrate ions in parts per million (ppm).

3 Record your results in a table.

4 Write a discussion of your findings and suggest further investigations which could be carried out to test any conclusions you reach.

Practical 25.2 To investigate the effects of fertilisers and detergents on *Lemna* (duckweed)

HARMFUL
Fertiliser solutions

Requirements
Jam jars, 8
Liquid fertiliser solution
Detergent
Lemna
Other equipment may be required by individual students

In this practical you need to design and carry out an investigation to see what effect fertilisers and detergents have on the reproduction of *Lemna*. *Lemna* (duckweed) is a small plant which floats on water. It reproduces quite rapidly, which means that two to three weeks should be long enough for your investigation. Here are some of the things you will need to think about before setting up your investigation:

- How many different concentrations of liquid fertiliser will you use?
- How many different amounts of detergent will you use?
- How can you separate out the effects of liquid fertiliser and detergent concentration?
- Can you clearly tell when one *Lemna* has split into two?
- What will be your controls?
- Do you need any replicates?
- Do you need to provide any extra lighting or warmth?
- Should you carry out a pilot investigation first?

SAFETY: Wash your hands after each occasion on which you come into contact with liquid fertiliser, detergent or the containers in which the plants are growing.

As you go along, keep a careful record of what you did and what you found out. Once you have completed the investigation, analyse your findings and write-up the entire investigation, possibly using the following headings: introduction, aim, methods, results, discussion, conclusion.

Summary

- The carbon cycle shows how carbon moves around ecosystems. Its chief features are photosynthesis, respiration, decomposition, combustion and the accumulation of carbon in fossil fuels and limestones.
- Human activity over the last two hundred years has led to a rise in atmospheric carbon dioxide levels. This is probably causing global warming and may have serious environmental consequences.
- The nitrogen cycle shows how nitrogen moves round ecosystems. Its chief features are nitrogen fixation, lightning, decomposition and the conversion of ammonia into nitrate ions by bacteria.
- The root nodules of legumes contain nitrogen-fixing bacteria.
- Ammonia can be made from nitrogen gas by the Haber process.
- The water cycle shows how water moves round ecosystems. Its chief features are precipitation, drainage, the flow of water, evaporation, transpiration and condensation.
- Humans have affected the water cycle through artificial drainage, deforestation and the construction of wells, dams and reservoirs.
- The harvesting of crops leads to a loss of nutrients from the soil.
- Soil fertility can be improved through planting legumes, spreading manure, leaving fields fallow and using artificial fertilisers.
- Fertilisers can greatly increase crop yields. However, run-off can lead to eutrophication.

Self check

See page 255

CHAPTER 26

Human population growth and environmental resources

In this chapter you will learn about the growth of human population size and about the consequences this has had both for ourselves and for the environment.

Human population growth

If a few individuals of a species find themselves in a new habitat with plenty of food and space, exponential growth often results. This is as true for humans as it is for bacteria, plants and other animals. A typical growth of population size against time is given in Figure 26.1. Note the following phases of population growth:

- **lag phase**
- **exponential growth**
- **population growth slows down**
- **population more or less constant.**

During exponential growth, the population doubles in numbers at regular intervals. For a bacterium, the doubling time might be as short as 20 minutes; for humans it is rarely less than 20 years.

Q1: Suppose a country in 1900 had 10 million people and was showing exponential growth with a doubling time of 30 years. How many people would you expect there to be in the country in (a) 1930; (b) 1960; (c) 1990?

Q2: Suggest four reasons why exponential growth cannot continue forever in human populations.

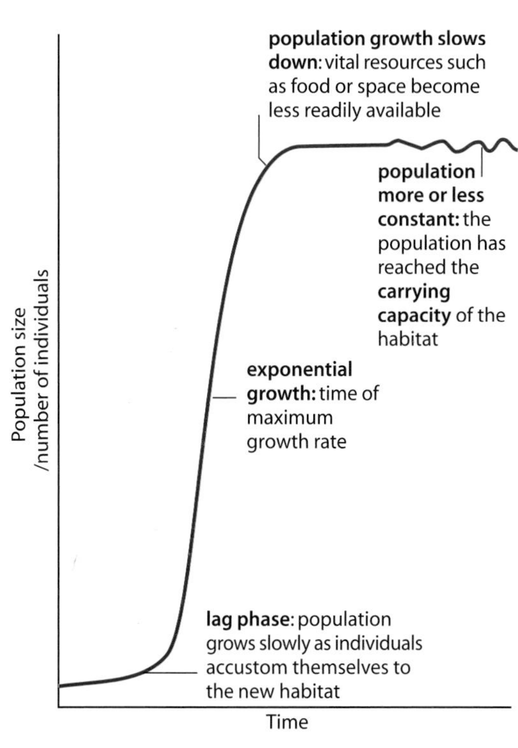

Figure 26.1 A generalised graph of population growth.

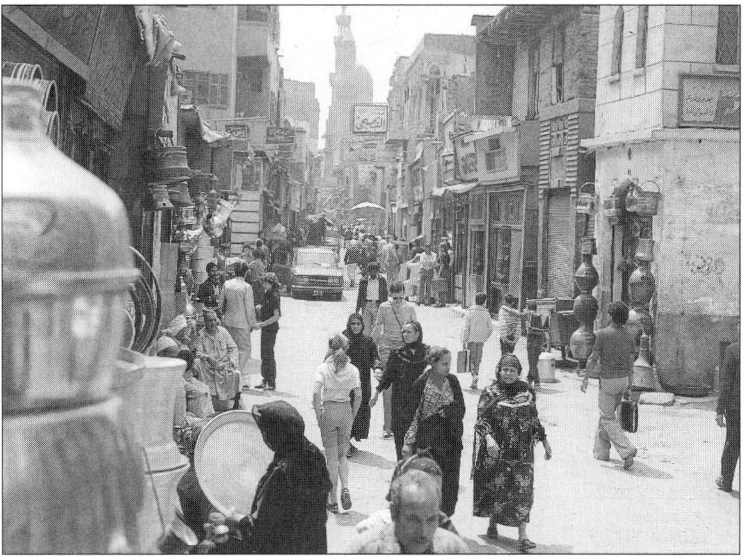

Figure 26.2 Nowadays many people live in towns and cities, whereas three hundred years ago the great majority of people lived in the countryside. This is modern-day Cairo, a city that dates back several thousand years but has grown hugely over the last hundred years.

World population growth

Human population size is affected by such things as:

- food and water supply
- health (nutrition, disease, medication, environmental health measures)
- birth control
- wars and other conflicts.

The number of people has increased hugely over the past few hundred years (Figure 26.2). In 1995 the total population of the world is thought to have been 5650 million, over five and a half billion. Each *day* the world's population increases by approximately 250 000 people.

Q3: By how much is the world's population increasing each year?

It is difficult to obtain accurate figures about the world's population at different times in the past, but Table 26.1 shows how the world's population is thought to have changed over the last 2000 years. There have probably been three periods in the human history of exponential growth, so-called 'population explosions':

- **tool-making revolution** – approximately 20 000 years ago tools began to be used for hunting and food-gathering techniques
- **agricultural revolution** – approximately 10 000 years ago animals and plants began to be domesticated
- **scientific–industrial revolution** – approximately 300 years ago the use of machines in industry really 'took off'.

We are still in the middle of the scientific–industrial revolution during which time there have been, in industrial countries, massive increases in food production and great improvements in physical health. The United Nations estimates that in the year 2020 the world's population will be approximately 8000 million people.

Table 26.1 World population size over the last 2000 years

Year	World population/millions
0	260
1000	280
1200	380
1500	430
1750	730
1900	1700
1950	2500
1960	3300
1970	3700
1980	4450
1990	5200
1995	5650

Q4: Plot the data in Table 26.1 on a graph. Compare your graph with Figure 26.1. Which of the four phases of Figure 26.1 is the world population size currently in?

Population growth in the UK

Figure 26.3 shows how the population of England is thought to have changed over the last 2200 years. If the other parts of the UK were included the shape would still be very similar.

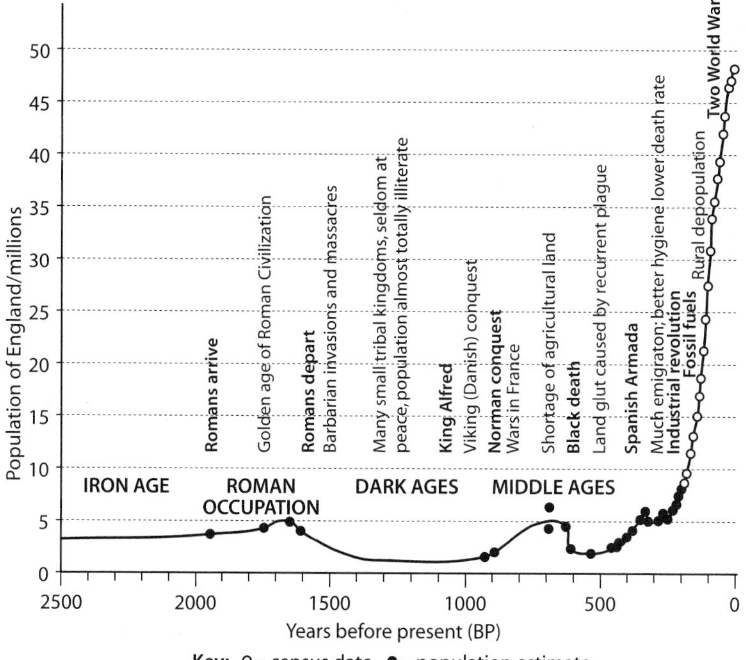

Figure 26.3 Changes in the population of England over the last 2200 years. In the 1st World War (1914–18) some 600 000 people in England died; in the 2nd World War (1939–1945) some 250 000 people in England died. Notice how, despite all these deaths, the two World Wars had almost no visible effect on the overall population size of England.

Q5: At which three times did the population of England decrease during the last 2200 years?

Q6: During which century has the population increase been greatest?

Birth rates and death rates

The size of a country's population is affected by:

- **births**
- **deaths**
- **immigration**
- **emigration.**

- The **birth rate** of a country equals the number of babies born in a year per 1000 people in that country.

Q7: (a) Which two of these factors lead to increases in the population size? (b) Which two of these factors lead to decreases in the population size?

- The **death rate** of a country equals the number of people who die in a year per 1000 people in that country.

Q8: What would happen to the population size if: (a) the birth rate and death rate were equal? (b) the birth rate was greater than the death rate? (c) the birth rate was less than the death rate?

Table 26.2 gives the birth rates and death rates of 16 different countries. The greater the difference between birth rate and death rate (i.e. birth rate minus death rate), the faster a population is growing.

Q9: In Table 26.2, which country: (a) is decreasing in size (b) has a stable population (i.e. no change in size over time)? (c) has the fastest growing population?

People in industrialised countries, such as Britain and Japan, sometimes blame those in less industrialised countries, such as Kenya and India, for the problem of the world's very large population.

Table 26.2 Birth rates and death rates for 10 countries in 1992

Country	Birth rate per 1000 people	Death rate per 1000 people	Country	Birth rate per 1000 people	Death rate per 1000 people
Bangladesh	37	13	Ireland	15	9
Brazil	26	7	Israel	21	6
China	20	7	Italy	10	9
Denmark	13	12	Kenya	45	9
Egypt	32	7	Nigeria	46	16
Germany	11	11	South Africa	34	8
Hungary	12	14	UK	14	11
India	30	10	USA	16	9

Actually, industrialised countries often have a *higher* density of people (number of people per unit area of land) than other countries. The UK, for example, has a population density of 230 people per square kilometre, while Uganda has 68, Kenya 37 and Brazil 16. Less industrialised countries are simply going through the type of scientific–industrial population explosion which countries in the West have already gone through.

Population pyramids

A **population pyramid** shows the composition of a population in terms of gender and age. Figure 26.4 shows the population pyramid for the UK in 1995. Each shaded block shows the number of people of that particular age and sex who were alive in the UK in 1995.

The UK population is still increasing in size, but only very slowly and more because of a low death rate than a high birth rate. Its population pyramid reflects this, as the blocks for people aged 0–4 and 5–9 are not especially wide. Figure 26.5 shows the population pyramid for India in 1995. Population pyramids of this shape are often found in countries with populations that are increasing rapidly.

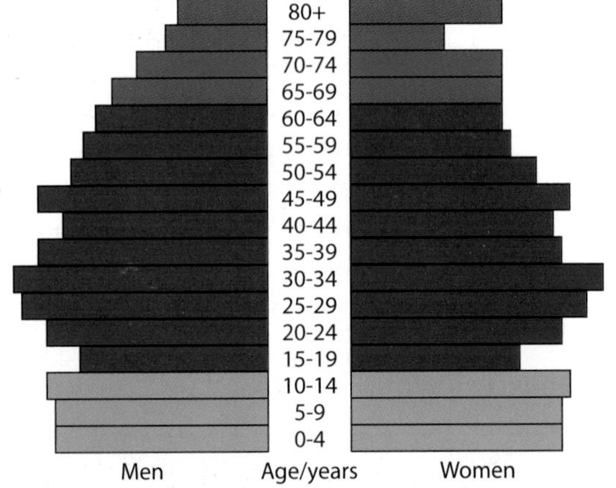

Figure 26.4 The population pyramid for the UK in 1995.

Q10: In the UK in 1995: (a) are there more people aged 10–19 or 20–29? (b) are there more men or women aged over 80? (c) which five year age block has the most people?

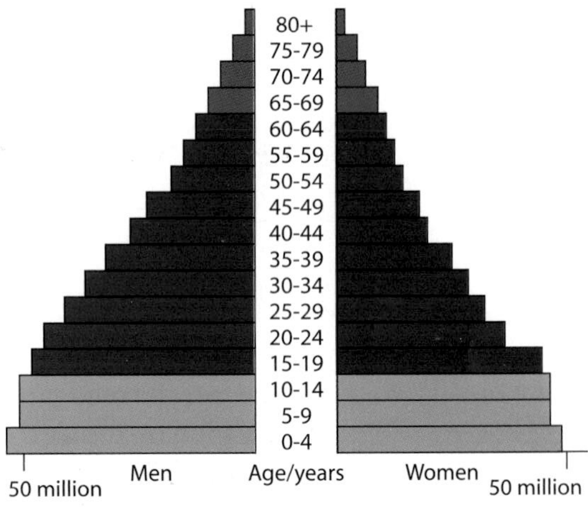

Figure 26.5 The population pyramid for India in 1995.

Q11: Approximately how many girls under the age of 10 were there in India in 1995?

Agriculture

The domestication of animals and plants seems to have happened independently around ten thousand to twelve thousand years ago in the Middle East, Indo-China and the Americas and has continued ever since (Table 26.3). With agriculture

Table 26.3 Dates and places for the domestication of some animals and plants

Organism	Date domesticated /years ago	Place domesticated	Organism	Date domesticated /years ago	Place domesticated
Dog	12 000	Iraq, Palestine	Potato	9 000	Peru
Goat	10 000	Iran, Afghanistan	Bean	9 000	Peru
Sheep	10 000	Iran, Afghanistan	Rice	9 000	Indo-China
Wheat	10 000	Palestine	Pumpkin	9 000	Central America
Barley	10 000	Palestine	Pig	8 000	Eastern Asia, China

Agricultural practices

A tremendous range of agricultural practices are used to increase yields.

- **Selective breeding** – for example, modern wheat has a shorter stem, more grains per stem, greater resistance to disease and greater tolerance to extreme environmental conditions than wheat did only a generation ago. Modern techniques of tissue culture, cloning and genetic engineering are revolutionising plant breeding (see page 169).
- **Optimal growing conditions** – for example, environmental conditions can be altered within glasshouses and polythene tunnels to optimise temperature, carbon dioxide, light and water levels (through irrigation). Plants can be grown by means of **hydroponics** (in water cultures) to allow precise control of mineral ions.
- **Fertilisers** and **pesticides** – for example, **insecticides**, or **natural predators** such as ladybirds, can be used to control aphids (which feed on plants and can carry virus diseases); **fungicides** can be used to control mildews and potato blight; **herbicides** can be used to get rid of weeds.

Industrialisation and urbanisation

Many cities have their origins thousands of years ago. However, it is only within the last few hundred years that vast numbers of people have moved to towns and cities either for employment or to live. This trend is known as **urbanisation** and is a consequence of **industrialisation.** Heavy industry requires a lot of people. For example, in the late eighteenth and early nineteenth century in northern England there was a shift in the way cloth was woven. Before then there was a cottage industry. Here each family was self-employed and wove its own cloth. With the Industrial Revolution, cloth weaving was done in huge mills situated in rapidly expanding towns. Most people involved in weaving became employees and only a few people owned mills.

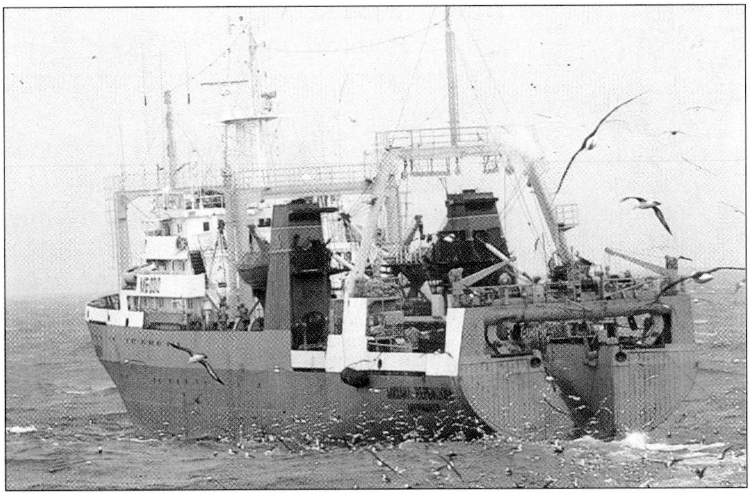

Figure 26.6 Modern trawlers and other fishing vessels are often equipped with radar and other sophisticated devices to find shoals of fish. They catch far more fish than the smaller fishing boats of a generation ago and have contributed to the problem of overfishing.

Depletion of resources and pollution

The enormous increase in the size of the human population over the last couple of hundred years has had unfortunate environmental consequences.

- More and more resources have become depleted. We have already seen how we are rapidly running out of oil and gas (page 202). The same is true of many other resources. For example, many fisheries have collapsed through **overfishing** (Figure 26.6). The harvesting of any natural biological resource, such as fish, may require careful regulation. If the organisms are removed more quickly than they can replace themselves through reproduction (or immigration), the population will decline and fewer of the organisms will be available for harvesting. Management may involve setting **quotas** (limits), avoiding breeding seasons or breeding areas, or selectively removing certain groups of organisms, such as non-breeding adults.

- The loss of tropical rainforests and other natural habitats is probably causing several species of animals and plants to become extinct *each day*. **Deforestation**, which takes place for timber, to provide land for agriculture and for new roads, houses and factories, has other consequences. In particular, it increases the release of carbon dioxide into the atmosphere. In the UK, farmers were, until the mid-1990s, being encouraged to remove hedges to increase the amount of land available for agriculture. However, this practice can reduce the diversity of organisms and make the countryside more barren as hedges are visually attractive and provide valuable habitats for many plants, insects, birds and small mammals. There can be a conflict between food production and the conservation of natural habitats. Ironically, by the 1980s Europe's farmers were so successful at producing food that vast amounts of money were being spent on storing grain, wine and other produce in so-called 'grain mountains' and 'wine lakes'. A **set-aside scheme** was therefore introduced in which farmers are paid not to grow food on some of their land.
- **Pollution** has become a serious problem. Pollution is the result of the release by humans of damaging materials or energy into the environment. The material or energy released is called a **pollutant**. A useful distinction can be made between pollutants that break down in nature (**biodegradable**) and ones that don't break down but accumulate (**non-biodegradable**). We shall now summarise briefly some of the causes and consequences of pollution before looking, in Chapter 27, at how pollution can be controlled.

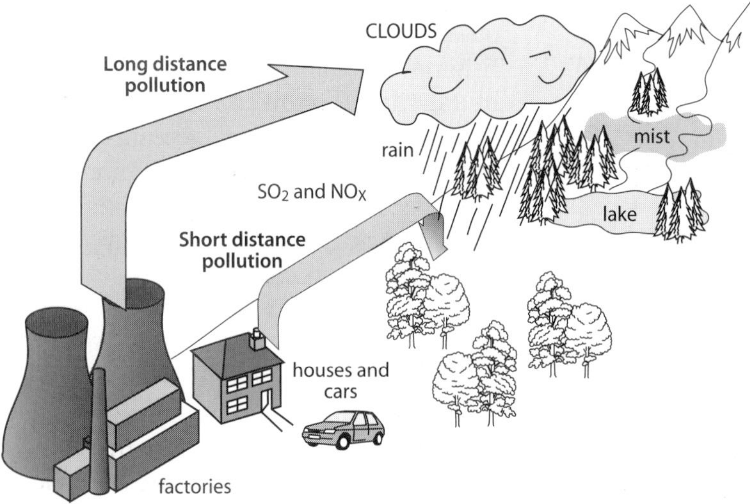

Figure 26.7 Acid rain results mainly from the release of sulphur dioxide (SO_2) and various oxides of nitrogen (collectively described as NO_X) into the air. Breathing in sulphur dioxide can also cause health problems for humans.

Global warming

We have already seen how the increase in the atmospheric concentration of carbon dioxide over the last two hundred years is probably causing the world's temperature to rise (page 207). This is an example of **air pollution**. However, global warming is also caused by:

- the release of hydrocarbons (chemicals made only from carbon and hydrogen), especially **methane** (CH_4), into the atmosphere. Quite a lot of the methane entering the atmosphere is produced by cattle kept for beef or milk; some comes from rice-fields
- chlorofluorocarbons (CFCs) (see 'Depletion of the ozone layer' on page 219)
- nitrogen dioxide, NO_2, largely produced by the burning of petrol in vehicles.

Possible consequences of global warming are considered on page 207.

Ways of minimising global warming are summarised on page 222.

Acid rain

Acid rain is the result of a number of processes which lead to rainwater having a pH of around 4 to 5, rather than its usual 5.6. The main problem is the burning of coal, oil and petrol in factories, houses, cars and other vehicles. This releases sulphur dioxide and nitrogen oxides into the atmosphere. These dissolve in rainwater, lowering its pH (Figure 26.7). Acid rain causes rivers and lakes to become acidic and has caused many lakes to lose their fish. This is because fish are particularly sensitive to low pHs. Conifer trees are also badly affected by acid rain, and lichens are killed by sulphur dioxide pollution. Acid rain therefore involves both **air** and **water pollution**.

Ways of reducing acid rain are summarised on page 222.

Q12: Sometimes sulphur dioxide and nitrogen oxides can be carried many hundreds of miles by the wind. In Europe, westerly winds are more common than easterly ones. Which is more important: acid rain in the UK caused by air pollution in Scandinavia or acid rain in Scandinavia caused by air pollution in the UK?

Practical 26.1 To simulate the effect of acid rain on the growth of plants

Wear eye protection

A simulation is an artificial situation set up to model or imitate reality. In this practical we shall investigate the effect of buffers of different pHs on the germination and growth of cress as a simulation of the effect of acid rain on the growth of plants.

Requirements
- Petri dishes, 6
- Filter paper, 6
- Eye protection
- Cress (*Lepidium sativum*) seeds, 60
- 10 cm^3 of buffer solution of pH 2
- 10 cm^3 of buffer solution of pH 3
- 10 cm^3 of buffer solution of pH 4
- 10 cm^3 of buffer solution of pH 5
- 10 cm^3 of buffer solution of pH 6
- 10 cm^3 of buffer solution of pH 7

1. Set up six Petri dishes, each with a piece of filter paper inside.
2. Label the Petri dishes pH 2, pH 3, pH 4, pH 5, pH 6 and pH 7.
3. Onto each filter paper place 10 cress seeds.

SAFETY: Wear eye protection for steps 4 and 5.

4. Water the Petri dish labelled pH 2 with buffer solution of pH 2 so that the filter paper is wet, but not sodden. Similarly, water the other Petri dishes with the appropriate buffer solutions.
5. Over the next few days add the appropriate buffer solution whenever a filter paper starts to dry out.
6. After a week, record the percentage germination in each Petri dish and measure the length of any seedlings from the tip of the shoot to the tip of the root.
7. Is there a relationship between the pH and the percentage germination?
8. Is there a relationship between the pH and the length of any seedlings?
9. Explain the relevance of this practical to the problem of acid rain.

Depletion of the ozone layer

Ozone, O_3, is found at low concentrations in the Earth's stratosphere, 15 to 50 km above the Earth's surface. One effect it has is to absorb much of the ultraviolet radiation from the Sun which would otherwise reach the Earth's surface, damaging our genetic material (DNA) and causing cancers.

During the 1980s measurements above the Antarctic showed that a 'hole' was appearing in the ozone layer and getting bigger each year. Intensive scientific research has shown that **CFCs** (**chlorofluorocarbons**) are responsible. These catalyse the destruction of ozone. Until recently, CFCs were widely used as refrigerator coolants, in aerosol sprays and in fast-food packaging.

Ways of protecting the ozone layer are discussed on page 223.

Eutrophication

We have already seen (page 210) how fertiliser run-off can result in eutrophication (a rise in the nutrient content of water). Eutrophication can also result from the movement of each of the following into waterways:

- farmyard slurry – i.e. the semi-liquid

manure formed from the faeces of cattle or sheep
- untreated sewage
- concentrated organic solutions, e.g. waste from sugar factories.

In each case the resulting dramatic rise in the concentrations of nitrate and phosphate ions can lead to algal blooms and the death of fish (Figure 26.8).

Ways of tackling eutrophication are discussed on page 223.

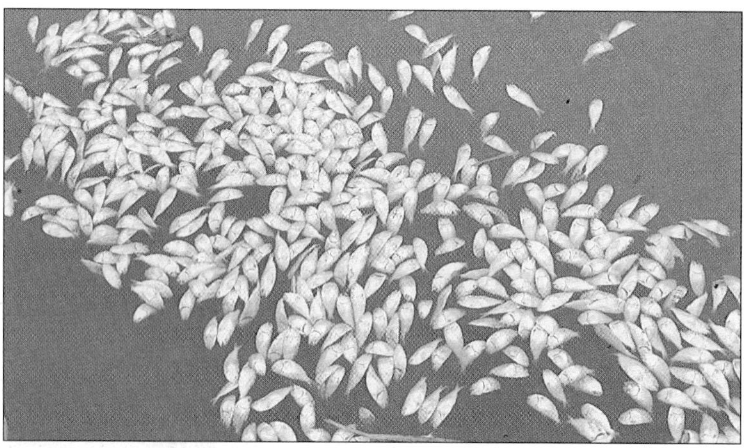

Figure 26.8 The drop in the amount of dissolved oxygen in a river as a result of eutrophication can be enough to kill large numbers of fish.

Q13: Are farmyard slurries, sewage and concentrated organic solutions biodegradable or non-biodegradable?

Radioactivity

The great majority of the **radioactivity** the average person in the UK receives each year is natural (Figure 26.9). Natural radiation comes either from outer space (cosmic rays) or from rocks in the Earth's crust that contain radioactive materials (e.g. radon gas). However, the situation in some countries is very different. For instance, the explosion at the Chernobyl nuclear power station on 26 April 1986 led to hundreds of thousands of people in the former Soviet Union receiving high radiation doses. Around 10 000 people are thought to have died as a result.

Ways of dealing with radioactive waste are examined on page 223.

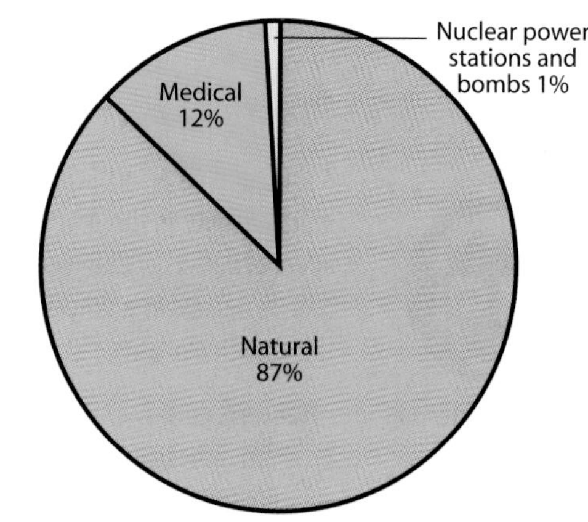

Figure 26.9 Sources of radioactivity for the average person in the UK.

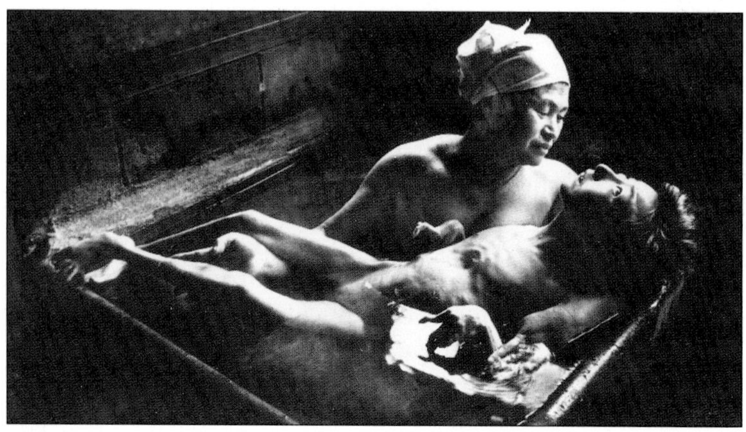

Heavy metals

Heavy metal toxicity occurs when elements such as mercury, lead, zinc and selenium are present in high levels. Mercury is used in a variety of industrial processes, and so mercury poisoning in humans can occur unless safety precautions are taken (Figure 26.10). Heavy metals tend to become concentrated as they pass up through food chains (known as **bioaccumulation**). This means that long-lived, top-level carnivores, such as eagles and hawks, are particularly susceptible to such pollutants. This is also the case for non-biodegradable pesticides such as DDT.

Ways of dealing with heavy metal toxicity are considered on page 223.

Figure 26.10 A 16 year-old woman suffering from congenital (i.e. from birth) mercury poisoning being bathed by her mother. The young woman is unable to see and cannot talk. She was one of many people who suffered mercury poisoning as a result of methyl mercury waste being dumped into the Minimata Bay, Japan in the 1950s. The mercury was consumed by fish and subsequently by women who then gave birth to deformed babies.

Q14: Are heavy metals biodegradable or non-biodegradable?

Carbon monoxide

Carbon monoxide (CO) is an invisible gas with no smell. It is poisonous if inhaled in large amounts. As discussed on page 28, this is because carbon monoxide binds very tightly to haemoglobin, thus reducing the oxygen-carrying capacity of the blood. Carbon monoxide is found in the fumes from:

- car exhausts
- badly fitting gas fires
- burning cigarettes.

Ways of reducing carbon monoxide emissions are listed on page 224.

Carbon monoxide emissions are often accompanied by the release of tiny particles of carbon. It is now known that these pose severe health risks, especially to the elderly and those with asthma. Some experts believe that several thousand deaths a year in the UK are the result of the damage that these carbon particles do to our lungs.

Noise

We may not think of **noise** as a pollutant but it can be.

- Loud noises, e.g. in people using pneumatic drills or standing too close to loudspeakers at rock concerts, can cause loss of hearing (Figure 26.11).
- Simply living near to a major airport or in a noisy city can cause stress and headaches.

It may only be when we are away from too much artificial noise, in the countryside for example, that we realise how noise can damage our health.

Ways of reducing noise pollution are summarised on page 224.

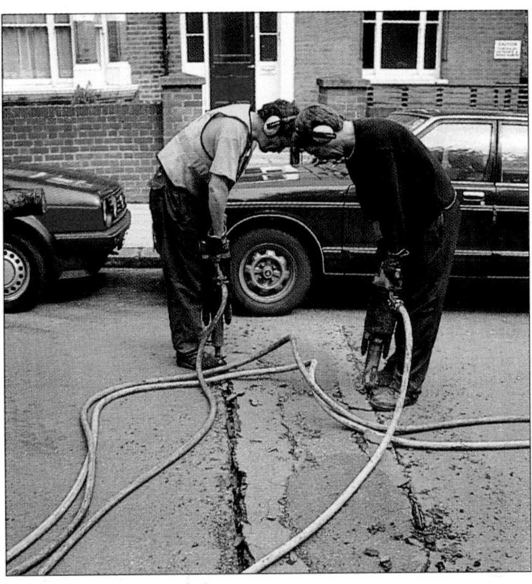

Figure 26.11
People using pneumatic drills are required to wear ear protection. This can protect their hearing as the delicate sensory hairs in the inner ear can be damaged by loud noises.

Summary

- The human population has probably grown exponentially on several occasions in its history.
- In 1995 there were approximately 5650 million people alive.
- A population increases in size if the birth rate exceeds the death rate.
- Population pyramids show the composition of populations in terms of gender and age.
- The increase in the number of people world-wide has led to depletion of resources and to pollution.
- Human activity is causing global warming, acid rain, damage to the ozone layer, eutrophication and pollution by radioactivity, heavy metals, carbon monoxide and noise.

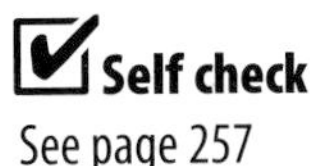

Self check
See page 257

CHAPTER 27

Management of planet Earth

In this chapter you will learn how the effects of pollution can be minimised and how sewage can be treated and drinking water purified.

Pollution control

There are three fundamental ways in which pollution can be controlled:

- each person can produce less pollution, either through being more careful or through lowering their standard of living and so making fewer demands on the environment
- technological improvements can help us either to prevent pollution or to deal with it more effectively
- if there were fewer people, less pollution overall would be produced.

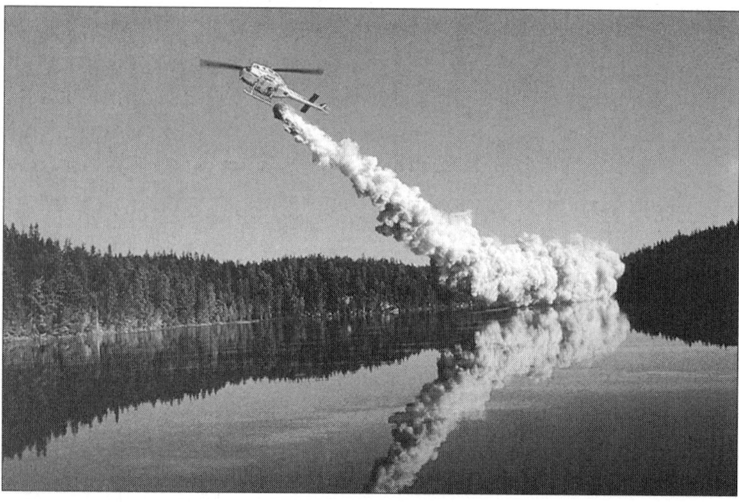

Figure 27.1 Limestone can be added to lakes affected by acid rain. This may help populations of sensitive organisms, such as fish, snails and plants, to recover. However, the only long-term solution to the problem of acid rain is to reduce its production.

Global warming

The main ways of reducing global warming are to:

- use fewer fossil fuels
- plant more trees.

Use of fossil fuels can be reduced by:

- switching to other power sources, e.g. solar, wind, nuclear, hydroelectric
- using fossil fuels more efficiently, e.g. using a car that does more miles to the gallon
- people changing their lifestyles, e.g. wearing a thick pullover instead of turning the heating up, travelling by public transport rather than by private car.

Acid rain

Acid rain can be reduced by:

- using natural gas and low-sulphur coals rather than high-sulphur coals
- fitting sulphur dioxide 'scrubbers' to reduce sulphur dioxide emissions from coal-fired power stations.

The effects of acid rain on affected lakes can be reduced by adding large amounts of calcium carbonate (limestone) to them (Figure 27.1).

Q1: Why would adding limestone to a lake affected by acid rain help to reduce the problem?

Depletion of the ozone layer

In 1987 pressure by environmentalists (people who campaign on behalf of the environment) and scientists led to the signing of the **Montreal Protocol** by over 30 countries. This convention laid down targets to ensure that fewer CFCs are released into the atmosphere. In the early 1990s there was a significant reduction in the use of CFCs, though the 'holes' in the ozone layer continued to get worse. This is because CFCs persist for many years high in the atmosphere.

Eutrophication

The only long-term solution to the problem of eutrophication is to prevent large amounts of nitrate ions, phosphate ions and organic matter entering rivers and lakes. This can mainly be achieved by:
- encouraging farmers to apply fertilisers at the most appropriate times of year
- prosecuting farmers and industrialists who allow large spills of organic matter into freshwater habitats
- building better sewage treatment works (see page 224).

In 1995 a group of biologists in Australia found that a bacterium (called *Sphingomonas*) could detoxify the poisons sometimes released by the algal blooms that result from eutrophication. These poisons can cause deaths of dogs, farm animals and even people. The intention is to grow the bacterium in bulk, freeze-dry it and release it when needed into affected waterways.

Radioactivity

There is no way in which radioactivity can be 'treated'. The only way that radioactive waste can be dealt with is to store it (Figure 27.2). Some radioactive elements have a short half-life, of only days or weeks. The half-life is the time taken for the amount of radioactivity to fall to half its original level as a result of radioactive decay. Unfortunately, some of the radioactive elements that are found in radioactive waste have a half-life of many thousands of years. To all intents and purposes, this waste will last for ever. Various ways of dealing with radioactive waste have been tried:
- seal it above ground in containers of lead, concrete or glass
- deposit it in sealed containers in deep, underground stores
- dump it in sealed containers in the sea.

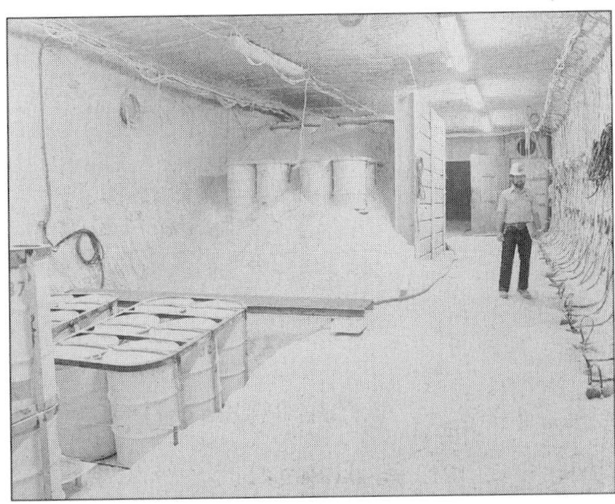

Figure 27.2 The only way of dealing with radioactive waste is to store it. Some people argue this merely postpones the problem of what to do with it.

Q2: Give (a) one advantage and (b) one disadvantage of dumping radioactive waste in the sea.

Some nuclear fuel is reprocessed. This means that some of the uranium and plutonium it contains is recovered. However, reprocessing produces its own radioactive waste and involves the transportation of radioactive materials around the country, or even overseas. This could be dangerous and is controversial.

Heavy metals

By far the best way of dealing with heavy metal pollution is to prevent it from happening. This involves the strict enforcement of environmental legislation. Most industrialised countries, including the UK, have state-funded employees who monitor health and safety at work and the pollution generated by industry. In the

UK, pollution is monitored by environmental health officers and other **pollution inspectors**.

In the case of lead, it has long been known that its slow accumulation can be poisonous. It is now also known that high lead levels can harm children's brains. These are the reasons why:
- lead paints are now rarely used (and are illegal on toys)
- lead is no longer used for pipes that supply drinking water
- the tax on unleaded petrol is less than on leaded petrol (to encourage people to switch to unleaded petrol).

Carbon monoxide

Carbon monoxide emissions can be reduced by:
- fitting **catalytic converters** to vehicles
- checking the installation of gas fires and boilers regularly
- ensuring that the combustion of carbon-based compounds (e.g. petrol) takes place with enough oxygen present.

Q3: What gas will be produced instead of carbon monoxide if enough oxygen is present when a carbon-based compound is burnt?

Oil pollution

Vast volumes of oil are carried around the world in supertankers. Oil pollution can occur in oil spills and in accidents at oil refineries. Oil is lighter than water and does not easily dissolve in it. As a result, large oil slicks form on the surface of the water. Slicks can kill many organisms, notably oceanic birds. Ways of tackling oil pollution include:
- trying to prevent accidents from happening
- using floating booms to prevent slicks from reaching the shore
- setting fire to the oil
- adding bacteria to digest the oil
- adding oil spill cleansers that are relatively non-toxic and biodegradable.

Noise

Noise pollution can be reduced by:
- restricting noise emissions
- better sound insulation
- wearing ear protectors.

Sewage treatment

Sewage contains:
- faeces and urine from toilets
- dirty water from sinks and baths
- rain water that runs into the drains
- waste from industry, hospitals and abattoirs.

(Agricultural sewage is not allowed to mix with domestic and industrial waste, and is treated separately.)

Sewage usually flows through **sewers** (underground pipes) to **sewage treatment works**. However, small amounts of sewage, for example that produced by the people living in an isolated house, may be dealt with in a **septic tank**.

The principles of sewage treatment centre around:
- the initial removal of large waste items (plastic bottles, condoms, twigs, etc.)
- the use of microorganisms to remove much of the organic matter from the sewage
- the production of water which is sufficiently unpolluted to be passed into a river or the sea.

The essential design of a typical sewage treatment works is shown in Figure 27.3. The following products result:
- **grit** and **sand** – used for landfill
- **sludge** – some of this is digested at the sewage works in anaerobic digesters by anaerobic bacteria which make methane (CH_4). This is then used as a fuel at the sewage works. The rest of the sludge is either turned safely into **agricultural fertiliser** or dumped at sea
- **effluent** – which is discharged into a river or the sea.

Sewage treatment is a form of biotechnology since microorganisms (bacteria

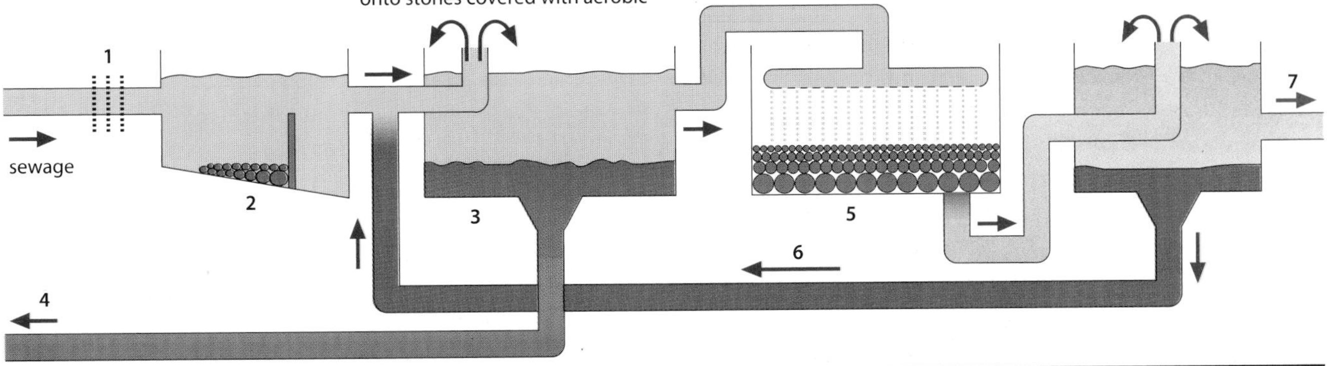

1 **Screening**: removes large objects

2 **Grit settling tank:** grit and sand settle out, are collected and used for landfill

3 **1st sedimentation tank**: large particles settle and become sludge

4 Sludge taken off to be treated

5 **Aeration tank**: sewage sprayed onto stones covered with aerobic bacteria and protozoa which feed on the organic matter and convert ammonium compounds into nitrates

6 Sludge recycled for settlement

7 Fairly clean water (effluent)

sewage

Figure 27.3 Diagrammatic representation of a sewage treatment works. There are different types of sewage treatment works, but the fundamental principles are as shown.

and protozoa) are being used to benefit humans. In the activated sludge process there are activated sludge tanks where these microorganisms use the organic matter and nutrients in sewage for their own growth and reproduction. The resultant liquid goes into sedimentation tanks where the remaining organic matter settles to the bottom. Figure 27.4 shows a photograph of a sewage treatment works that uses the activated sludge process.

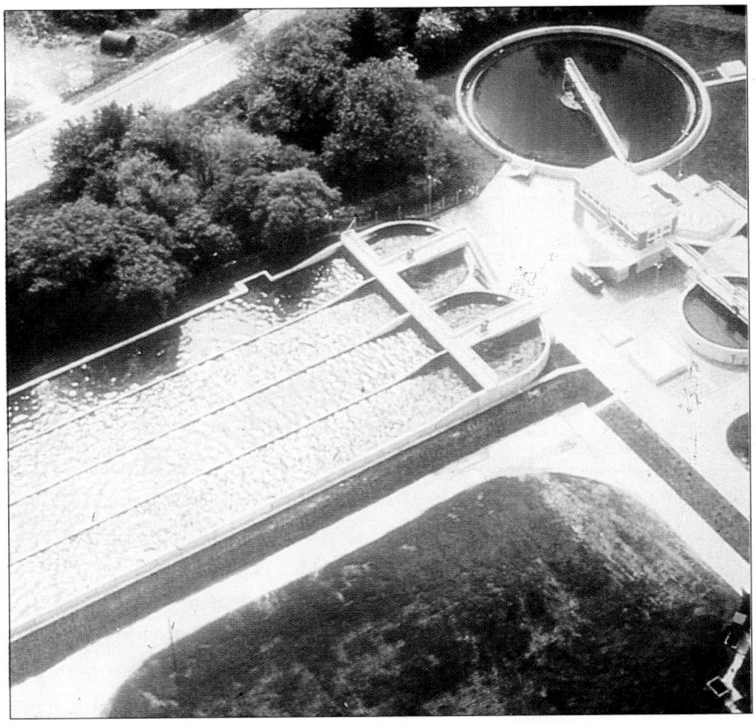

Figure 27.4 An aerial view of a sewage treatment works that uses the activated sludge process.

Q4: Why doesn't the effluent from a successful sewage treatment works cause eutrophication when it enters a river?

Water treatment

Pure water is 100% H_2O. Water doesn't need to be that pure for drinking purposes; indeed absolutely pure water tastes rather bland. Water must be clean enough to be acceptable to the community. In practice, this means that it must be safe for people (including babies) to consume, should look clear (rather than being discoloured) and should have an acceptable taste (so, for example, chlorine levels must not be too high). For these reasons, drinking water is constantly monitored to check its quality. The essential principles of water purification are shown in Figure 27.5. Notice the following processes:

- **screening** to remove large debris
- **sedimentation** to remove soil particles
- **filtration** to remove fine particles
- **digestion** by saprotrophs and protozoa to get rid of organic matter and most bacteria
- **chlorination** to kill any remaining bacteria (e.g. those that cause cholera, typhoid, dysentery and food poisoning).

In addition, iron or aluminium salts may be added at the sedimentation stage to cause the smaller particles to **flocculate** (clump together) and so settle out more quickly.

Q5: Why are fluorides sometimes added to drinking water?

1 Lake, reservoir, well, river or spring

2 **Screens:** to remove fish, logs, etc.

3 Pump

4 **Settlement tank:** to remove soil particles, etc.

5 **Filter bed:** has layers (from the top) of sand, fine gravel, coarse gravel, small stones, large stones. Organic matter is trapped by the sand and decomposed by saprotrophs. Most disease-causing bacteria are consumed by protozoa

6 Pipes collect clean water

7 Chlorine added to kill any remaining bacteria. Fluorides may also be added (fluoridation)

8 Water tower or covered reservoir

9 Stopcock

10 Covered domestic tank in roof

11 Tap

12 Running water

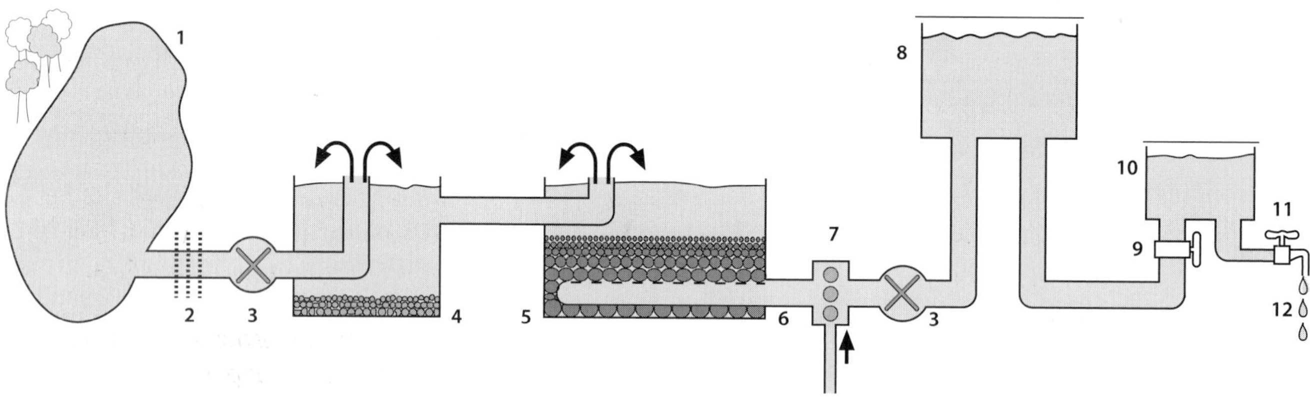

Figure 27.5 Diagrammatic representation of water purification.

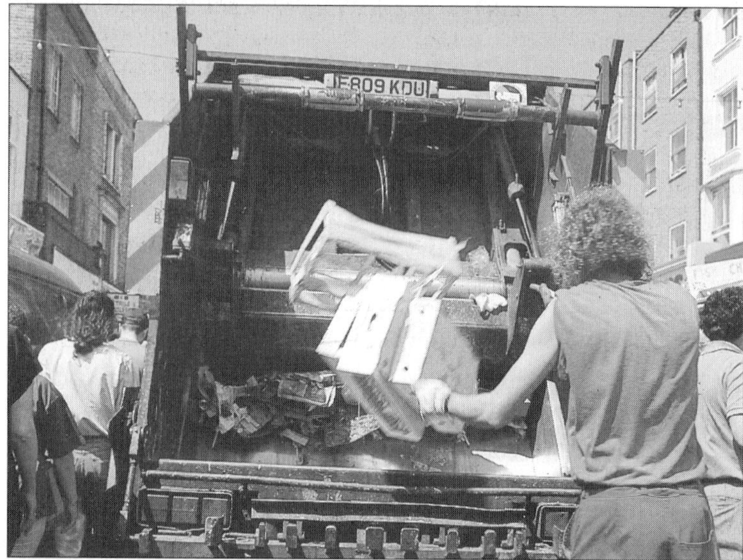

Figure 27.6 The mechanical rams at the back of a dust cart reduce the volume of the rubbish, but fail to kill fly larvae.

Refuse disposal and recycling

Domestic refuse contains such things as ash, remains of food, metals, plastics, paper and glass. To prevent it accumulating, which would be inconvenient, unsightly and would spread disease, it is collected by **dust carts** (sometimes called **refuse collection vehicles**). These usually have mechanical rams (Figure 27.6) which compress the rubbish and therefore allow the dust cart to carry more. Most refuse is tipped into hollowed-out areas called **refuse tips** or **landfill sites**. These are normally situated at least a mile from any residential areas. They are often surrounded by fences to keep blown rubbish in and children out.

Q6: Suggest three reasons why refuse tips are normally placed well away from houses.

At a refuse tip, the compressed waste is buried under about 0.5 m of soil. Burying the refuse reduces the numbers of rats, mice, birds (e.g. gulls) and flies that can feed at the site. Instead, soil bacteria and fungi decompose the organic component of the rubbish. As a result, gases are given off and the volume of rubbish decreases. Once decomposition is completed, the tip can be grassed over and used for agriculture, building or recreational purposes.

Recycling

Recycling is the reusing of products or materials which would otherwise be thrown away. It includes:

- reusing items in their original form
- sending items off to be pulped or melted down before new products are made.

Many items can be reused:

- glass milk bottles
- jars (for home-made marmalades and jams)
- carrier bags (for shopping)
- paper that has only been used on one side
- clothes (resold or redistributed by charities).

Examples of items that can be sent off to be pulped or melted down include:

- glass bottles
- paper
- cans
- some plastics
- corks.

Recycling can not only make scarce resources last longer, but can reduce the energy requirements of the manufacturing industry. For example, it takes twenty times less energy to make an aluminium can from recycled aluminium than from aluminium ores. However, for recycling to become widespread it must be economically viable. Companies will only recycle if at least one of the following three conditions is fulfilled:

- their products are cheaper than if they didn't use recycling
- people are prepared to pay more for recycled products
- they receive subsidies from central or local government for manufacturing products using recycled materials.

Q7: Which natural resource do we use less of if we recycle paper?

Composting

Compost heaps are constructed to allow the aerobic decay of material of plant (and animal) origin. A successful compost heap needs a good range of microorganisms, a supply of oxygen (so it should not be too compact), moisture (so it should not be situated in full sunlight) and warmth.

Inside the compost heap, the microorganisms feed by secreting digestive enzymes (external digestion) and then absorbing the nutrients. The heat they release warms up the compost heap, speeding up the breakdown of the organic matter to more compost. The microorganisms also produce carbon dioxide. The end result is the formation of a rich compost which can be used for gardening. This compost is usually high in organic matter and mineral ions.

Summary

- Pollution can be reduced by people being more careful, by lowering their standards of living, by technological improvements or by there being fewer people.
- Specific steps can be, and sometimes have been, taken to reduce global warming, acid rain, the depletion of the ozone layer, eutrophication, and pollution by heavy metals, carbon monoxide or noise.
- The only way to deal with radioactive waste is to store it until it decays. This can take a very long time.
- Sewage treatment relies on the decomposition of organic matter by microorganisms.
- A sewage treatment works produces fertiliser, methane and relatively clean effluent.
- Water purification produces water fit to drink and involves screening, sedimentation, filtration, digestion and chlorination.
- Domestic refuse is carried by dust carts to refuse tips, where organic waste is decomposed.
- Recycling is the reusing of products or materials which would otherwise be thrown away.

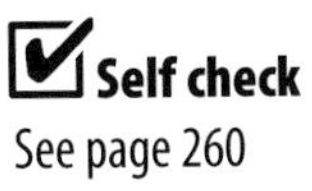

See page 260

Self-check questions

Chapter 1

1 (a) Draw an animal cell and label the following structures:
cell surface membrane, cytoplasm, mitochondrion, ribosome, rough endoplasmic reticulum, smooth endoplasmic reticulum, nucleus, nucleolus, chromosomes, nuclear envelope, nuclear pore. (6 marks)

(b) Make a table like the one below to give the function of each of the cell components listed in (a) above.

Cell component	Function
nucleolus	

(9 marks)

2. List three differences between the cells of an animal and a plant. (3 marks)

3. In your own words, describe what is meant by:
(a) tissue;
(b) organ;
(c) organ system. (3 marks)

Chapter 2

1. Define (a) anabolism (b) catabolism. (2 marks)

2. By means of drawing show the three states of matter. (3 marks)

3. Samples of red blood cells were placed in salt solutions of varying concentrations and examined under a microscope. The first sample was placed in solution A and there appeared to be little or no effect upon the cells. When a second sample was placed in solution B the cells appeared to swell up and eventually burst. A third sample was placed in solution C and these decreased in size.

(a) Which solution contained the greatest concentration of salt? (1 mark)
(b How do you know this? (1 mark)
(c) What process is responsible for the change in size of the red blood cells? State a precise definition of this process. (3 marks)
(d) Account for the changes when a sample of cells was placed in solution B. (3 marks)

4. Using a measuring cylinder and water the volume of 10 raisins was found. These were placed in a sugar solution for 24 hours. At the end of this time their volume was remeasured and recorded. A similar experiment was performed with 10 raisins in pure water. The results are seen below.

	Raisins in sugar solution	Raisins in water
Initial volume/cm³	10	10
Final volume/cm³	10	15

(a) How would you use the measuring cylinder and water to measure the volume of the raisins? (2 marks)
(b) Explain the results of the raisins in the sugar solution. (2 marks)
(c) Explain the results of the raisins in the water. (2 marks)
(d) What would you expect to happen to the volume of the raisins if they had been placed in a very strong sugar solution? (2 marks)

5. The graph below shows the rate of digestion of starch by amylase at various temperatures.

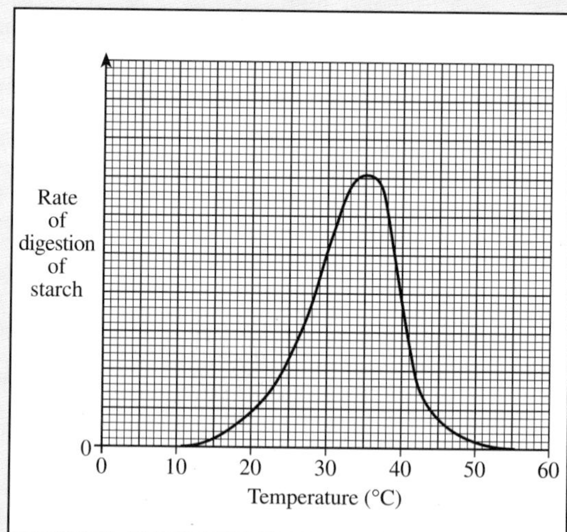

(a) What optimum temperature is indicated by the graph? (1 mark)
(b) Name three factors which should be kept constant in this investigation. (3 marks)
(c) The samples of starch and amylase originally incubated at 15°C and 70°C were all later incubated at 35°C. Suggest and explain what is likely to be found in each of these samples after an extra period of incubation. (5 marks)

Chapter 3

1. (a) List all seven requirements in the diet. (7 marks)
   (b) What elements do proteins contain? (2 marks)
   (c) Describe a food test for:
      (i) reducing sugar, e.g. glucose (3 marks)
      (ii) protein. (3 marks)
   (d) What substance can be used to detect vitamin C? (1 mark)

2. (a) Name one example of:
      (i) polysaccharide
      (ii) disaccharide
      (iii) monosaccharide. (3 marks)
   (b) What two substances is a lipid made up of? (2 marks)
   (c) What is the difference between:
      (i) globular and fibrillar protein (1 mark)
      (ii) essential and non-essential amino acids? (1 mark)
   (d) State one function of:
      (i) vitamin A
      (ii) vitamin D
      (iii) vitamin K. (3 marks)
   (e) State one function of:
      (i) calcium
      (ii) iron. (2 marks)

3. (a) Name the four types of teeth. (4 marks)
   (b) What is plaque? (1 mark)
   (c) What are:
      (i) dental caries (1 mark)
      (ii) periodontal disease? (1 mark)
   (d) List four ways to prevent tooth decay. (4 marks)

4. (a) The figure below shows part of the alimentary canal.

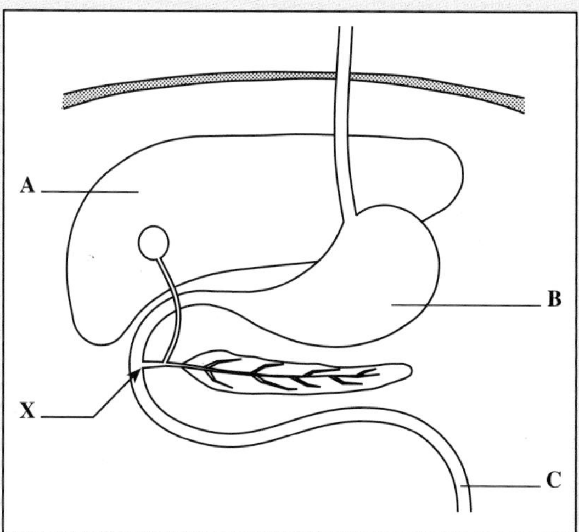

      (i) Name the parts labelled A, B and C on the above diagram. (3 marks)
      (ii) Name one chemical substance passed into the digestive system at the place marked X, and give one of its functions. (2 marks)
   (b) The experiment shown below was set up to investigate one factor which affects the action of an enzyme on the breakdown of starch. All the test tubes were kept at 30°C for 30 minutes from the start of the experiment.

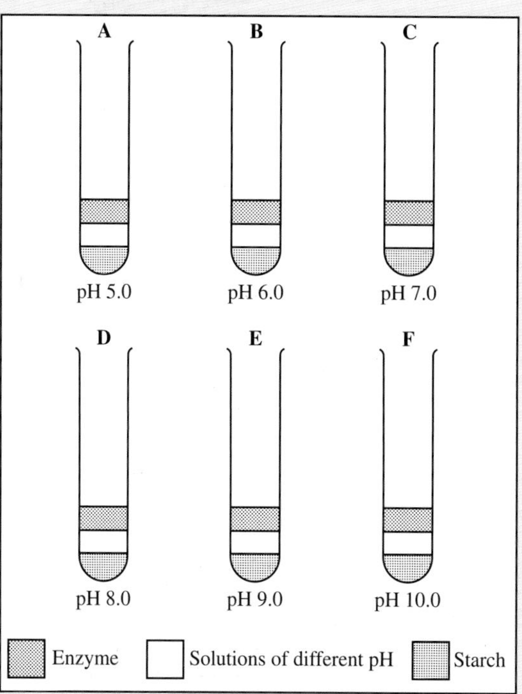

   After 15 minutes and 30 minutes each of the test tubes was tested for the presence of starch. The results are shown below.

Test Tubes

Time	A	B	C	D	E	F
15 mins	Starch	Starch	No Starch	No Starch	Starch	Starch
30 mins	Starch	No Starch	No Starch	No Starch	No Starch	Starch

      (i) Why were all the test tubes kept at a constant temperature? (1 mark)
      (ii) What do the results tell you about the activity of the enzyme? (3 marks)
      (iii) Describe how you would set up an experiment to test the hypothesis that the enzyme is deactivated by temperatures in excess of 50°C. (3 marks)
   (SEG 88)

Chapter 4

1. Looking at the diagrams of red blood cells and white blood cells below.

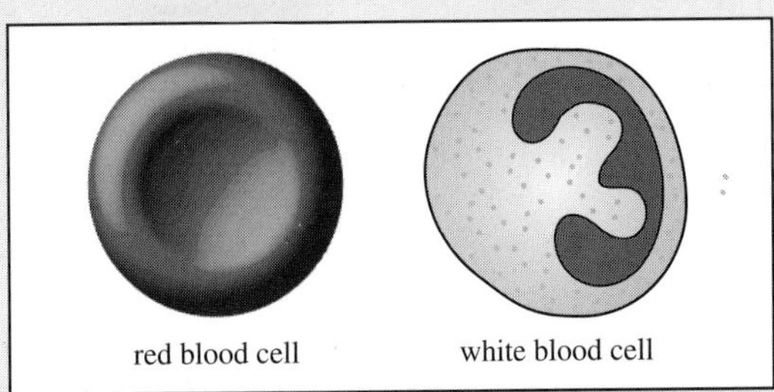

(a) State two structural differences between the two. (2 marks)

(b) State two functional differences between the two. (2 marks)

(SEG 89)

2. List the stages that occur in the body between the time of cutting your finger and the formation of a scab. (6 marks)

3. (a) What is serum? (1 mark)

(b) List the antigens and antibodies found in the following blood groups: A, B, AB and O. (4 marks)

(c) If blood group A is added to the serum of group B agglutination (clumping of the red blood cells) occurs. Explain. (3 marks)

(SEG 84)

4. Draw a series of diagrams to illustrate phagocytosis. (2 marks)

5. The diagram on the right shows a plan of the blood circulation.

(a) (i) Name the type of blood vessel labelled A. (1 mark)

(ii) Name the type of blood vessel labelled C. (1 mark)

(b) Name the type of blood vessel which connects the blood vessels A and C. (1 mark)

(c) Draw an arrow on the blood vessel labelled B to show the direction of blood flow. (1 mark)

(d) What is the function of the heart in the circulation of the blood? (1 mark)

(e) Read the following account and answer the questions which follow.

> ATHEROSCLEROSIS
>
> Atherosclerosis is a condition in which the smooth internal lining of the blood vessels becomes covered with fatty deposits. This causes a reduction in the diameter of the blood vessels. The fatty deposits often cause blood clots to form which further narrow the blood vessel and eventually block it completely. Family history is probably the most important factor in the development of atherosclerosis but the high incidence of the condition in developed countries suggests it is connected with some aspects of the Western way of life.
>
> The consequences of atherosclerosis such as coronary thrombosis (heart attack) are reaching epidemic proportions in some countries. Medical efforts and public health campaigns are aimed mainly at prevention.

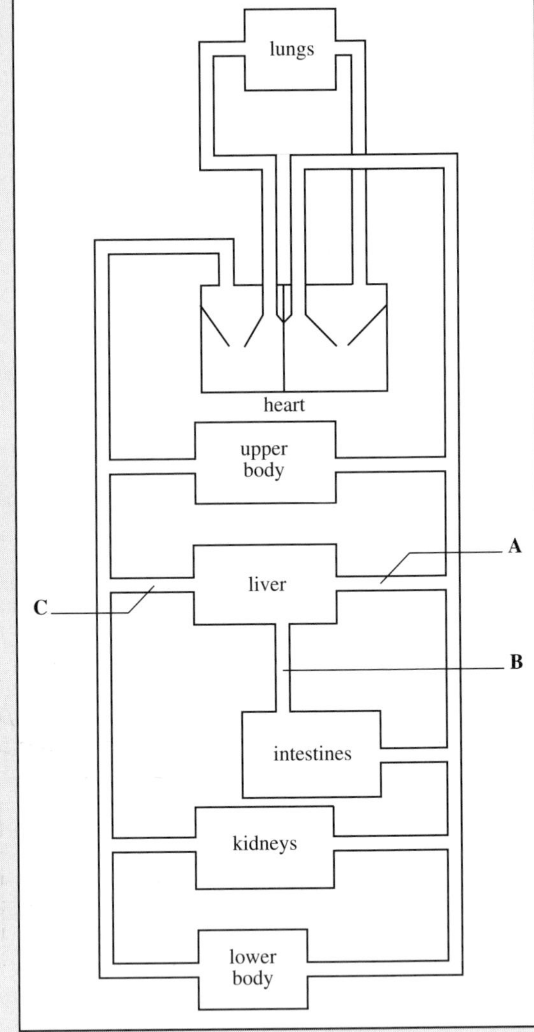

(i) What does the account suggest is the most important cause of atherosclerosis? (1 mark)

(ii) Explain how atherosclerosis can lead to a heart attack. (3 marks)

(iii) Outline TWO ways by which atherosclerosis may be prevented. (2 marks)

(MEG 94)

6. (a) The diagram (page 231, top left) shows the external view of the heart from the front.

(i) Choose a letter which best labels each of the structures named in the table. Enter the letter you choose in the second column of the table. (4 marks)

Structure	Letter
Aorta	
Left atrium	
Pulmonary vein	
Vena cava	

(ii) The vessel numbered 1 in certain conditions may become blocked. Explain why this blockage may cause a heart attack. (3 marks)

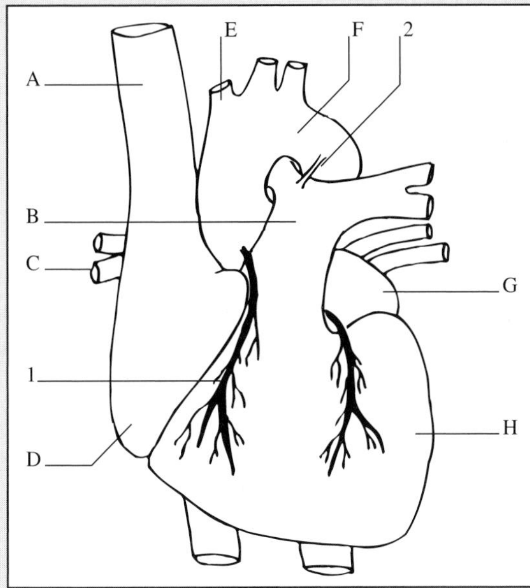

(iii) In a foetus the structure numbered 2 is an open blood vessel allowing blood to flow. In a foetus the pressure produced by the right ventricle is greater than that by the left ventricle. Which way will blood flow through this vessel in the foetus? (1 mark)

(iv) Shortly after birth vessel 2 closes. However, in some people it remains open allowing blood to continue to pass. In which direction will blood now flow in such people? Explain the reason for your answer. (2 marks)

(v) If this vessel remains open there will be a lack of oxygen reaching the tissues of the body. Briefly explain why this is so. (2 marks)

(b) The photograph below shows cross sections of an artery and a vein as seen with a microscope. Give three reasons why it is possible to know that A is an artery. (3 marks)

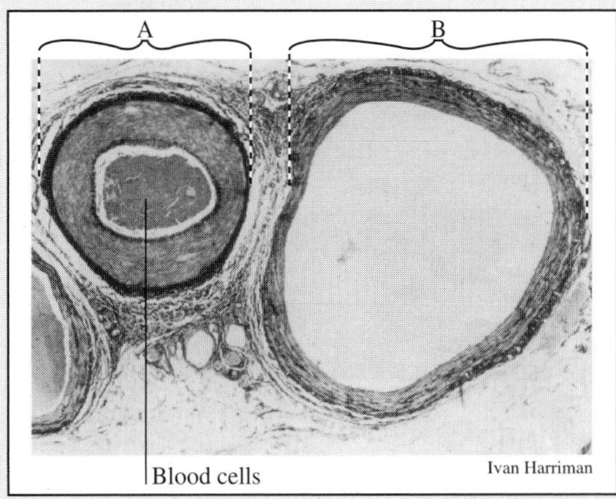

(SEG 92)

7. Describe the route blood will take from entering the heart at the right atrium until it reaches the left ventricle. (8 marks)

Chapter 5

1. (a) The diagram below shows an apparatus which may be used to demonstrate some of the features of the mechanism of breathing.

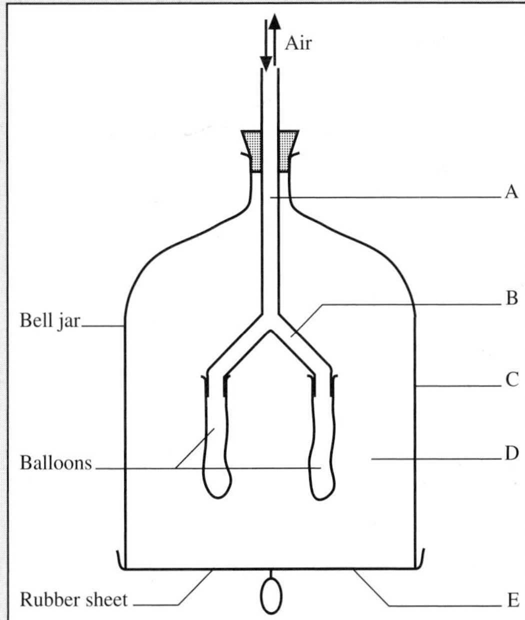

(i) When the rubber sheet is pulled down, a small amount of air enters the balloons, causing them to inflate slightly. Explain the reason for this. (4 marks)

(ii) Name those structures of the thorax which are represented in the apparatus by the letters A to E. (5 marks)

(iii) Briefly describe five ways in which the apparatus is a poor representation of the structure of the thorax. (5 marks)

(b) (i) State two effects which 10 minutes of vigorous exercise will have on breathing. (2 marks)

(ii) Athletic training, involving regular exercise over a period of several weeks, will affect breathing. State one effect which may be produced. (1 mark)

(AEB 81)

2. The graph below represents the lung volume changes based on a number of spirometer readings during various breathing actions.

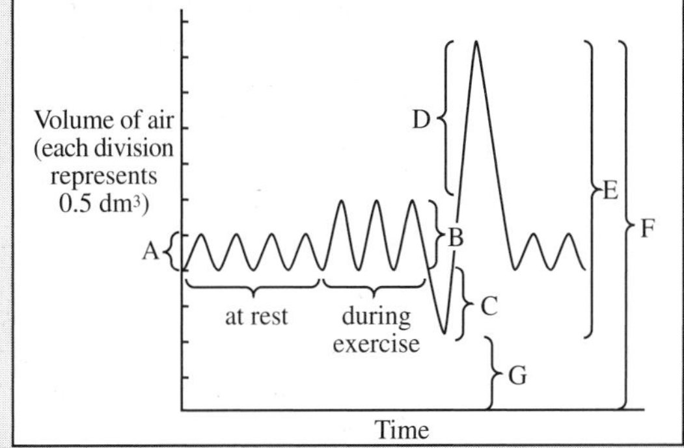

(a) (i) What is meant by the term "tidal volume"? (2 marks)
(ii) Describe concisely an experiment which may be used to measure the volume of a person's tidal air. (3 marks)
(b) State the letter labelling:
(i) Residual air volume
(ii) Vital capacity
iii) Inspiratory reserve volume
(iv) Total lung capacity. (4 marks)
(c) At rest the subject breathes at a rate of 16 breaths per minute. During exercise the subject breathes at a rate of 21 breaths per minute. What volume of air will the subject breathe during:
(i) 5 minutes at rest?
(ii) 2 minutes at exercise? (4 marks)
(d) Describe clearly the role of the diaphragm, ribs, external intercostal muscles and abdominal muscles in bringing about an inflow of air into the lungs during inspiration. (9 marks)
(AEB 82)

3. Describe an experiment you could perform to show that there is more oxygen in the air you breathe in than there is in the air you breathe out. (6 marks)

4. (a) (i) Name the main tube which brings air from the atmosphere to the lungs. (1 mark)
(ii) Name the blood vessel which brings blood to the lungs from the heart. (1 mark)
(b) The diagram shows part of the respiratory (breathing) system and its blood supply.

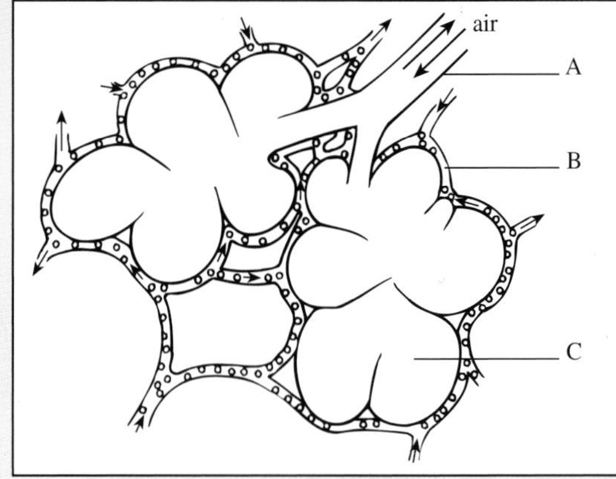

Use the guidelines to label the parts of the respiratory system given below.

alveolus (air sac) bronchiole blood capillary (3 marks)

(c) Use the following terms to complete the table below to show the difference between air breathed in and air breathed out:
more less the same (4 marks)

Type of air	Percentage amount of gas			
	oxygen	carbon dioxide	nitrogen	water vapour
breathed in	20.7	0.04	78.0	low
breathed out				

(MEG 94)

Chapter 6

1. Explain the difference between excretion and defecation. (2 marks)

2. Why would the loop of Henlé in a desert animal be longer than in a human? (2 marks)

3. What is the difference between urea and urine? (2 marks)

4. Explain how the urine composition might vary with:
(a) hot, dry weather. (2 marks)
(b) exercise. (2 marks)
(c) high protein diet. (2 marks)

5. List three differences in blood composition between the renal artery and renal vein. (3 marks)

6.

Substance	Percentage composition	
	Urine	Plasma
Water	96	90
Protein	0	8
Waste nitrogenous compound	2	0.0004
Salts	1.5	0.8
Glucose	0	0.1

(a) Using the table answer the following:
(i) What two items in the table support the view that the kidney is an organ of osmoregulation? (2 marks)
(ii) Why is there 8% of protein in the blood yet none in the urine? (2 marks)
(iii) Name the compound labelled waste nitrogenous compound. (1 mark)
(iv) Where in the body is this produced? (1 mark)
(v) What is the process called that produces it? (1 mark)
(vi) How do the kidneys function to maintain the blood glucose level at approximately 0.1%? (2 marks)
(b) Draw a large fully labelled diagram to show the urinary system plus associated blood vessels. (6 marks)
(c) The diagram (page 233, top left) shows the structure of a nephron.
State the letter which most accurately indicates the position of:
(i) a region of ultra-filtration
(ii) the main region of water re-absorption
(iii) the region controlling the amount of water re-absorbed
(iv) the region of amino acid re-absorption. (4 marks)
(d) Name the parts E and G (2 marks)
(AEB 80)

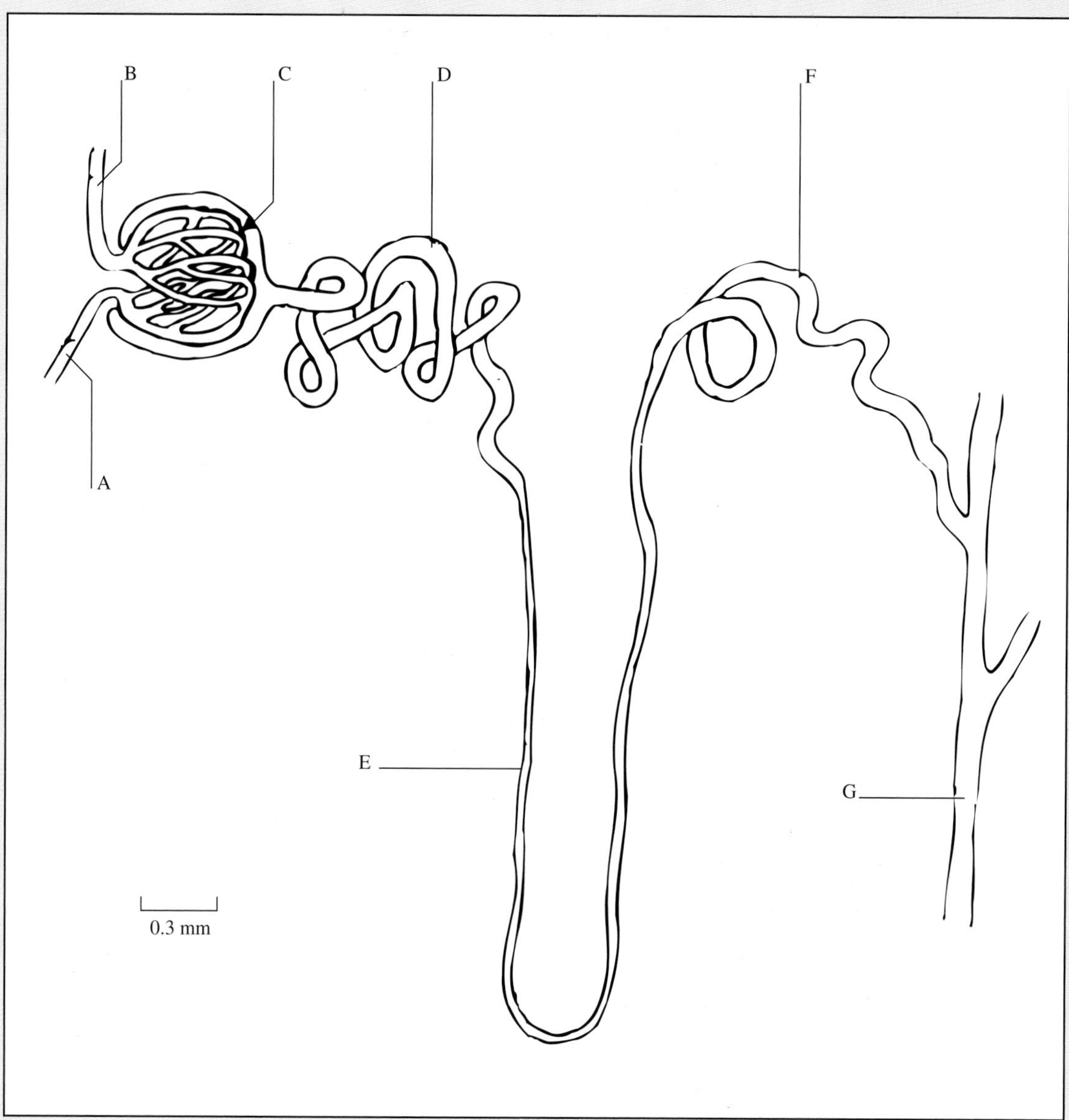

7. (a) Explain briefly how a dialysis machine works. (4 marks)
   (b) Under what circumstances might glucose diffuse from the patient's blood into the dialysis fluid? (1 mark)

8. (a) Draw a fully labelled nephron. (5 marks)
   (b) Using annotations explain how it works. (5 marks)

Chapter 7

1. (a) One of the main functions of the skin is protection. Explain concisely how the skin protects the body against:
   (i) the entry of bacteria
   (ii) dehydration
   (iii) ultra-violet radiation. (6 marks)

   (b) The diagram below represents a 'Heat balance' for the human body.

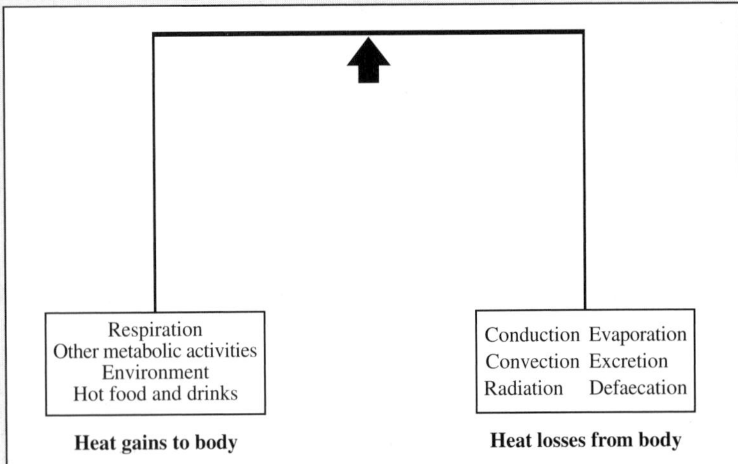

Heat losses and heat gains by the body must be balanced.
   (i) Explain why the maintenance of this balance is essential. (3 marks)
   (ii) Explain how the skin can reduce heat loss by radiation. (3 marks)
   (iii) On a very hot summer's day the skin produces a lot of sweat. Explain the value and consequence of this action. (5 marks)

   (c) Explain why the hands should be washed before handling food. (3 marks)
(AEB 82)

2. The diagrams below show the structure of the upper region of a person's skin (as seen in section). The diagrams show the skin under two different external conditions A and B.

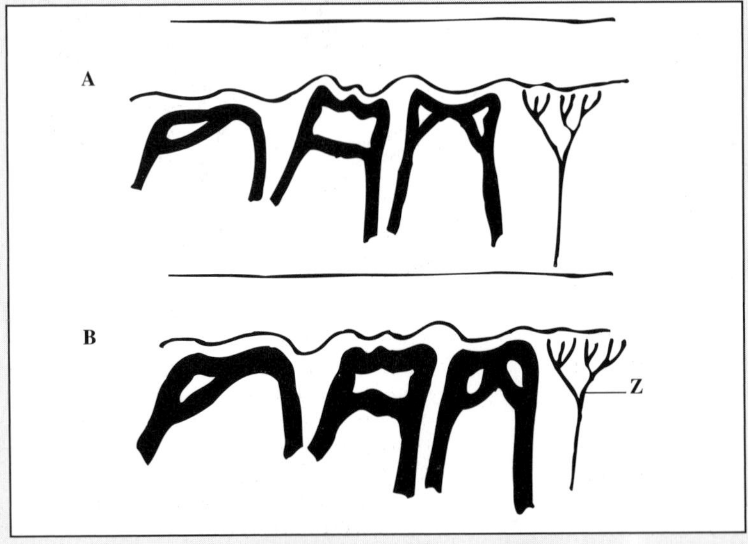

   (a) (i) In which condition does the skin contain the most blood?
   (ii) Explain the reason for your answer. (2 marks)

   (b) One diagram shows the skin at an external temperature of 5°C and the other at a temperature of 25°C.
   (i) Which diagram shows the skin at 5°C?
   (ii) Explain the reason for your answer. (2 marks)

   (c) What part does the structure labelled z have in causing the skin to change as shown in the diagrams? (1 mark)
(SEG 89)

3. The graph below shows how the rate of metabolism of a person varied with the external temperature over a year.

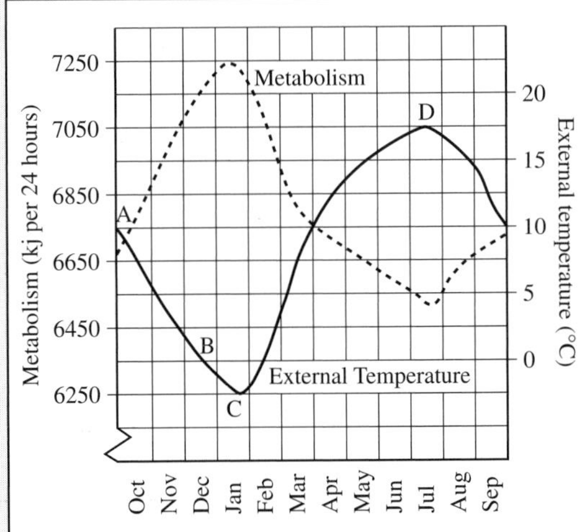

   (a) What general observations may be made about the relationship of the rate of metabolism and external temperature? (1 mark)
   (b) When the external temperature is –2°C, what is the value for the rate of metabolism? (2 marks)
   (c) Suggest the reason for the change in the rate of metabolism as the external temperature falls between points A and B. (2 marks)
   (d) State four ways in which the body may attempt to maintain a constant body temperature when the external temperature is at point C. (4 marks)
   (e) What is the value for the minimum rate of metabolism? (2 marks)
   (f) State and briefly explain one way in which the body may attempt to maintain a constant body temperature when the external temperature is at point D. (3 marks)
(AEB 81)

4. Read the following passage on diabetes and insulin:

Diabetes is an illness in which the body does not produce the hormone insulin. Insulin is a protein which limits the glucose level in the blood. Lack of insulin allows too much stored glycogen to change into glucose. This leads to a high glucose level in the blood. This results in the symptoms of diabetes, which include extreme thirst, passing a lot of urine, blurred vision and weight loss.

Diabetes cannot be cured, but it can be controlled. In cases of severe diabetes, regular injections of insulin are given. The aim is to keep glucose levels as near normal as possible. It is important to control diabetes because, over a long period, a high glucose level can cause problems such as heart disease, gangrene and blindness. However, if too much insulin is injected, a person may become unconscious.

Use your own knowledge and information in the passage to answer the questions below.

(a) Which organ normally produces insulin? (1 mark)
(b) Which organ stores most glycogen? (1 mark)
(c) Which TWO symptoms of diabetes mentioned in the passage could be due to a low level of water retention hormone (ADH) in the blood? Explain your answer. (3 marks)
(d) Suggest why insulin has to be injected rather than taken by mouth. (1 marks)
(e) Suggest an explanation for the effect of injecting too much insulin. (2 marks)

(ULEAC specimen paper)

5. The amount of heat lost from the skin of a naked person depends upon the surrounding temperature. A sudden increase in the amount of heat lost occurs when the person begins to sweat. The diagram shows a section of human skin.

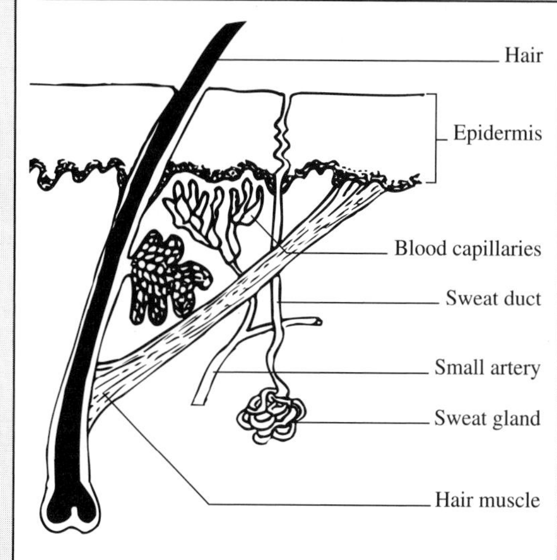

(a) Use the information in the diagram to help explain how sweating causes heat loss from the skin. (5 marks)
(b) Use information in the diagram to help explain how heat loss from the skin can help to cool the body's internal organs. (3 marks)

(ULEAC specimen paper)

Chapter 8

1. (a) The diagram below shows a synovial joint in the skeleton.

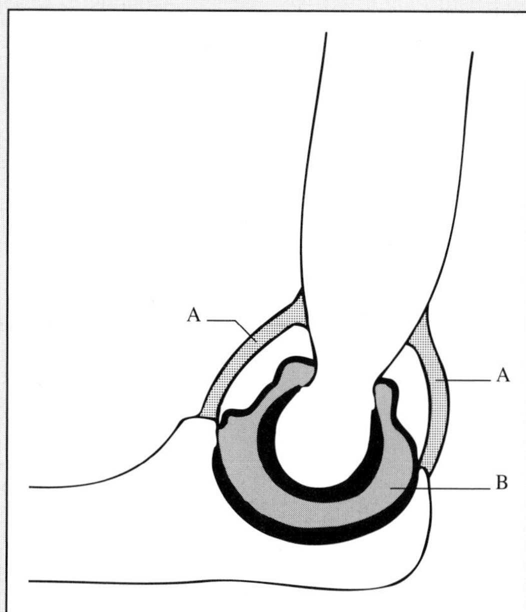

(i) Give one property of the tissue which protects the articulating surfaces. (1 mark)
(ii) What is the function of the material which fills the space labelled B? (1 mark)
(iii) Give two properties of the tissue labelled A. (2 marks)

(b) The diagram shows two lumbar vertebrae as they would be joined in the vertebral column.

(i) What passes through the cavity labelled X in the living body? (1 mark)
(ii) What is the function of the projection labelled Y? (1 mark)
(iii) What is the function of the structure labelled Z? (1 mark)

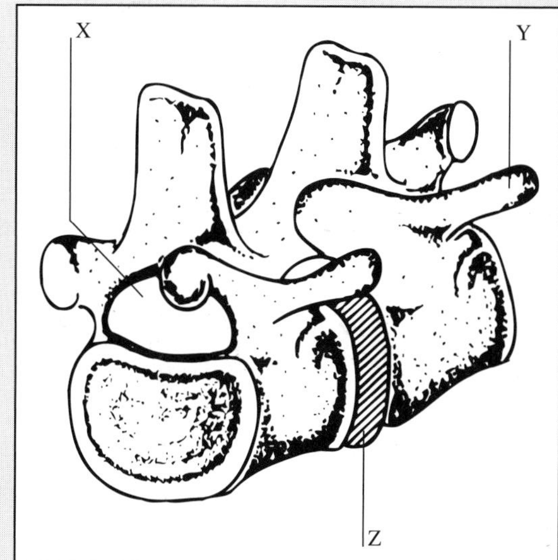

(c) The diagram (page 236, top left) the outline of a runner with the main arm and leg bones shaded. The letters refer to the position of pairs of muscles in the legs and arms.

(i) Describe how the pairs of muscles have brought about the positions of the left arm and right and left legs. (4 marks)

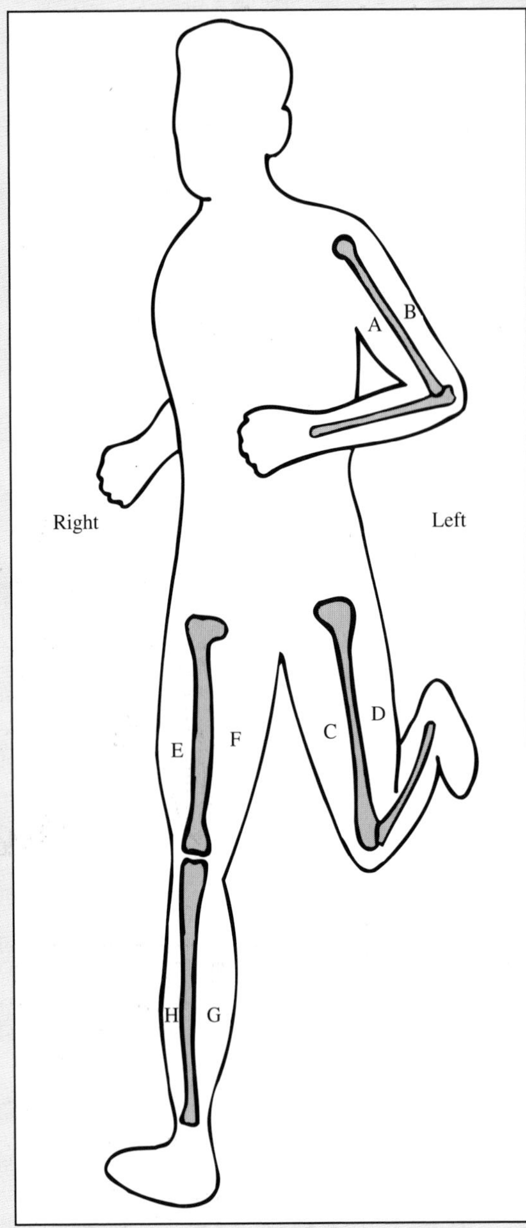

(ii) Which muscle must contract to move the body forward from the runner's position in the diagram? (1 mark)
(SEG 88)

2. The diagram below represents a generalised vertebra.

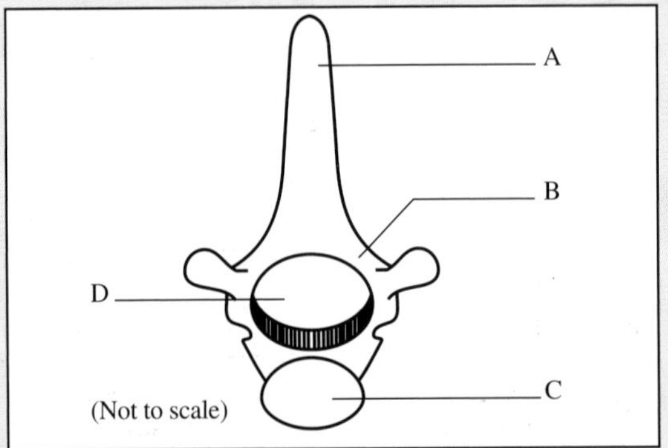

(a) State the skeletal functions of A, B and C. (3 marks)

(b) Which organ occupies space D? (1 mark)
(AEB 87)

3. (a) The photograph below shows an X-ray of a hip which has had an artificial replacement of the joint.

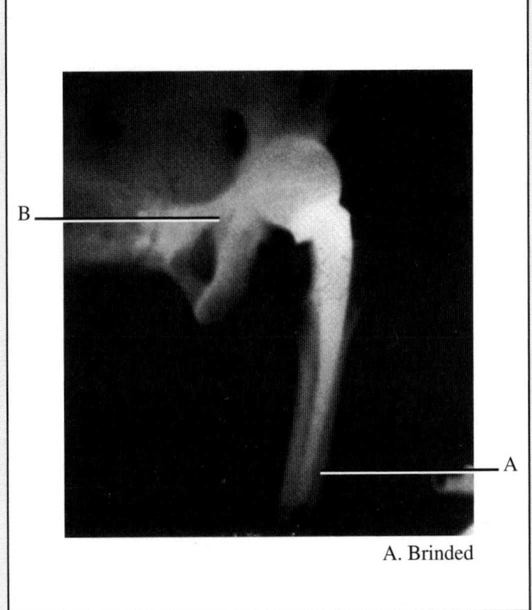

A. Brinded

(i) Name bones A and B. (2 marks)

(ii) State one of the functions of bone A. (1 mark)

(iii) What two substances are usually present at the hip joint to reduce friction and allow easy movement? (2 marks)

(iv) Suggest a reason why a person's hip joint may need to be replaced in old age. (1 mark)

(b) The diagram below shows the artificial hip (ball and socket) in detail.

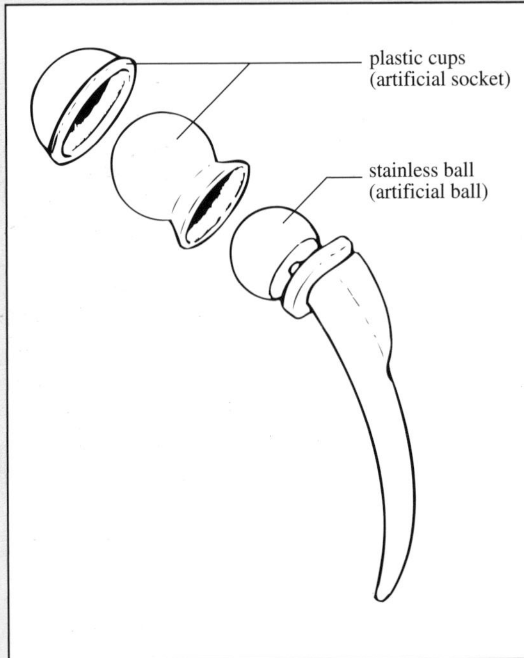

(i) Suggest three reasons why the ball and socket are made from materials such as metal and plastic. (3 marks)

(ii) How is the degree of movement allowed by the ball and socket at the hip different to movement at the elbow? (2 marks)

(c) Read the passage below carefully and then answer the questions that follow:

'Kim was a very active 12-year old when her hip problem was discovered. She had inherited a condition which causes the ends of the bones in her hips to be shaped abnormally. This means that the ball does not move smoothly in the socket. It is a painful condition and will probably get worse. Her doctors decided that a hip replacement was necessary but they did not want to operate immediately.'

(i) Give two reasons why hip replacement was felt to be necessary. (2 marks)

(ii) Using your biological knowledge, explain why the operation needs to be delayed. (2 marks)

(SEG 93)

4. The drawing below shows the bones in the right hand of an adult human. Two muscles are shown, both of which can move the thumb.

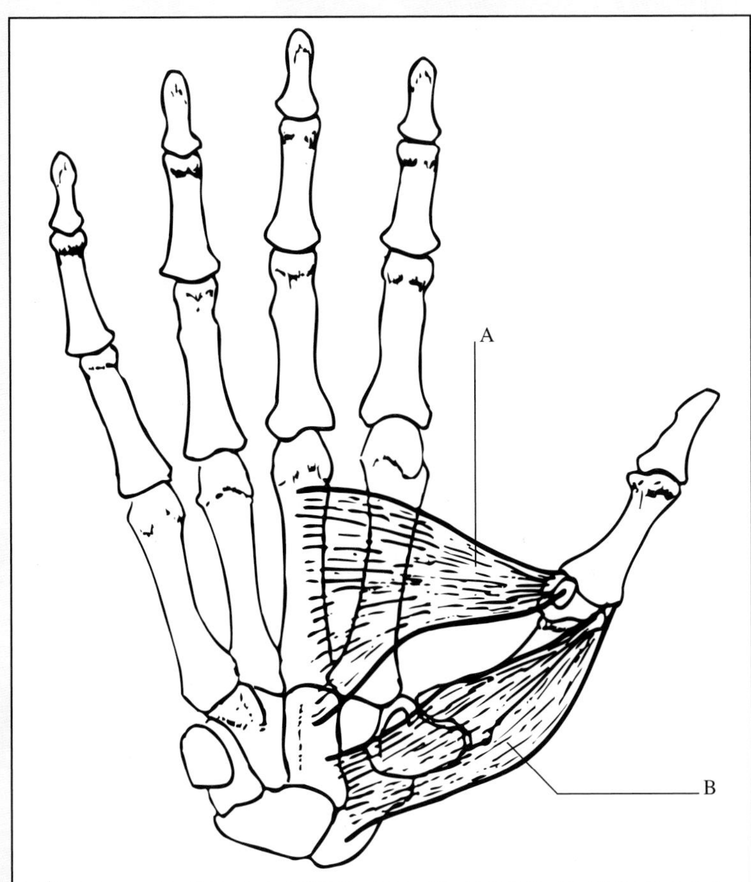

(a) (i) Which of the muscles shown will pull the thumb towards the fingers? (1 mark)

(ii) What will the other muscle do whilst this is happening? (1 mark)

(b) Explain why there must be two muscles to move the thumb. (2 marks)

(SEG 89)

5. (a) The diagram below shows the position of the human foot bones whilst wearing high-heeled shoes. Examine the picture carefully, and then answer the questions that follow.

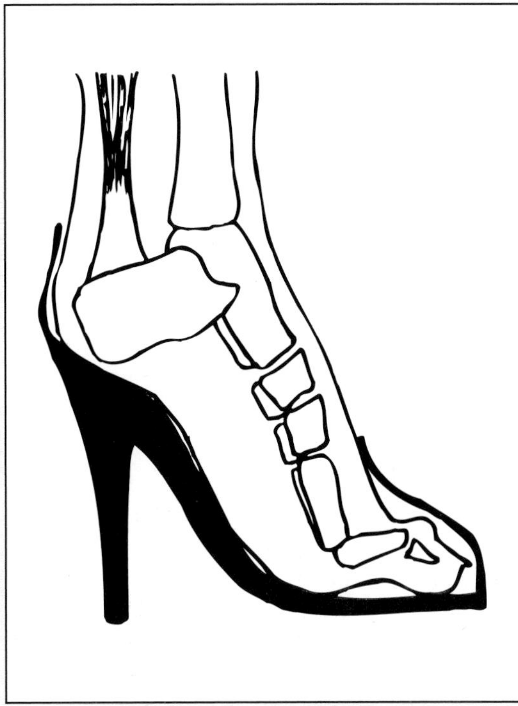

(i) Suggest two ways in which high-heeled shoes can damage feet. (2 marks)

(ii) What damage can wearing high-heels cause to the wearer's body other than to the feet? (2 marks)

(iii) Why is it important for young children to wear shoes that fit correctly? (2 marks)

(b) When lifting a heavy object, the back should be kept as straight as possible. This can be achieved by bending the knees, grasping the object firmly and straightening the legs. Explain how a failure to do this can damage the vertebral column and spinal cord. (3 marks)

(c) Draw and label a typical synovial joint. State the function of two of the parts you have labelled. (6 marks)

(SEG 90)

6. (a) What is muscle tone? (1 mark)

(b) What are the benefits of good muscle tone? (2 marks)

(c) What are the advantages of correct posture? (3 marks)

(d) Why should you lift heavy objects as close to the body as possible? (2 marks)

(e) State three other rules for safe lifting. (3 marks)

7. Copy the blank skeleton (page 238) and label:

(a) as many bones as you can. (5 marks)

(b) (i) two hinge joints

(ii) two ball and socket joints. (4 marks)

Chapter 9

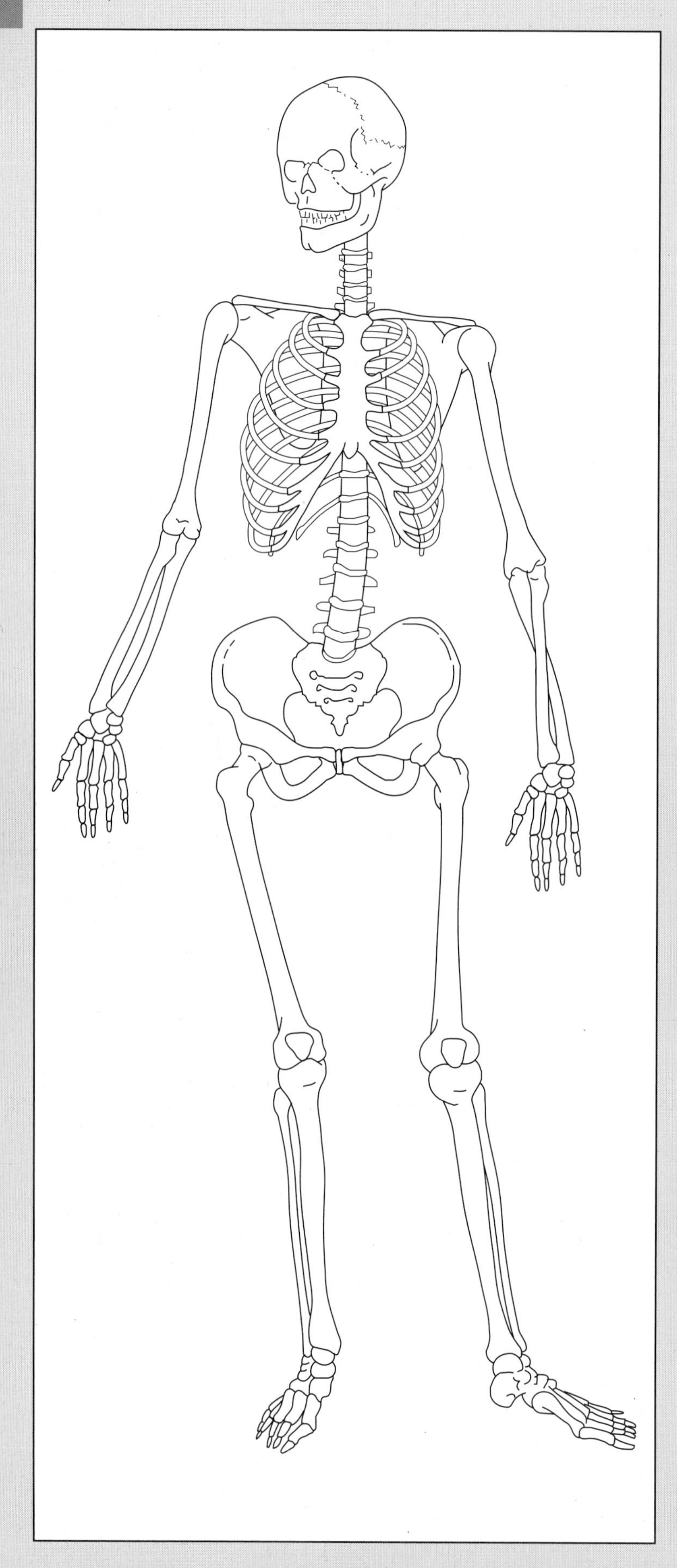

1. (a) The diagram (page 239, top) represents a simple reflex arc.
   Which letter is the label for:
   (i) the grey matter
   (ii) the ventral root
   (iii) a mixed nerve
   (iv) an effector
   (v) a motor neurone? (5 marks)

   (b) (i) When the finger is pricked by the pin the stimulus sets up a nerve impulse. Explain briefly how this impulse passes from the receptor to neurone F. (4 marks)
   (ii) If the subject had consumed a quantity of alcohol before pricking their finger how would this have affected their response? (2 marks)

   (c) The diagram below is a sectional view of the brain.

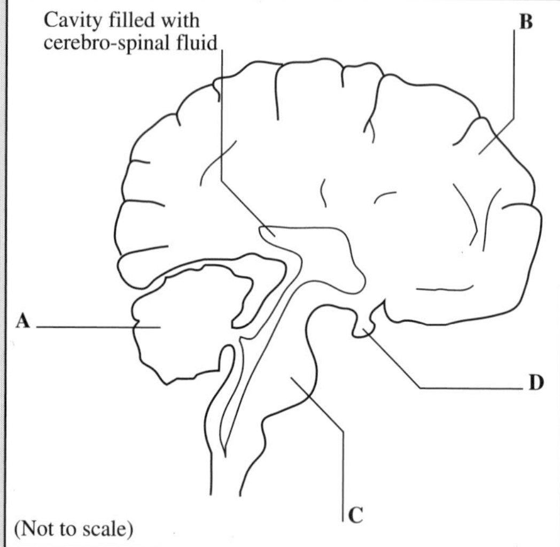

   (i) Briefly describe the main functions of the parts labelled A, B and C. (3 marks)
   (ii) Name the part labelled D. (1 mark)
   (iii) Briefly describe the ways in which the brain is protected from physical damage. (3 marks)
   (iv) The region labelled B is deeply folded. What advantage does this feature have? (2 marks)
   (AEB 87)

2. (a) Explain what is meant by a reflex action. (2 marks)
   (b) A primitive reflex found in a new-born baby is called the rooting reflex which occurs when the baby's cheek is touched: the baby turns its head in the direction of the touch. Suggest how this may benefit a new-born baby. (2 marks)

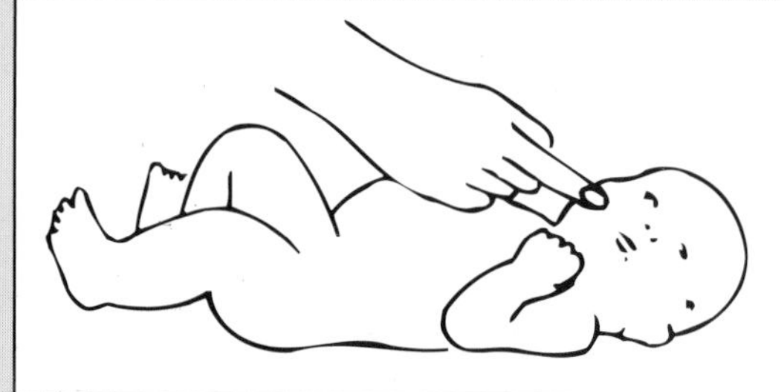

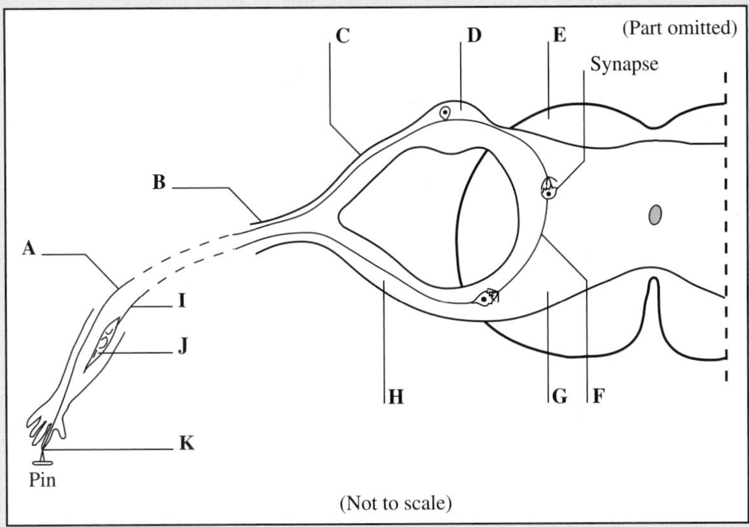

(c) Describe, without the aid of diagrams, the pathway of the knee-jerk reflex from stimulus to response. (6 marks)

(d) The following information was recorded at a hospital before and after a patient had brain surgery. The chart shows the size of the patient's pupils and whether or not they react to light (+ or –); it also shows the amount of limb movement (a dot is for both limbs).

(i) What happens to the size of the pupils after the operation? (2 marks)

(ii) Which arm loses power after the operation? (1 mark)

(iii) Why is it necessary to record the left side of the body separately from the right side? (2 marks)

			TIME 10.00	18.00	Operation	14.00	14.30	15.00	15.30	16.00	16.30	17.00	17.30	18.00			
PUPILS	right	Size (mm)	3	3		4	4	3	3	3	3	3	3	3			+ reacts – no reaction c. eye closed by swelling
		Reaction	+	+		+	+	+	+	+	+	+	+	+			
	left	Size (mm)	3	3		4	4	3	3	3	3	3	3	3			
		Reaction	+	+		+	+	+	+	+	+	+	+	+			
LIMB MOVEMENT	ARMS	Normal power	●	●		●	●	●	R	R	R	R	●	●			Record right (R) and left (L) separately if there is a difference between the two sides
		Mild weakness							L	L	L	L					
		Severe weakness															
		Spastic flexion															
		Extension															
		No response															
	LEGS	Normal power	●	●		●	●	●	R	R	R	R	●	●			
		Mild weakness							L	L	L	L					
		Severe weakness															
		Extension															
		No response															

(SEG 91)

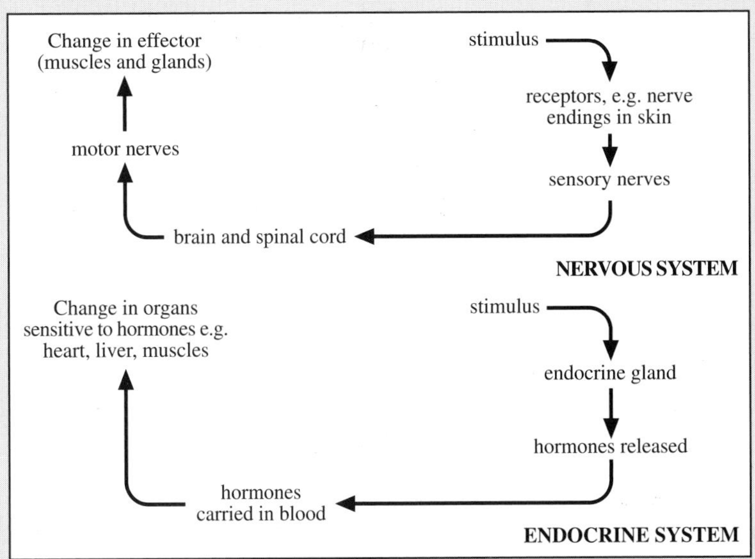

3. The body is controlled and co-ordinated by the nervous system and by the endocrine (hormone) system. The diagrams show the main features of these two systems.

Using the information from the diagrams only:

(i) give two ways in which these systems are similar; (2 marks)

(ii) give one way in which these systems are different. (1 mark)

(SEG 90)

Chapter 10

1. (a) The diagram below shows a vertical section through part of the human eye.

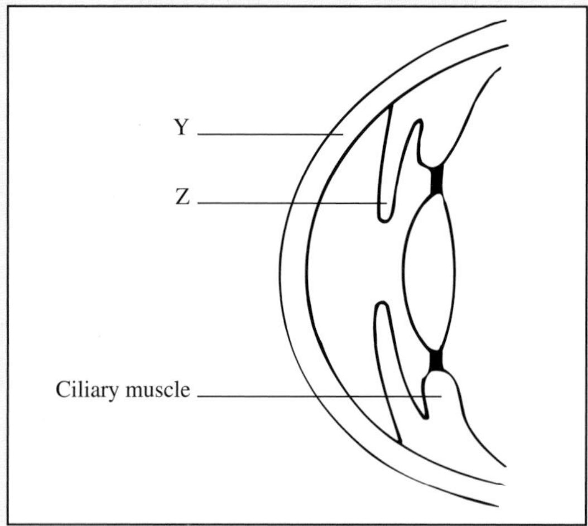

(i) Name parts labelled Y and Z. (2 marks)
(ii) Describe how the ciliary muscle brings about changes in the shape of the lens. (4 marks)

(b) Read the passage and then answer the questions that follow:

'Sometimes the eye lens becomes clouded – a disease called a cataract. This causes blurred vision and eventually blindness. The problem usually occurs in old age and is particularly common in developing countries. In India 5.5 million people are unable to see because they have cataracts. The cure is simple – remove the clouded lens and fit the patient with glasses. However, there are few eye hospitals in India and most patients cannot afford the treatment.

One solution to this problem has been the setting up of Eye Camps, where a tent or local building is turned into a clinic. A temporary operating theatre is set up and patients are examined and treated. Surgeons may operate on up to 200 patients in a day, removing a diseased lens in five minutes. Ten days later the bandages are removed and the patient is fitted with glasses – their sight restored.'

(i) What is a cataract? (1 mark)
(ii) Explain how a cataract causes blurred vision and blindness. (2 marks)
(iii) State two reasons why India still has a large percentage of its population suffering from cataracts. (2 marks)
(iv) What action is being taken to reduce the number of people suffering from cataracts? (2 marks)
(v) Why are glasses needed after an operation to remove a cataract? (2 marks)

(SEG 92)

2. (a) A person is reading the programme at a football match and looks up to watch a player score a goal.

(i) Explain the changes that take place in the person's eye so that a focused image of the goal can be formed on the retina. (4 marks)
(ii) Explain the functions of the retina and the optic nerve in communicating information about the goal to the brain. (3 marks)

(b) The graph below shows the number of rod and cone cells in the human retina at different distances across the retina.

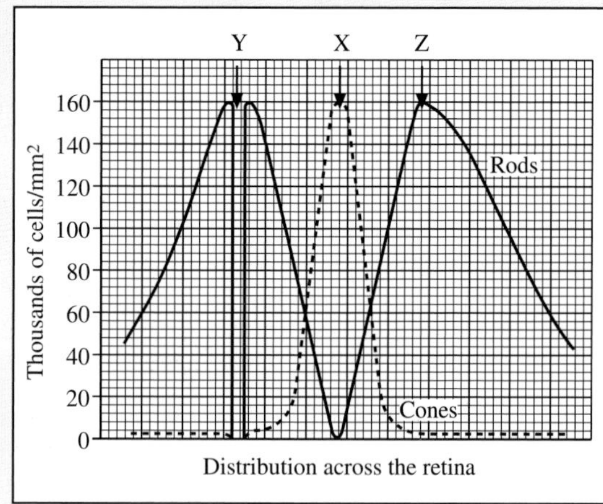

(i) What is the density of cones found at point X on the retina? (1 mark)
(ii) What is the name given to part of the retina that has this high density of cones? (1 mark)
(iii) At point Y on the retina there are neither rods nor cones. What is this point called and why are there no light detecting cells here? (2 marks)
(iv) A person wishes to see a very faint star and looks slightly to the side of the star so that the image falls on point Z on the retina. Why does this give the best chance of seeing the star? (2 marks)
(v) Explain why it would not be possible to tell the colour of the star if viewed in this way. (2 marks)

(SEG 94)

3. (a) Draw a large clearly labelled diagram of the middle and inner ear. (7 marks)
(b) Explain concisely how vibrations of the oval window lead to nerve impulses being transmitted along the auditory nerve. (6 marks)
(c) Explain why an infection in the auditory tube (Eustachian tube) may lead to temporary deafness. (4 marks)
(d) The figure below represents a sectional view of an ampulla. Explain concisely how the structures shown detect movement of the head. (3 marks)

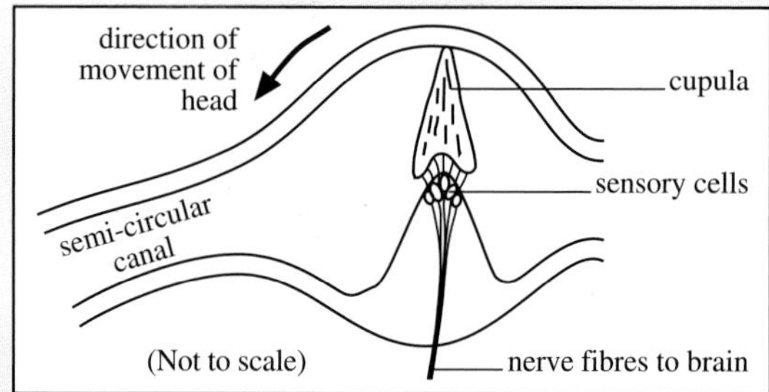

(AEB 83)

Chapter 11

1. The following passage is based on the instructions that accompany a commonly used combined oral contraceptive pill. Read it and answer the questions that follow.

Combined oral contraceptives reduce the risks of cancers of the ovary and the lining of the womb (endometrium) by up to a half. Benign (non-malignant) breast disease is greatly reduced. Generally, irregular periods are replaced by regular bleeding, and heavy periods by lighter bleeding. Painful periods are in most cases abolished. The symptoms that often make the last few days before a period so unpleasant (known as the premenstrual syndrome) are commonly eliminated.

There is a general opinion, based on statistical evidence, that users of combined oral contraceptives experience more often than non-users various disorders of the circulation of blood, including strokes (blood clots in, and haemorrhages from, the blood-vessels of the brain), heart attacks (coronary thromboses) and blood clots obstructing the arteries of the lungs (pulmonary emboli). There might not be full recovery from such disorders and it should be realised that in a few cases they are fatal. How often these disorders occur in users of modern low-dose oral contraceptives is not known, but there are reasons for suggesting that they may occur less often than with older pills.

(a) Give four benefits of taking a combined oral contraceptive pill. (4 marks)

(b) Why do you think taking the pill generally causes irregular periods to be replaced by regular ones? (2 marks)

(c) Rewrite the first sentence of the second paragraph so as to make it easier to understand. (4 marks)

(d) Imagine you are the parent of a 14 year-old who has exceptionally painful periods. How would you feel if her GP suggested she went on the pill to reduce the pain? (2 marks)

2. (a) The diagram (below left) shows a sectional view of the male reproductive system.

(i) Explain how the structure labelled W changes to allow sexual intercourse to take place. (3 marks)

(ii) List the following structures in increasing order of size, as shown on the diagram:
BLADDER
PROSTATE GLAND
TESTIS (2 marks)

(iii) What evidence does the diagram give about the age of the person whose reproductive system is drawn? Explain your answer. (2 marks)

(iv) Name part Z. (1 mark)

(b) The diagram below shows a sperm cell and an egg cell (ovum).

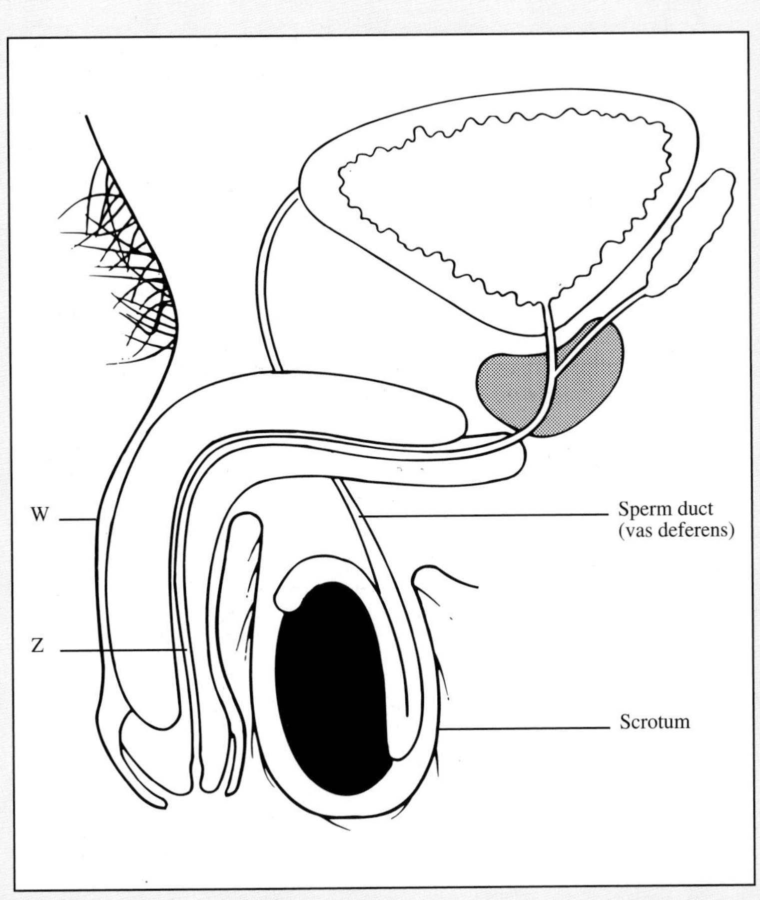

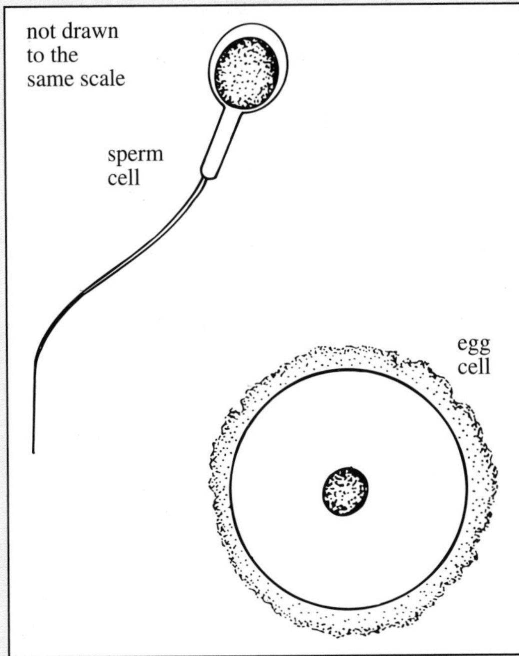

(i) State two differences, visible in the diagram, between the two cells. (2 marks)

(ii) State one similarity, not visible in the diagram, between the two cells. (2 marks)

(c) Explain the term 'fertilisation'. (3 marks)

(SEG 93)

3. (a) State one function for each of the following parts

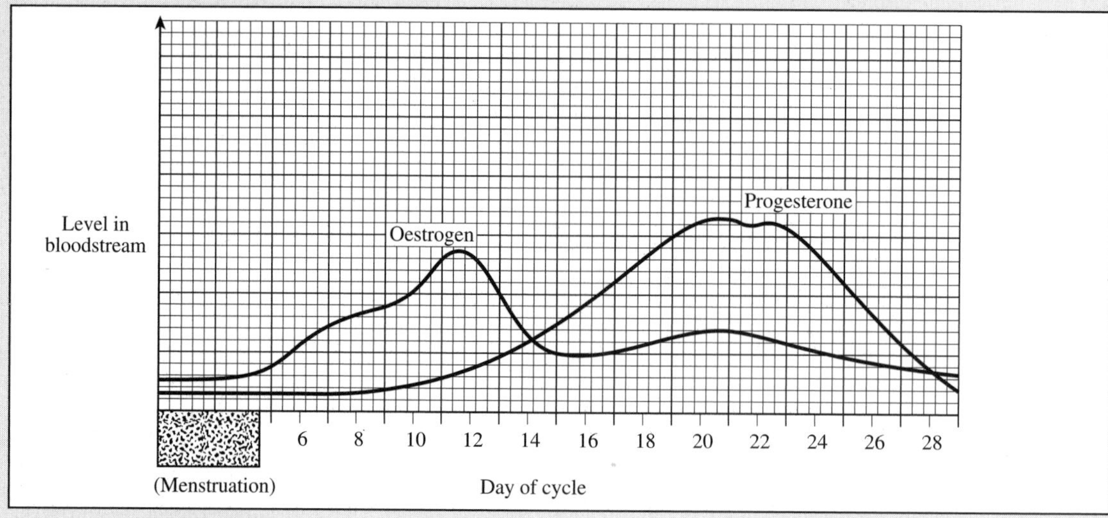

of the male reproductive system:
(i) the scrotum
(ii) the prostate gland
(iii) the penis. (3 marks)

(b) The graph above shows how the levels of oestrogen and progesterone change throughout the female menstrual cycle.
(i) What term describes both oestrogen and progesterone? (1 mark)
(ii) What happens to the level of progesterone immediately after day 14? Explain what causes this. (3 marks)
(iii) State the effects of these changing levels of oestrogen and progesterone in the menstrual cycle. (4 marks)

(c) The diagram shows a vertical section through the uterus lining. Using only features from the diagram, explain how its structure makes it suitable to receive a fertilized ovum (egg cell). (4 marks)

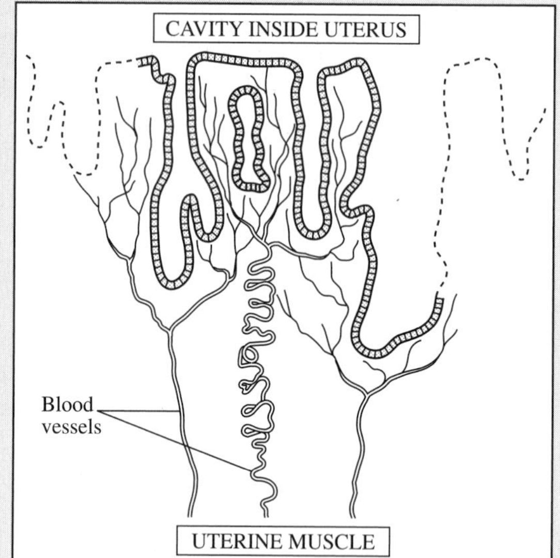

(SEG 91)

Chapter 12

1. (a) The diagrams (page 243, top)show three of four stages in the process of amniocentesis.
Stage one also shows ultra scanning taking place. This instrument uses sound waves to create an image of the inside of the uterus. This image is shown on a television monitor.
(i) What is visible, apart from the embryo (fetus), on the television monitor screen? (1 mark)
(ii) Describe in the order shown each stage in the process of amniocentesis. Draw a labelled diagram if it helps you to describe stage 3. (8 marks)

(b) The drawings (page 243, bottom) show the chromosomes of two nuclei, A and B, of embryo cells removed from the uterus of a woman at the same time.
(i) What is the normal diploid number of chromosomes in a human nucleus? (1 mark)
(ii) Do the drawings show a normal or an abnormal number of chromosomes for each human nucleus? (1 mark)

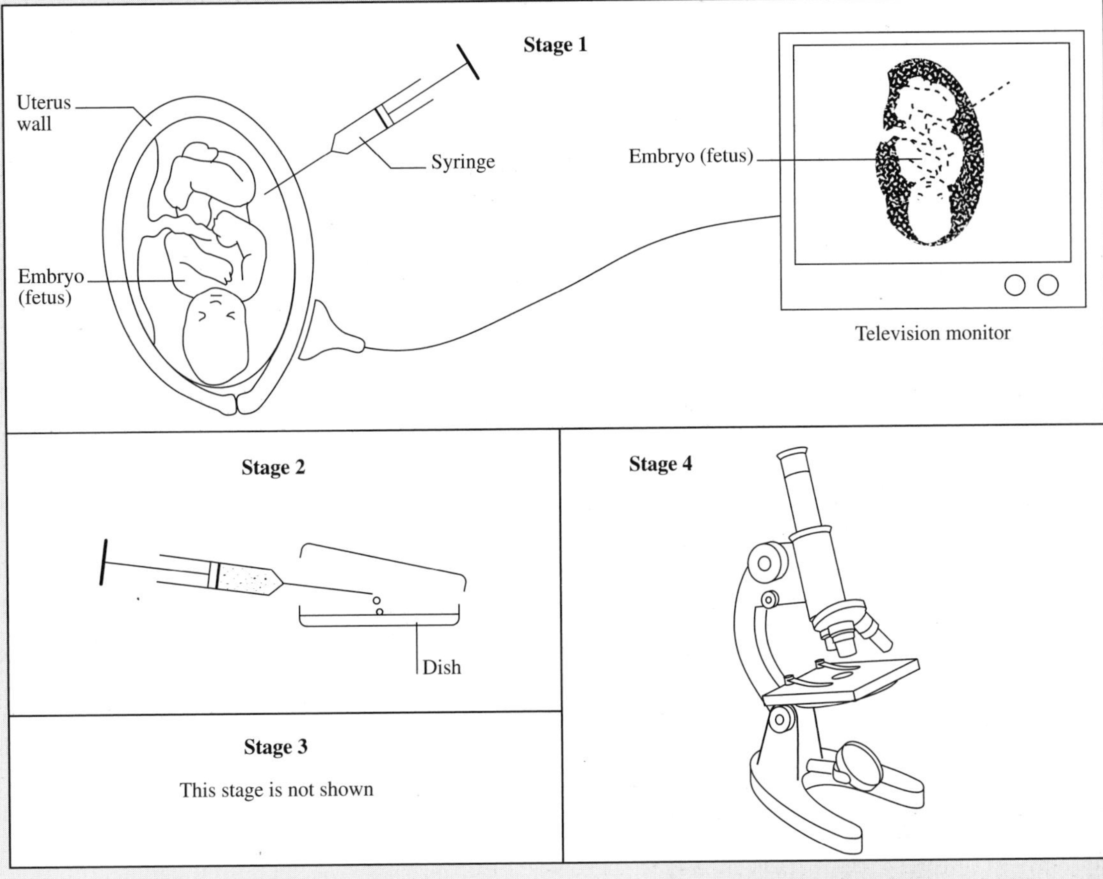

(iii) Name ONE condition in which a human has one extra chromosome in each nucleus. (1 mark)

(iv) Which other important facts about this pregnancy are evident in the drawings? (2 marks)

(v) State the number of sperm and ova involved in fertilisation leading to this pregnancy. (1 mark)

(ULEAC 93)

Chromosomes of nucleus A	Chromosomes of nucleus B
X X	X Y

Chapter 13

1. Some students decided to investigate growth in humans by recording the heights of males and females at different ages. Their results are shown in Tables 1 and 2.

TABLE 1

Heights of 12 year old students					
student	sex	height/cm	student	sex	height/cm
1	male	157	11	male	146
2	female	151	12	female	158
3	male	142	13	female	146
4	male	155	14	female	153
5	female	158	15	male	155
6	female	143	16	male	141
7	male	162	17	female	159
8	male	139	18	female	158
9	female	159	19	female	149
10	male	154	20	male	147

(a) (i) What was the height of the shortest student? (1 mark)

(ii) What was the sex of the tallest student? (1 mark)

(iii) Using data from Table 1, calculate the average (mean) height of the 12 year old girls. Use your answer to complete Table 2. (4 marks)

TABLE 2

Age/years	Average heights of students/cm	
	males	females
12	149.8	-----
14	166.7	163.1
16	176.4	167.4
18	181.1	170.2

(b) (i) Using the data in Table 2 draw line graphs, on the single set of axes provided, to show the average heights of males and of females between the ages of 12 and 18 years old. Use the scales indicated. (5 marks)

(ii) At which age are males and females the same height? (1 mark)

(iii) Between which ages do females seem to be growing fastest? (1 mark)

(c) Suggest a reason why the average height of twelve year old females is greater than the average height of males of the same age. (1 mark)

(MEG 93)

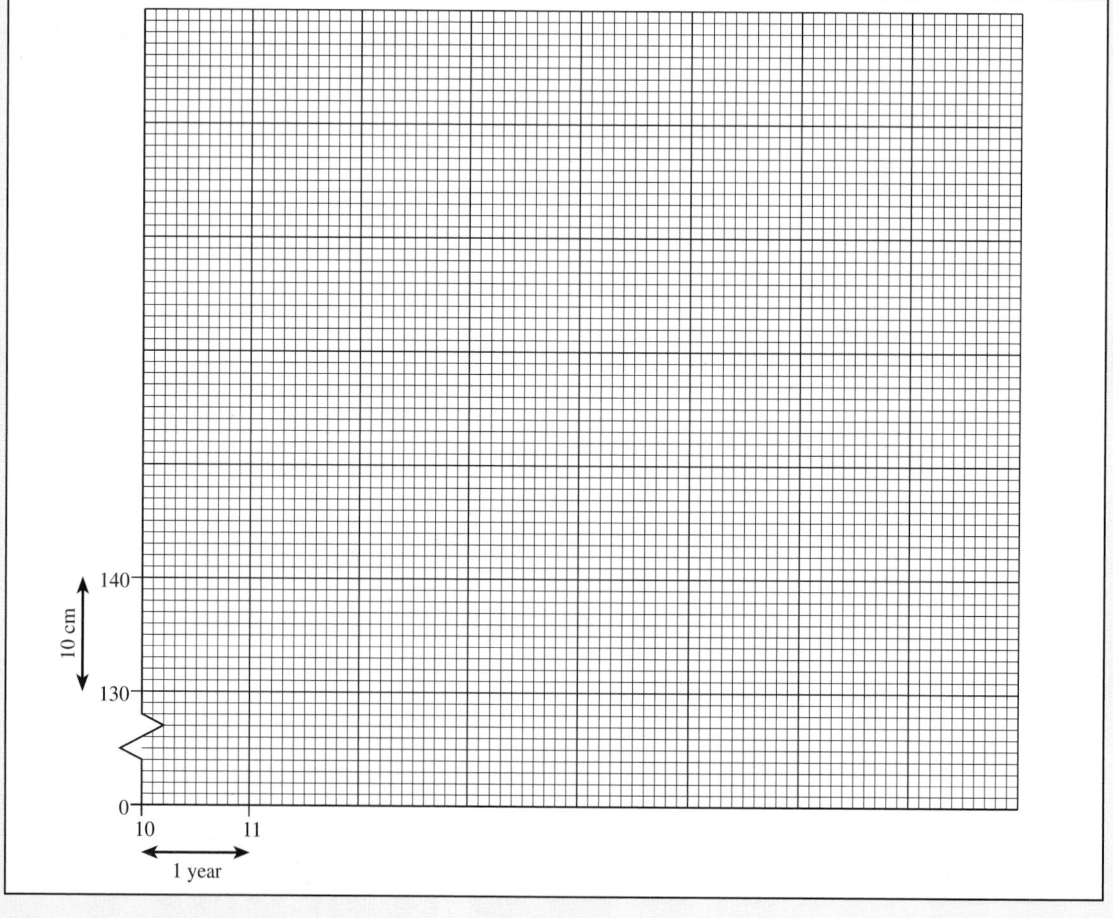

Chapter 14

Note: Some questions require knowledge of the appropriate parts of Chapters 3, 4 and 5.

1. Table 1 gives some information about the nutritional content of a traditional beefburger and of a similar non-meat vegetable burger. Vegetable burgers are made from a mycoprotein, coloured and flavoured to taste like beef.

TABLE 1

Contents per 100g	Beefburger	Vegetable burger
energy	1192 kJ	970 kJ
protein	15.0 g	18.5 g
carbohydrate	3.7 g	11.7 g
fat	23.8 g	12.7 g
sodium **	0.5 g	1.3 g
fibre	0.4 g	4.5 g

** mostly as sodium chloride

(a) (i) Which 'burger' has the higher protein content per 100 g? (1 mark)
(ii) How much protein is present in 120 g of beefburger? (1 mark)
(iii) In which organ of the body are carbohydrates stored? (1 mark)
(iv) Name the carbohydrate which is stored in this organ. (1 mark)
(b) State TWO reasons why a person who is anxious to eat a healthy diet might choose the vegetable burger rather than the beefburger. Give an explanation for the choice in each case. (4 marks)
(MEG 94)

2. The table below shows the energy needed each day by members of the Smith family. Tom and Lucy are twins.

Smith family	Energy needed in kilojoules per day
Cindy (new born baby)	1 800
Tom (10 years)	8 200
Lucy (10 years)	9 400
Mrs Smith (breast feeding mother)	11 400
Mr Smith (coal miner)	15 000

Use the information given to help you answer the following.
(a) Which member of the family needs the most energy per day? (1 mark)
(b) Which food supplies Cindy with her energy? (1 mark)
(c) How much energy would Mrs Smith need when not breast feeding? Show your working. (2 marks)
(d) Suggest two reasons why Lucy needs more energy than Tom even though they are twins. (2 marks)
(e) If Mr Smith takes in approximately 17 000 kilojoules per day, what effect may this have? (1 mark)
(ULEAC 93)

3. (a) The table below compares cigarette smoking by British men and women between the years 1972 and 1984, based upon a survey of about 20 000 people each year. All figures given are percentages. Use the table to answer the questions which follow.

MEN:	1972	1974	1976	1978	1980	1982	1984
Regular cigarette smokers:							
Light (under 20 per day)	28	25	22	22	21	20	20
Heavy (more than 20 per day)	24	26	24	23	21	18	16
Total regular cigarette smokers	52	51	46	45	42	38	36
Ex-regular cigarette smokers	23	23	27	27	28	30	30
Non smokers or occasional smokers	25	25	27	29	30	32	34
WOMEN:	**1972**	**1974**	**1976**	**1978**	**1980**	**1982**	**1984**
Regular cigarette smokers:							
Light (under 20 per day)	30	28	24	23	23	22	22
Heavy (more than 20 per day)	11	13	14	13	13	11	10
Total regular cigarette smokers	41	41	38	36	36	33	32
Ex-regular cigarette smokers	10	11	12	14	14	16	17
Non smokers or occasional smokers	49	49	50	49	49	51	51

(i) Which group regularly smoked the most – men or women? (1 mark)
(ii) Compare the results for light and heavy smoking. (3 marks)
(iii) What has happened to the number of male regular smokers between the years 1972 and 1984? Suggest a reason for your answer. (3 marks)
(b) Name two smoking related illnesses. (2 marks)
(c) Describe how smoking can have an adverse effect on other people who are non-smokers. (1 mark)
(SEG 95/96 Sample papers)

4. The figure below shows activities commonly carried out in a laboratory. Identify the hazard in each situation and say what the student should have done before starting the activity.
Activity A (2 marks)
Activity B (2 marks)
Activity C (2 marks)
Activity D (2 marks)
(MEG 94)

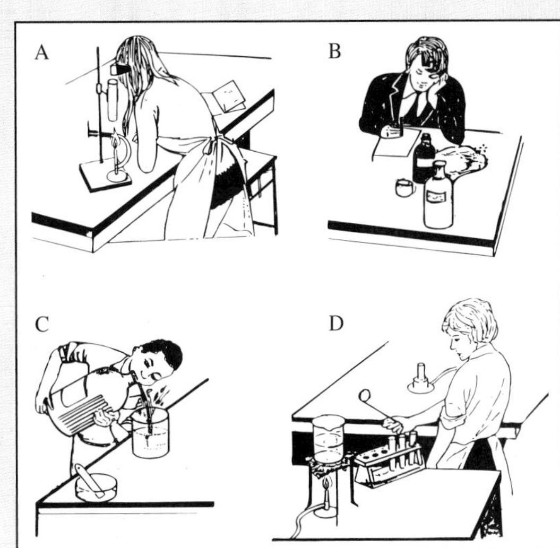

Chapter 15

1. Nadia and Peter showed the symptoms of an illness caused by Bacterium X. The graph below shows the average number of Bacteria X per 10 cm³ of blood in these two people over two weeks.

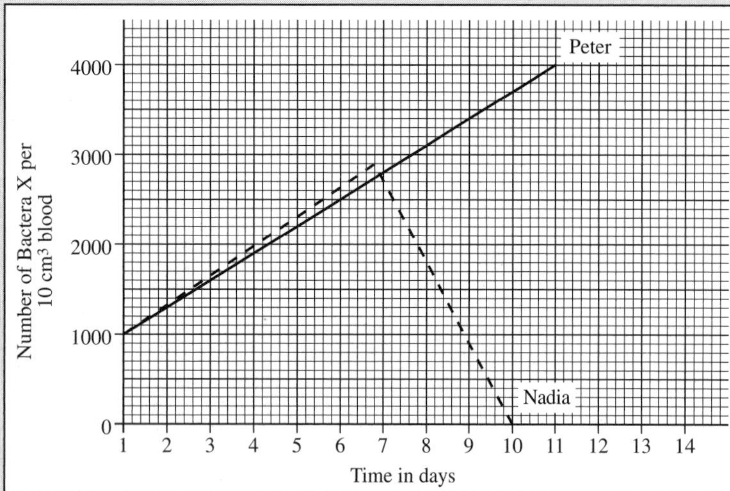

Use the information in the graph and your own knowledge to answer the following questions.

(a) (i) How many Bacteria X were there in 10 cm³ of Peter's blood on day 3? (1 mark)

(ii) When did both patients have the same number of Bacteria X? (2 marks)

(b) (i) Which blood cells can defend the body from invading bacteria? (1 mark)

(ii) Describe how they defend the body. (2 marks)

(c) One of the patients was suspected of having AIDS. Name this patient. Give a reason for your answer. (2 marks)

(d) (i) Which type of microbe causes AIDS? (1 mark)

(ii) Describe ONE way in which AIDS is transmitted. (1 mark)

(ULEAC 93, Biology (Human), Paper 1)

2. Fig. 1 shows *Plasmodium*. It lives in the salivary glands of a mosquito. When humans become infected with this organism they may develop malaria.

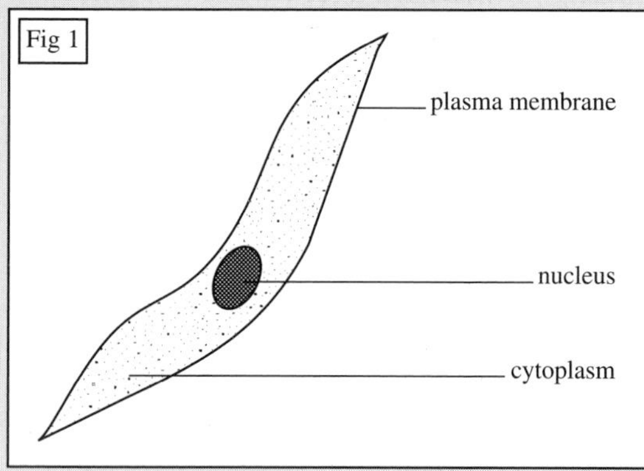

(a) (i) To which group does *Plasmodium* belong? (1 mark)

(ii) Give a reason for your choice. (1 mark)

(b) What type of nutrition is used by *Plasmodium*? Explain your answers. (2 marks)

(c) Female mosquitoes need blood. Suggest how *Plasmodium* gets into the human body. (2 marks)

Fig. 2 is a map of Africa showing where malaria is found.

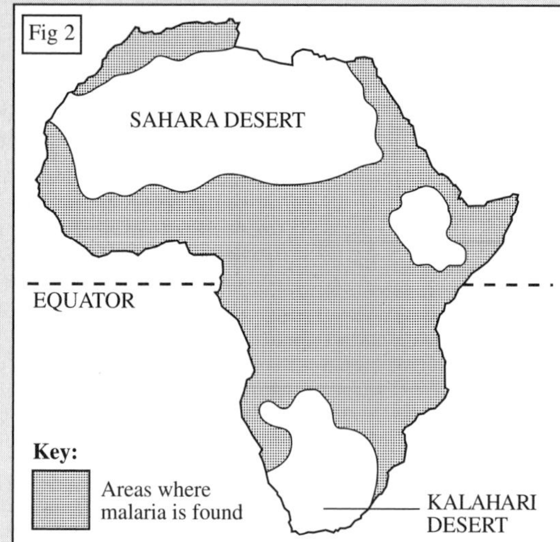

(d) Suggest why a person is unlikely to be infected with malaria in a dry area such as the Sahara desert. (2 marks)

(MEG 94)

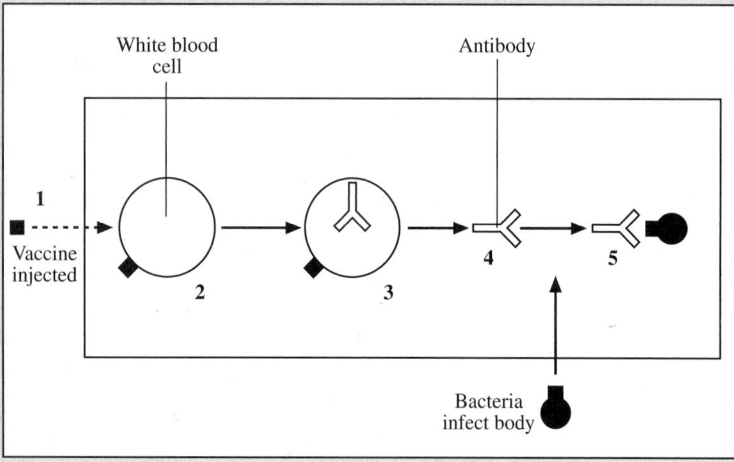

Chapter 16

1. (a) Several stages are involved when a person is immunised against a disease. Some of these stages are shown here in a very simple way.

(i) What is a vaccine? (1 mark)

(ii) Briefly describe, using information shown in the diagram, what happens following the vaccine to make the person immune to a disease. (6 marks)

(b) Certain diseases, such as the common cold and influenza, are spread by droplet infection. Frequently large numbers of people have to work together in the same room. Suggest three ways in which droplet infection in such a situation can be reduced. (3 marks)

(SEG 95/96 Sample papers)

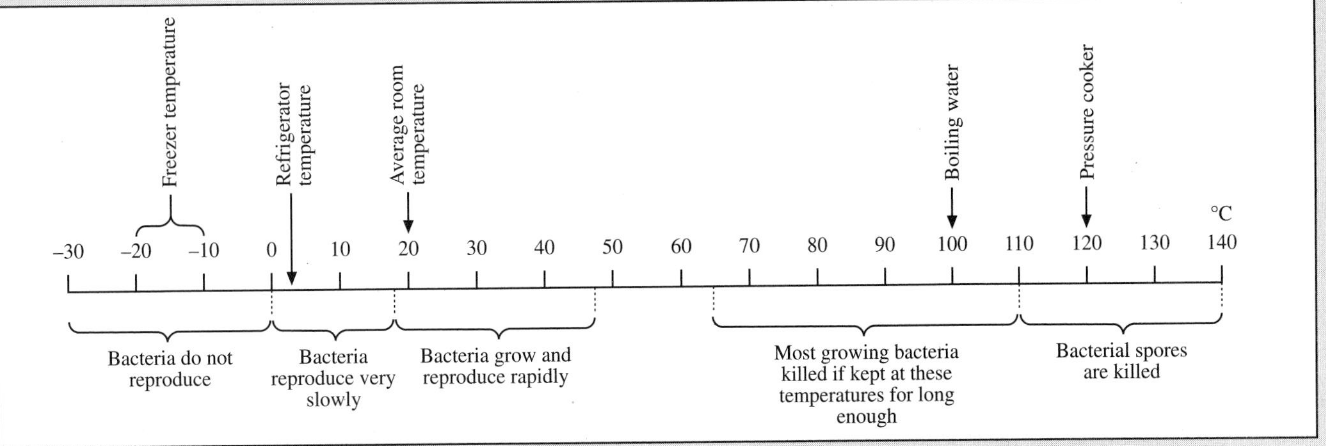

2. The diagram above shows the effect of different temperatures on bacteria.
Use information from this diagram to help explain each of the following.
(a) Milk which has been pasteurised (heated to 70°C) stays fresh for a few days but eventually goes sour. (2 marks)
(b) UHT milk has been heated to 132°C. It remains drinkable for a very long time. (1 mark)
(c) A freezer preserves food for much longer than a refrigerator. (2 marks)
(SEG 95/96 Sample papers)

3. Malaria is still one of the commonest tropical diseases causing over 2 million deaths each year. This is in spite of measures to control its vector and the introduction of several new drugs to destroy the pathogen.
(a) (i) What is meant by the term pathogen? (1 mark)
(ii) What is meant by the term vector? (1 mark)
(iii) To which group of organisms does the malarial pathogen belong? (1 mark)
(iv) State and explain ONE way in which knowledge of the life cycle of the vector has been used to reduce the occurrence of malaria. (2 marks)
(b) Since the 1960s the pathogen has shown increasing resistance to drugs.
(i) Explain the effect the increasing resistance of the pathogen will have on the numbers of patients suffering from malaria. (2 marks)
(ii) Resistance is passed on from one generation of the pathogen to another. Suggest what is the likely cause of this resistance. (1 mark)
(c) Scientists have recently been able to isolate a number of antigens from the surface of the malaria pathogen. What is an antigen? (1 mark)
(d) Genes coding for the formation of these antigens have recently been identified. These genes can be transferred into bacteria which will produce large quantities of the antigens when grown in a culture solution. Suggest how these techniques could be used to provide a method for giving people long term protection against malaria. (3 marks)
(MEG 93)

4. A number of diseases can be transmitted by sexual contact.
(a) Name ONE such disease and explain the physical effects and social problems associated with this named disease. (6 marks)
(b) Suggest TWO ways in which the risk of transmission of such diseases can be reduced. (2 marks)

5. The following list describes methods of food preservation which prevent microorganisms from spoiling food.
A Food is heated to a high temperature, which destroys the microorganisms
B Microorganisms are prevented from reproducing due to a low temperature
C Food is dried so that enzymes produced by micro-organisms cannot work
D Microorganisms have their water removed by osmosis
E An acid pH prevents the reproduction of micro-organisms
Complete the table below by writing ONE letter for each method.
The first one has been done for you.

Method of food preservation	Letter
Pickling	E
Dehydration	
Canning	
Salting	
Freezing	

(4 marks)
(ULEAC 93)

6. An experiment was set up to investigate the effectiveness of various treatments on milk. A 10 cm^3 sample of milk was placed in each of six test tubes with 1 cm^3 of an indicator dye. This dye is coloured blue and changes through pink to colourless as oxygen is removed from any solution in which it is present. The test tubes were all incubated at 35°C and the colour of the sample was recorded at intervals. Samples 2, 3, 4 and 5 were taken from freshly opened bottles of milk which had been stored for the times indicated.

	Tubes					
	1	2	3	4	5	6
Time from start of experiment	Raw milk	Sterilised milk 1 Day old	Sterilised milk 4 Days old	Pasteurised milk 1 Day old	Pasteurised milk 4 Days old	Sterilised milk kept in an open jug for 4 Days
0.5 hour	Pink	Blue	Blue	Blue	Blue	Blue
1.0 hour	White	Blue	Blue	Blue	Pink	Blue
1.5 hours	White	Blue	Blue	Pink	White	Pink

(a) Explain the colour changes which occurred in tube 1.

(b) Explain the differences in the results between tubes 4 and 5.

(c) Explain the differences in the results between tubes 3 and 6.

(d) Why is it advisable that the test tubes should not be shaken during the experiment? (14 marks)

(AEB 84)

Chapter 17

1. The diagram below shows five small organisms. The detail of the structure of them can be seen only by using a microscope.
   (a) Name the two structures in organism E which are also present in a leaf mesophyll cell. (1 mark)
   (b) When compared with most plant and animal cells what is the most unusual feature of organism A? (1 mark)
   (c) Give one way in which organism D is similar to a plant and one other way it is similar to an animal. (2 marks)
   (d) Organisms A and C are classified in the same group. Give one way in which they can be seen to be related to each other when compared with the other organisms in the diagram. (1 mark)
   (e) (i) Use the key below to identify organisms C and D. (2 marks)

1 Chloroplast present 2
No chloroplast present 3

2 Chloroplast ribbon-like and in a spiral ......*Spirogyra*
Chloroplast U-shaped ....*Chlamydomonas*

3 Cell wall present 4
No cell wall ....*Amoeba*

4 Body thin and branching ....*Rhizopus*
Body consists of rounded parts joined together ....*Saccharomyces*

(SEG 94)

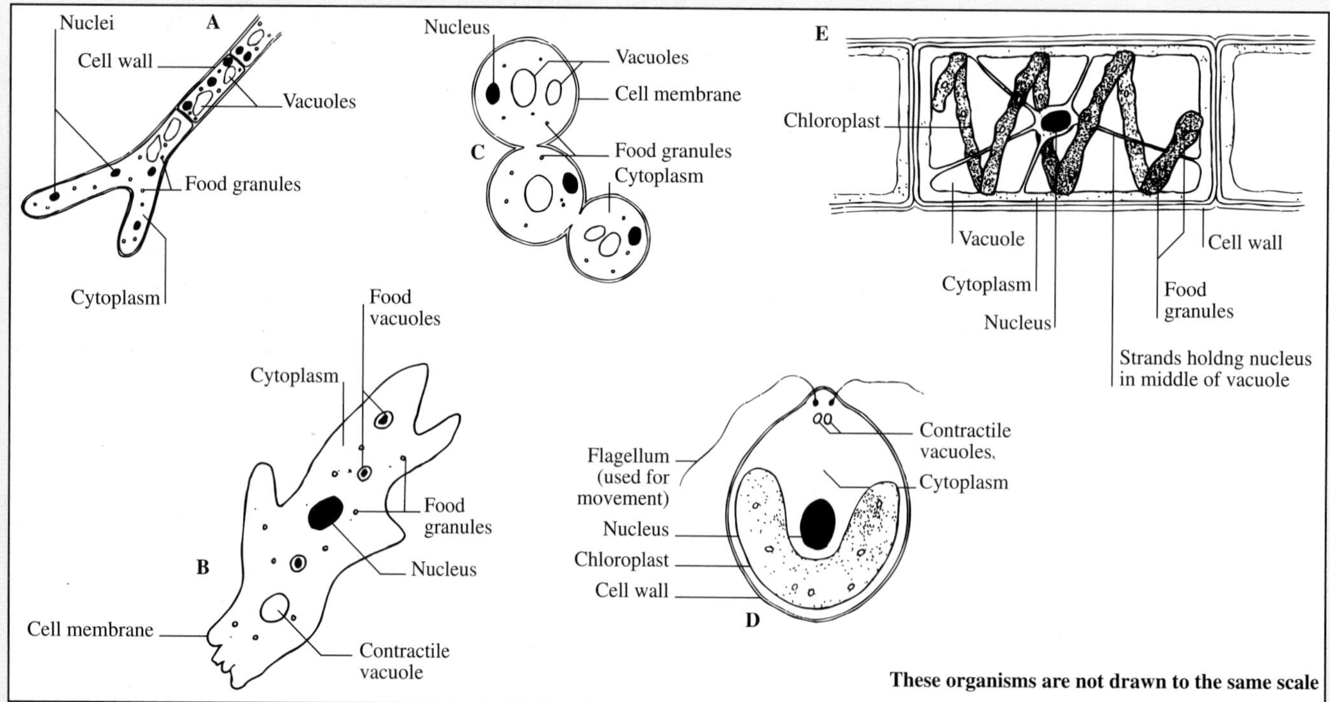

Chapter 18

1. The following organisms are helpful in processes which are useful to humans.

   Bacteria
   Fungi
   Insects

   Complete the table below by writing in the names of the correct organisms. You may use each organism once, more than once or not at all. The first one has been done for you.

Process	Organism(s)
Making alcohol	Fungi
Making cheese	
Making bread	
Making vinegar	
Making yoghurt	
Pollination	
Sewage disposal	

(Total 6 marks)
(ULEAC 94)

Chapter 19

1. The diagram shows a simplified cell with four chromosomes in the nucleus.
   Draw the results that would be produced if this cell divided by:
   (a) mitosis (ordinary cell division).
   (b) meiosis (reduction division which occurs in the ovary and testis). (5 marks)
   (SEG 90)

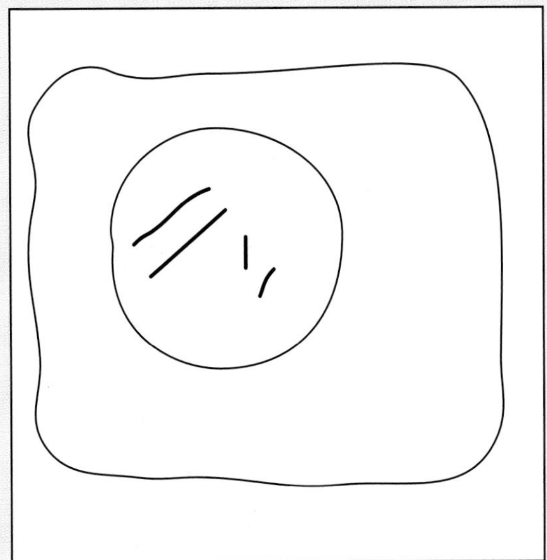

2. (a) A student prepared a piece of living tissue so that the chromosomes were deeply stained and easy to see. He then examined the prepared tissue with a microscope. The diagram shows the appearance of the tissue under the microscope.
   (i) What are chromosomes? (2 marks)
   (ii) The student decided that some of the cells had been dividing to produce new cells. Give one way in which this decision is supported by the diagram. (1 mark)
   (iii) He also decided that the cells had been dividing by mitosis. Give two ways in which the appearance of this tissue shows that this conclusion was correct. (2 marks)
   (iv) Name two structures in the bodies of humans where meiosis occurs. (2 marks)

   (b) Woolly hair is dominant to straight hair. The diagram (page 250, top) shows a family pedigree for the inheritance of these two types of hair. The genotypes of some members of the family are also shown.
   (i) What relationship is Vera to Darren? (1 mark)
   (ii) What percentage of the children and grandchildren of Sam and Vera were males with woolly hair? (1 mark)
   (iii) Vera is heterozygous for hair type. What does this mean? (1 mark)
   (SEG 94)

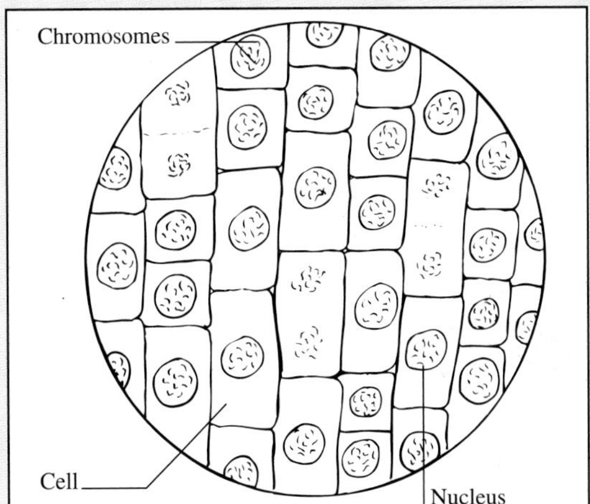

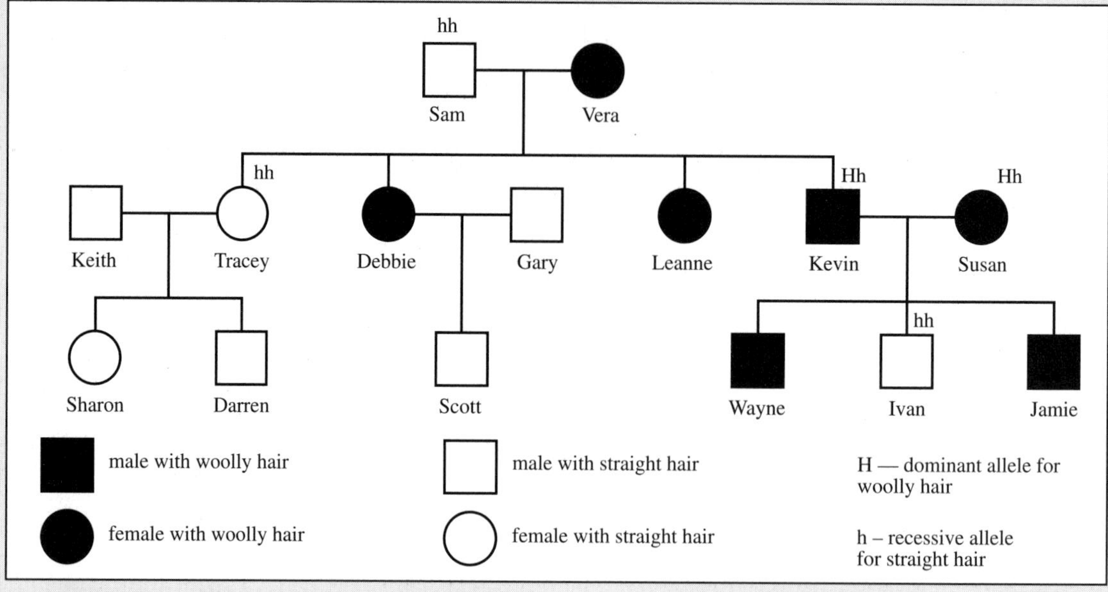

3. Mr and Mrs Wright have curly hair. Their two daughters, Carmen and Lucinda have straight hair. Their son, Darren, has curly hair. Mr Wright, Carmen and Darren have brown eyes. Mrs Wright and Lucinda have blue eyes. The body masses are: Mr Wright 76 kg, Mrs Wright 64 kg, Carmen 55 kg, Lucinda 51 kg and Darren 35 kg. Mr Wright and Lucinda have blood group AB, Mrs Wright and Darren have blood group B and Carmen has blood Group A.

(a) Give one feature of this family which shows discontinuous variation. Briefly explain the reason for your answer. (2 marks)

(b) The diagram below shows the pedigree for another family for the inheritance of hair colour.

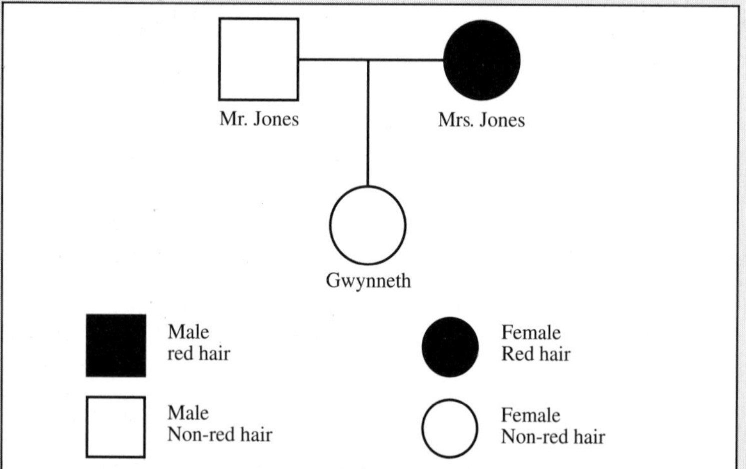

Draw a similar pedigree for the Wright family showing the inheritance of eye colour. (4 marks)

(c) (i) Complete the diagram (above, right) to show the possible inheritance of blood groups of the ABO system in the Wright family. (2 marks)

(ii) What are the possible genotypes of Carmen and Darren? (2 marks)

(d) (i) Using graph paper, draw a bar chart of the body masses of the Wright family. (4 marks)

(ii) State one other factor you would need to know about Mr Wright before you could decide if he was overweight. (1 mark)

(SEG 92)

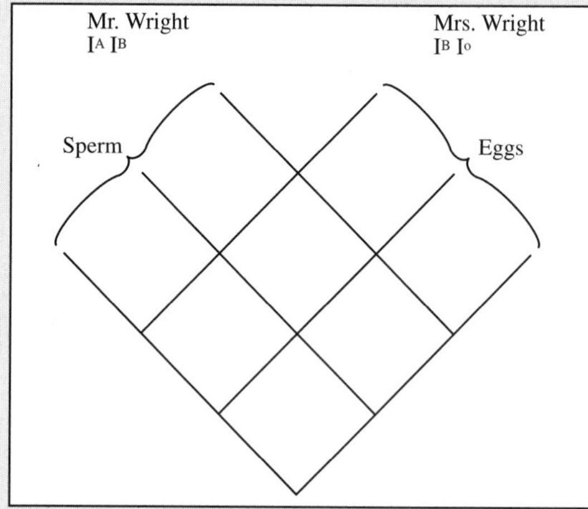

4. (a) Read through the following passage on chromosomes. Write on each dotted line an appropriate single word to complete the passage.

A chromosome is a strand of .... in the cell nucleus. Most human cells contain 46 chromosomes but the nucleus of ....contain only 23 chromosomes. This smaller number is known as the .... number of chromosomes. During cell division for body growth, cell nuclei exactly duplicate their chromosome. Eggs and sperm are produced by a different type of cell division, called .... in which the chromosome number is changed. Sex chromosomes, called X and Y, determine whether a .... develops into a male or female offspring. One X and one Y chromosome are present in the cell nuclei of ....offspring, while .... offspring carry two X chromosomes. (6 marks)

(b) Mrs Smith has blue eyes and Mr Smith has brown eyes although his mother had blue eyes. In humans, the allele for brown eye colour is dominant to the allele for blue eye colour.

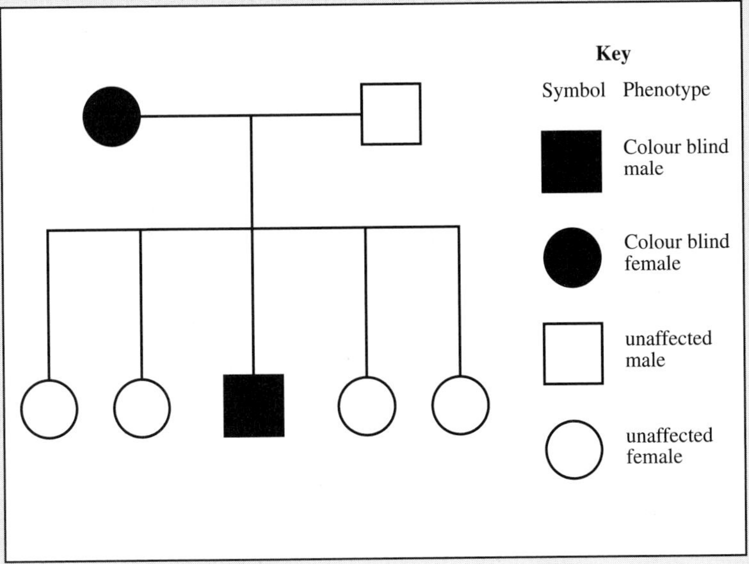

(i) The letter B is used for the allele for brown eyes and the letter b is used for the allele for blue eyes. What are the genotypes of Mrs and Mr Smith? Choose an answer from the following alternatives.
Mrs Smith BB Bb bb
Mr Smith BB Bb bb (2 marks)

(ii) If Mr and Mrs Smith had several children, what eye colour would you expect in each of their offspring? Explain your answer. (4 marks)
(ULEAC specimen paper)

5. The pedigree on the left shows the inheritance of colour blindness in a family.

Colour blindness is the result of a recessive, sex-linked allele.Explain how, although the mother is colour blind, all her daughters have normal vision. (Use the symbol N for normal vision and n for the allele for colour blindness). (5 marks)

Chapter 20

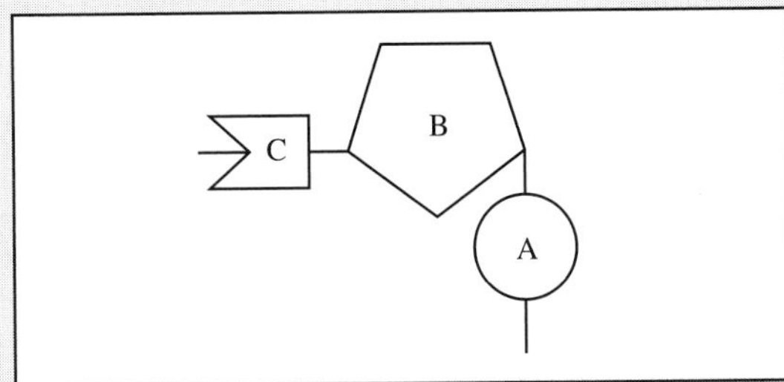

1. (a) Label A, B and C in the figure above. (3 marks)
   (b) What is this called? (1 mark)
   (c) What nitrogen base is found in DNA but not RNA? (1 mark)
   (d) What nitrogen base is found is RNA but not DNA? (1 mark)
   (e) What is transcription? (2 marks)
   (f) What is translation? (2 marks)

2. List the three stages in recombinant DNA technology. (3 marks)

3. What name is given to the enzymes that:
   (a) cut DNA into pieces
   (b) join DNA pieces together? (2 marks)

4. Give an advantage of using immobilised enzymes. (1 mark)

5. The figure below shows the effects of three antibiotics penicillin (Pe), streptomycin (St) and tetracycline (Te) on the bacterium *Bacillus subtilis*.

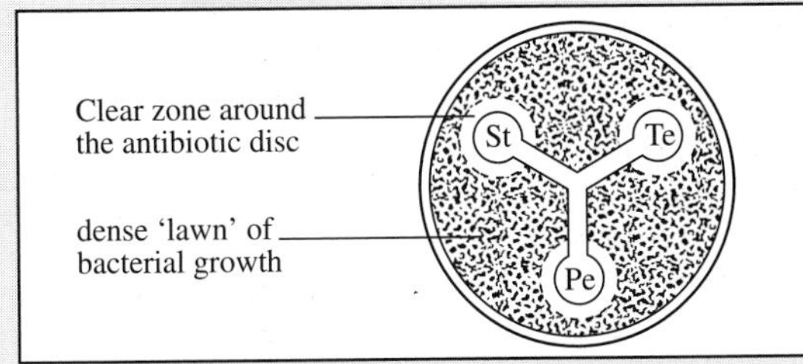

Which antibiotic is most effective?
Explain your answer. (2 marks)

6. Give three advantages of plant tissue culture over more traditional methods of growing plants. (3 marks)

7. The diagram below shows a wire loop carrying bacteria being drawn across an agar plate.

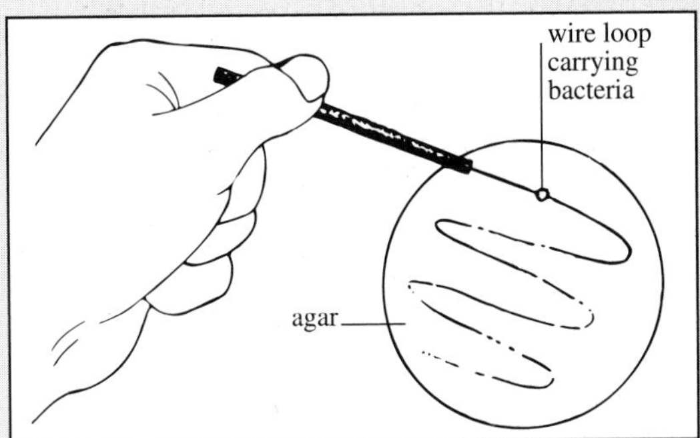

   (a) Which one of the following processes is being carried out?
   inoculation **sterilisation**
   disinfection **incubation** (1 mark)
   (b) Explain why viruses can not be grown on agar plates. (2 marks)
   (NEAB Specimen paper)

8. The antibiotic penicillin is produced by the fungus *Penicillium*. In the commercial production of penicillin the fungus is grown in nutrient broth inside a large container called a fermenter, as shown in the diagram (page 252, top).
   (a) The motor is used to turn the paddles inside the fermenter. Explain why this stirring is needed. (2 marks)
   (b) *Penicillium* grows best at a particular temperature. From information in the diagram, suggest how the correct temperature of the nutrient broth is achieved. (3 marks)

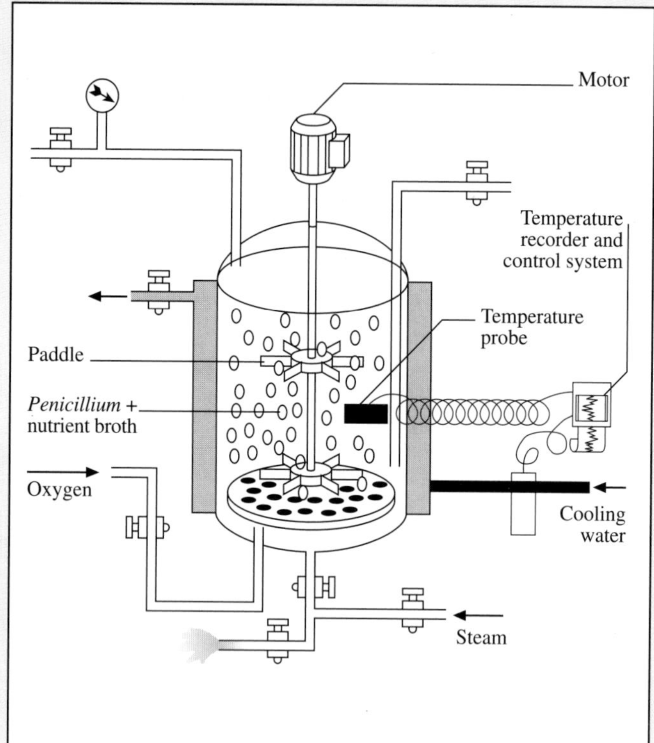

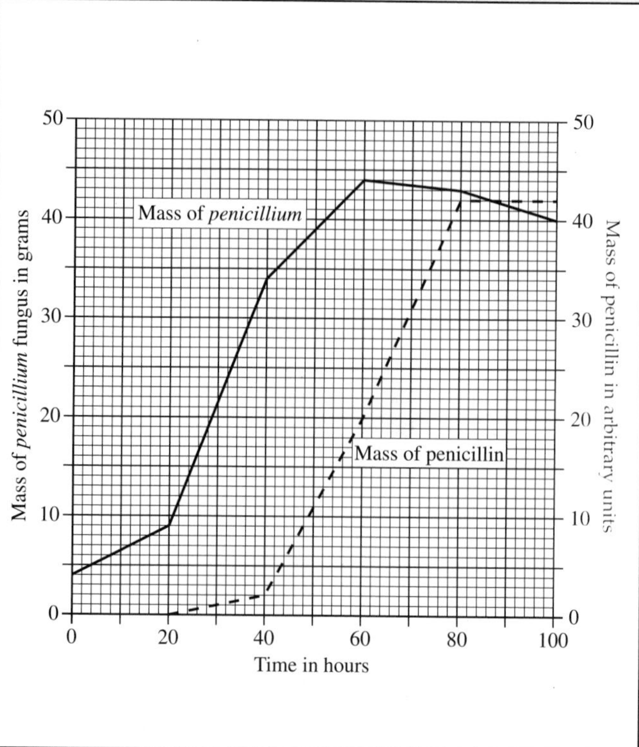

(c) In a trial run of the fermenter some penicillin fungus and nutrient broth were added. The mass per litre of *Penicillium* and the mass per litre of penicillin produced were recorded over a hundred hours. The results are shown in the graph above.

(i) How much *Penicillium* had grown after 30 hours? (1 mark)

(ii) Describe the pattern of growth of *Penicillium*. (3 marks)

(iii) How is the production of penicillin related to the pattern of growth of the *Penicillium* fungus? (1 mark)

(iv) For how many hours should the fermenter be allowed to run in order to produce the maximum amount of penicillin? (1 mark)

(ULEAC specimen paper)

9. Sometimes members of a family need to prove that they are related. One way in which scientists can help is by DNA fingerprinting.

(a) Describe the functioning of DNA in a cell. (3 marks)

(b) In a fingerprint test, cells were taken from the mother, the husband and the child. The cells were broken open and DNA fragments were extracted. The DNA fragments in each sample were separated into a column of bands, called a DNA fingerprint.

The diagram opposite shows the DNA fingerprint of each member of the family. The bands have been numbered to help you to answer the questions which follow.

(i) Which of the bands in the child's DNA fingerprint are in exactly the same position as bands in the mother's DNA fingerprint? (1 mark)

(ii) Suggest why some of the bands in the mother's DNA fingerprint are absent from the child's DNA fingerprint. (2 marks)

(iii) The bands in the child's DNA fingerprint which are absent from the mother's DNA fingerprint must have been inherited from the child's natural father. Does the husband's DNA fingerprint show that he is the child's father? Explain your answer. (2 marks)

(ULEAC specimen paper)

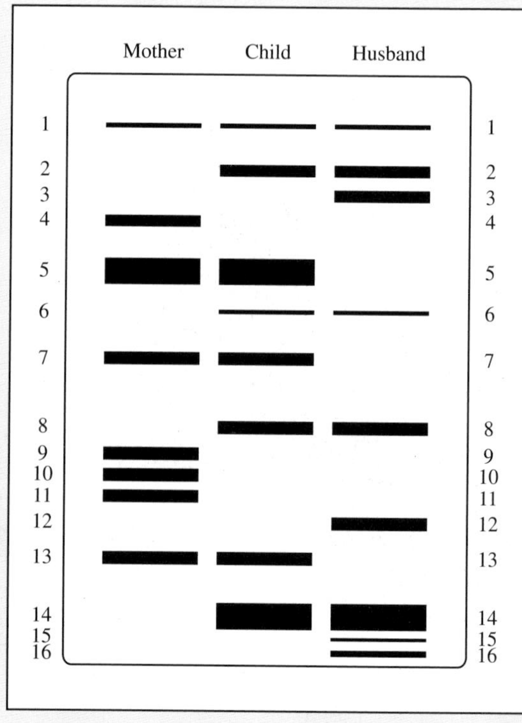

Chapter 21

1. Students in a school vary from each other in many ways. Some of these variations are caused by differences in genes and some by differences in environment as well as genes.

   (a) Decide the cause of each difference listed in the table below and then place a tick in the correct column. The first one has been done for you.

Variation between students	Cause of variation	
	Genes only	Genes and environment
Hair colour	✔	
Sex		
Overall height		
Blood group		
Eye colour		
Thickness of arm muscle		

(5 marks)

   (b) In what special case would variation between two people be due to environment only? (1 marks)

(ULEAC specimen paper)

2. Penicillin is an antibiotic which attacks actively dividing bacteria. However, some bacteria have become resistant to this. Explain how Darwin would have tried to explain this. (5 marks)

Chapter 22

1. The following passage and figure are taken from a booklet published by the Forestry Commission. The aim of the booklet is to help people who plant forests to manage them for the benefit of wildlife. Read the passage, examine the figure and then answer the questions that follow.

   In general, management of road edges seeks to provide a variety of habitats for plants and their associated butterflies. This is best achieved by grading the edge in stature from tall trees, down through shrubs and scramblers to grass and finally to bare ground that acts as a seed bed. There should be gaps in the shrub belt and some variety in the species. These features are shown in the figure.

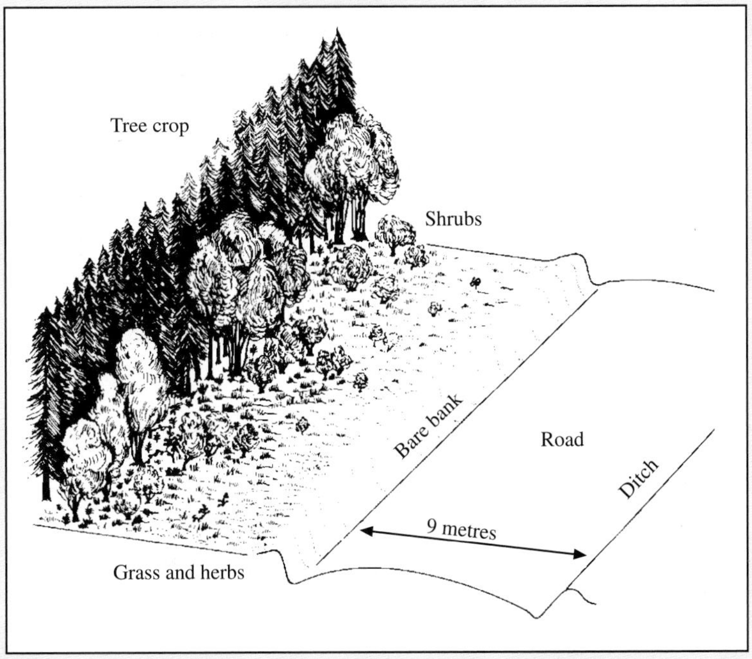

   (a) What effect will this management have on the number of habitats at the edge of the wood? (1 mark)

   (b) What effect will this management have on the number of species seen by people at the edge of the wood? (1 mark)

   (c) Suggest how one abiotic factor might differ at ground level between the tree crop and the area with grass and herbs. (2 marks)

   (d) What is likely to happen if the grass and herbs are left untended for many years? (2 marks)

   (e) Suggest one advantage of managing road edges in this way in addition to allowing more species to occur at the edge of a commercial wood. (2 marks)

   (f) Suggest one disadvantage of managing road edges in this way. (1 mark)

Chapter 23

1. The table below shows the results of an investigation to find the effect of carbon dioxide concentration on the rate of photosynthesis.

Concentration of carbon dioxide in air (%)	Rate of photosynthesis (Arbitrary units)
0.0	0
0.2	35
0.4	70
0.6	105
0.8	115
1.0	120
1.2	120
1.4	120

(a) Draw a line graph of these results. (4 marks)
(b) Use the graph to describe the effect of carbon dioxide concentration on the rate of photosynthesis. (2 marks)
(c) The rate of photosynthesis may be affected by factors other than carbon dioxide concentration. Give two of these factors. (2 marks)
(d) Plants in greenhouses grow faster than those planted outside. Give two reasons why. (2 marks)
(NEAB 93)

2. Read the following account and answer the questions which follow.

THE SCOTTISH MOORS
The Scottish moors cover thousands of hectares of land. The main type of vegetation is heather and grass. These may grow to a height of 0.5 metres.

The heather and grass provide food for grouse.

The moors are also home to small mammals, called voles. These also feed on the heather and grass.

The main predators on the moors are foxes which feed on both the grouse and the voles.

During certain times of the year, the grouse are shot for food by grouse hunters. During the shoot, loud noises are made to frighten the grouse and make them fly. The hunters use guns to shoot them down.

(a) Draw a food web for the organisms mentioned above, including humans. Your food web should make clear the direction of energy flow. (5 marks)
(b) Suggest what the heather and grass provide for the grouse, other than food. (1 mark)
(c) Gamekeepers try to reduce the number of foxes by shooting them.
(i) What would happen to the population of grouse if hunting and shooting foxes were banned? (1 mark)
(ii) How would this change affect the vegetation on the moor? (1 mark)
(NEAB 94)

Chapter 24

1. (a) Study the information provided and answer the questions that follow:

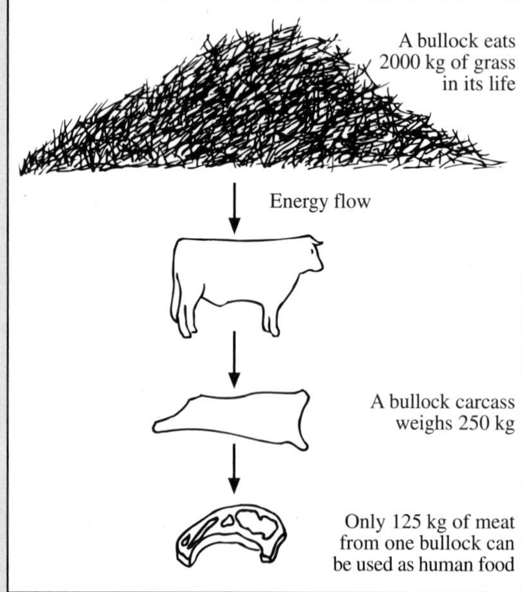

(i) What happens to the sun's energy after it has been trapped by the producers in the above chain? (4 marks)
(ii) What percentage of the mass of the grass eaten by the bullock is eventually available for humans to eat? (1 mark)

(b) Using farmland to raise animals is an inefficient use of land – since only a small part of the energy available in the grass gets converted into beef. If the land was used instead for growing vegetables, for direct human consumption, less energy would be lost from the chain. Why is less energy lost by growing vegetables for human consumption instead of producing beef? (2 marks)
(c) Graph A shows how Britain's 18 million hectares of agricultural land are used. Graph B compares the areas of agricultural land available to areas needed to support individuals on different diets.

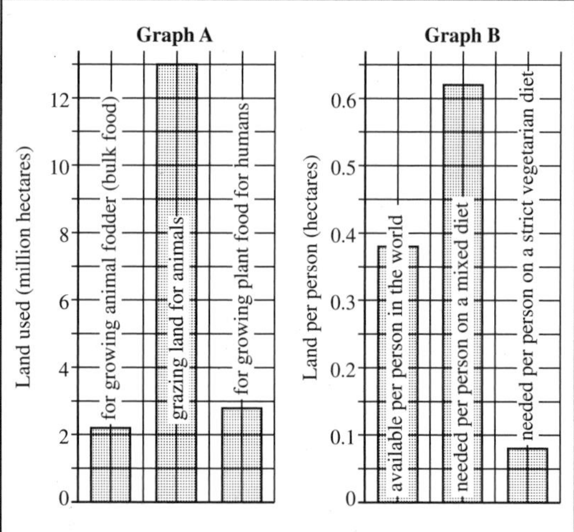

(i) How much of Britain's agricultural land is used for feeding 'animals' rather than for growing plant food for humans? (1 mark)
(ii) State the information given by Graph B. (3 marks)
(iii) What happens to column 1 of Graph B as the world population continues to grow? (1 mark)
(iv) If less meat were eaten, how could this change help to feed the world's growing population? (3 marks)
(SEG 92)

2. The organisms (right) form a food chain.
(a) Put arrow heads on the lines to show the direction of energy flow. (1 mark)
(b) Name the producer. (1 mark)
(c) Give ONE way in which energy is lost along a food chain. (1 mark)
(ULEAC 94)

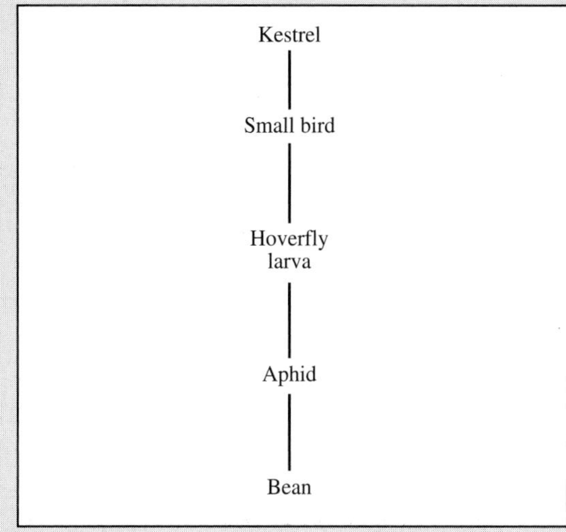

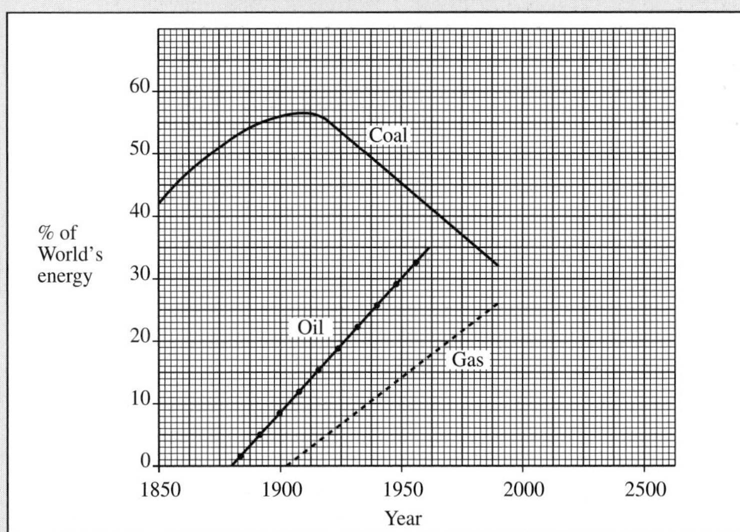

3. Coal, oil and gas provide a large proportion of the world's energy. The graph (left) shows how the percentage contribution to the world's energy from each fuel has changed between 1850 and 1990.
(a) What percentage of the world's energy came from coal in 1940? (1 mark)
(b) Extend the lines for coal and gas. Predict the year in which the amount of energy obtained from coal and gas will be the same. (2 marks)
(c) Scientists have estimated that the world's supply of oil will last only for another forty years, if it is used at the present rate. Name two infinite (renewable) energy sources that could be used instead of oil. (2 marks)
(d) The cost of building a new power station to produce electricity is very high. Despite the high costs, some Electricity Generating Companies are building new power stations which use gas as a fuel rather than coal. Suggest two reasons why such companies are using gas as a fuel rather than coal. (2 marks)
(NEAB 94)

Chapter 25

1. The graph below shows the changes in the level of carbon dioxide in the atmosphere of the northern half of the world since 1972.

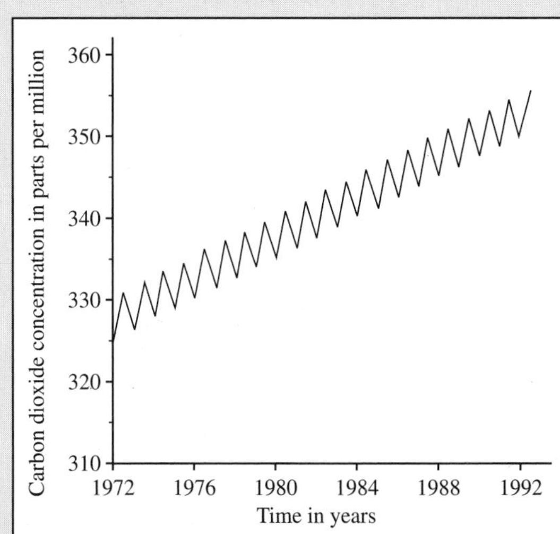

(a) Describe the overall trend of the carbon dioxide level in the atmosphere over the past 20 years. (1 mark)
(b) (i) Which group of organisms uses carbon dioxide? (1 mark)
(ii) In which process is this carbon dioxide used? (1 mark)
(c) Every year there is a high and low level of carbon dioxide. Suggest reasons for these changes. (4 marks)
(ULEAC 93)

2. The diagram (page 256, top) shows some features of the circulation of nitrogen in natural conditions.
(a) How many different types of bacteria are shown in this diagram? (1 mark)
(b) Give the name of one compound in the diagram which contains nitrogen. (1 mark)
(c) What process happens at the point marked X to cause the change shown? (1 mark)
(d) Crops such as potatoes or wheat are harvested and removed from the field. How does the

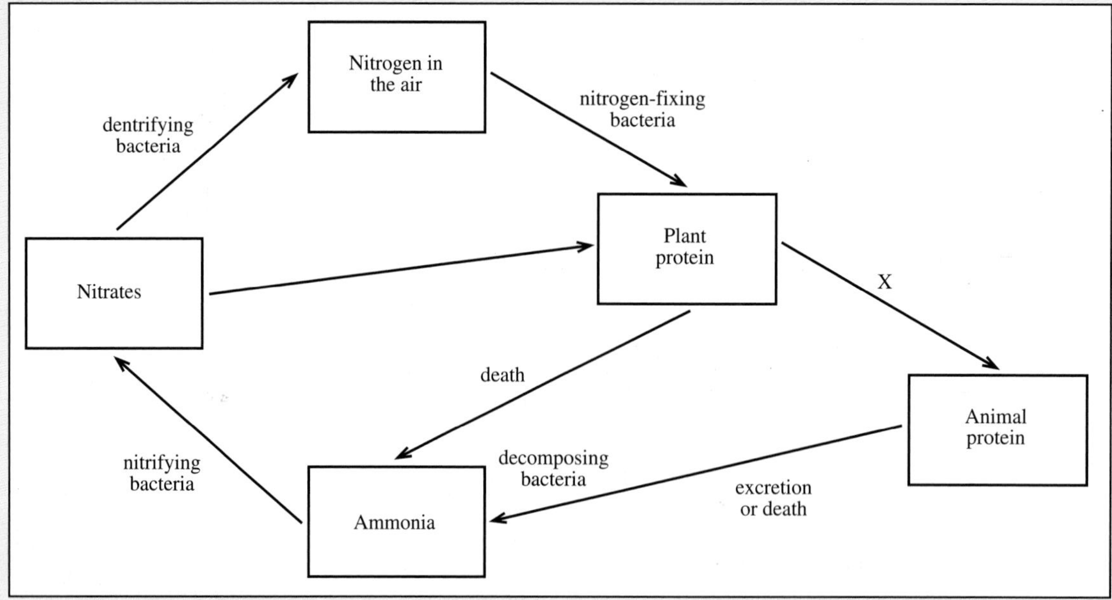

diagram help to explain why farmers need to add fertilisers or manure to the soil? (2 marks)

(SEG 94 Sample papers)

3. (a) The diagram below shows the connection between some living things and the water cycle.

(i) Fill in the missing words by naming the processes at A and at B. (2 marks)

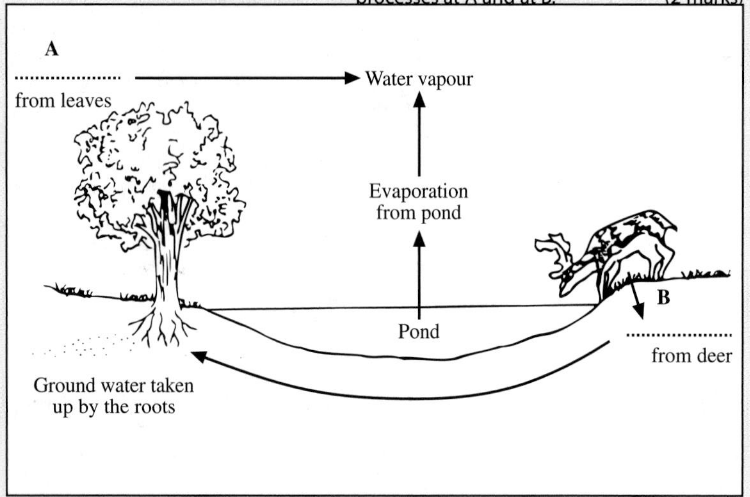

(ii) Suggest one way in which water vapour becomes pond water again, completing the cycle. (2 marks)

(b) The diagram below shows part of the carbon cycle on land.

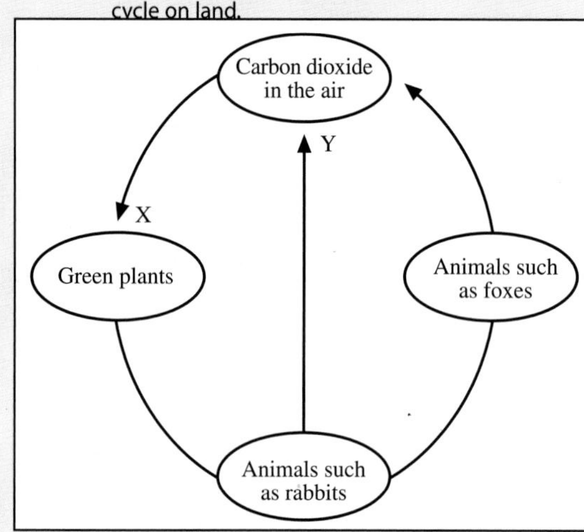

(i) Fill in the missing words by naming the processes at X and Y. (2 marks)

(ii) How is the carbon in the green plant passed to the fox? (2 marks)

(iii) What is the effect on the carbon cycle of cutting down a lot of trees? (2 marks)

(iv) The last two diagrams have shown the water cycle and the carbon cycle. Name one other element that is cycled. (1 mark)

Chapter 26

1. The diagram below shows a population pyramid for a small country.

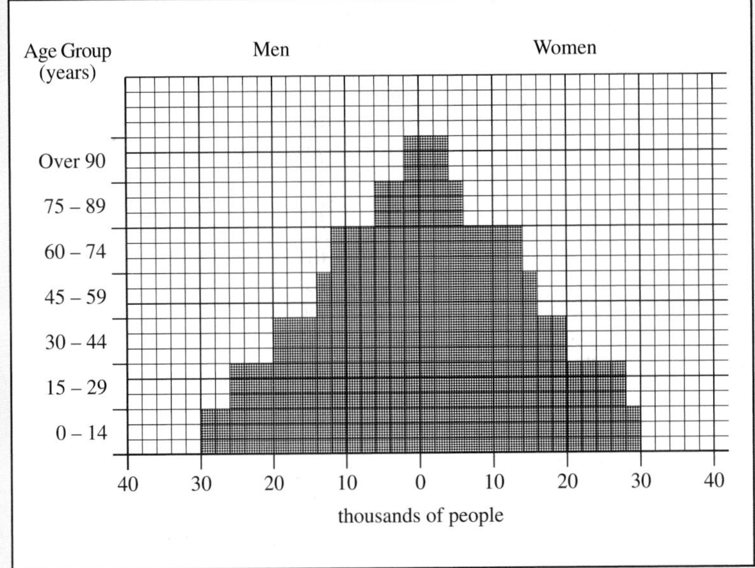

(a) How many women are aged 30 – 44 years? (1 mark)

(b) Calculate how many of the population are aged 75 years or older. (1 mark)

(c) Is the population of the small country likely to rise, fall or stay about the same over the next 20 years? Use information from the population pyramid to explain the reason for your answer. (3 marks)

(NEAB Sample material)

2. The table below shows some of the pollutants released by aluminium production and from car exhausts.

(a) Using information in the table, name TWO ways of reducing air pollution. (2 marks)

(b) A car without a catalytic converter travels 20 000 kilometres in a year at an average speed of 40 km per h. How many kg of carbon monoxide does it produce during this period? Show your working. (2 marks)

(c) Name ONE other source of sulphur dioxide pollution. (1 mark)

(d) (i) Carbon dioxide and sulphur dioxide contribute to the effects represented on the postage stamps in the table above, right. Write in the name of the gas which makes the major contribution in each case. (2 marks)

Postage stamp	Gas
Acid Rain Kills 24	
greenhouse effect 33	

Reproduced by permission of Royal Mail.

(ii) Suggest ONE advantage of showing examples of pollution on a postage stamp. (1 mark)

(iii) Give TWO possible effects when acid rain kills plants in a lake. (2 marks)

(ULEAC 94)

3. Biologists are able to estimate the amount of pollution in river water. They do this by counting the number of different types of animals in the water. The map (page 258, top) shows the River Leen and the levels of pollution at several sites measured on a 10 point scale (0 is very polluted; 10 is very clean).

(a) (i) Name a major source of pollution in this river system. (1 mark)

(ii) How do pollutants from this source get into the river? (1 mark)

(b) Describe and explain the overall pattern of pollution in this river system. Suggest its effect on number and types of animals in the water. (5 marks)

(c) (i) Mark on the map with the letter P, a point where it would be sensible to build a pumping station to extract water for drinking. (1 mark)

(ii) Explain why you would extract water from this point. (2 marks)

(d) Name TWO pollutants that are most likely to enter the River Leen as it flows through the city of Nottingham. (2 marks)

(MEG 94)

	Pollution released			
Air pollutant	during extraction from aluminium ore in g per tonne	during recycling of aluminium cans in g per tonne	from car exhausts without a catalytic converter in g per kilometre at average 40 km per h	from car exhausts with a catalytic converter in g per kilometre at average 40 km per h
Carbon monoxide	35 000	2500	10.0	1.0
Sulphur dioxide	88 600	886	0.6	0.05

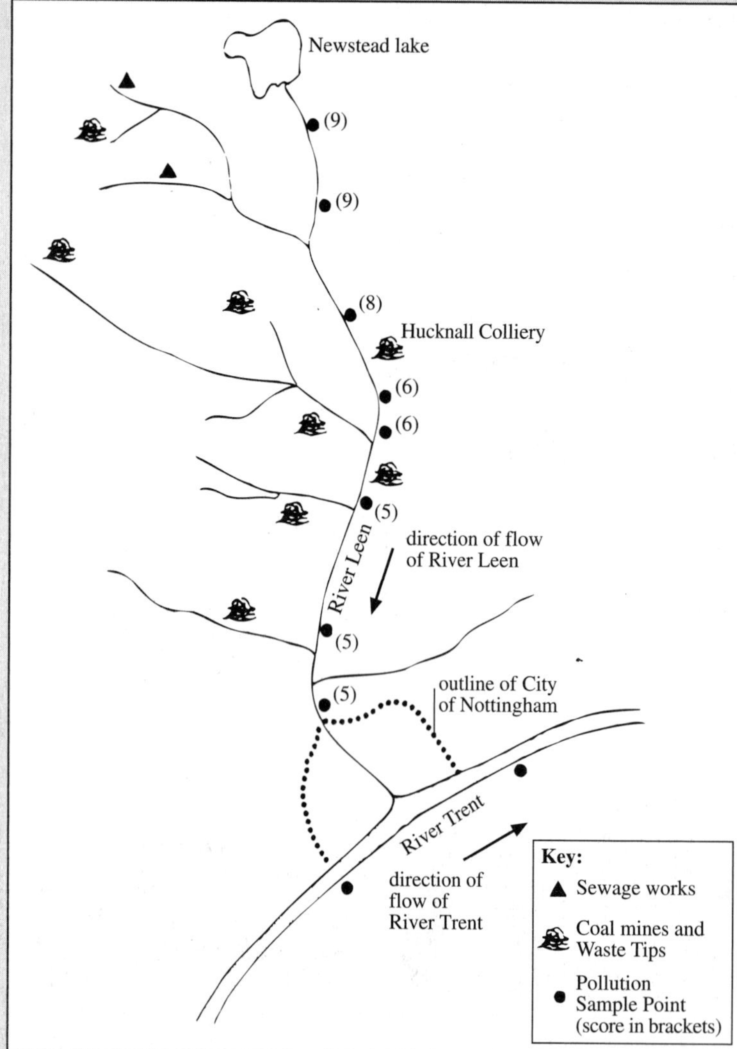

Chapter 27

1. (a) The diagram (below, left) shows the relative amounts of some of the pollutants released into the air of a large city during a year.
   (i) Which substance formed the greatest part of the pollution in the air of this city? Suggest an explanation for this. (2 marks)
   (ii) What percentage of this substance was present? (1 mark)
   (iii) What percentage of sulphur dioxide was present? (1 mark)
   (iv) In 1985 the generation of electricity by European power stations caused the release of 2.5 million tonnes of sulphur dioxide into the air. How does this help to explain the information shown in the diagram below? (3 marks)

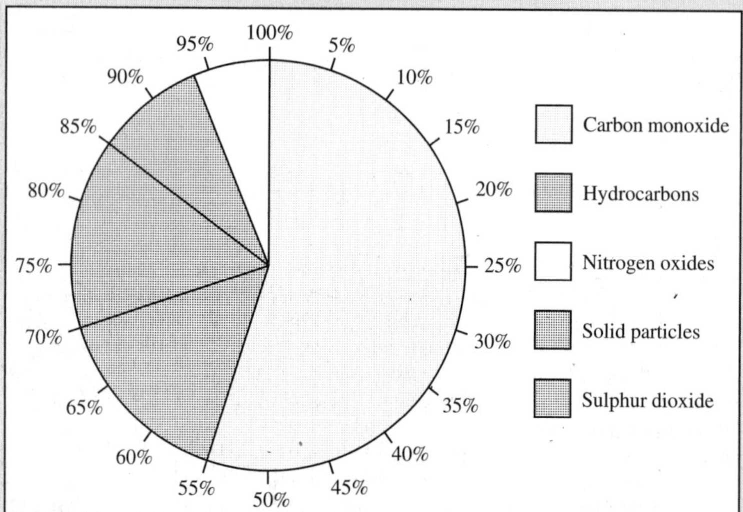

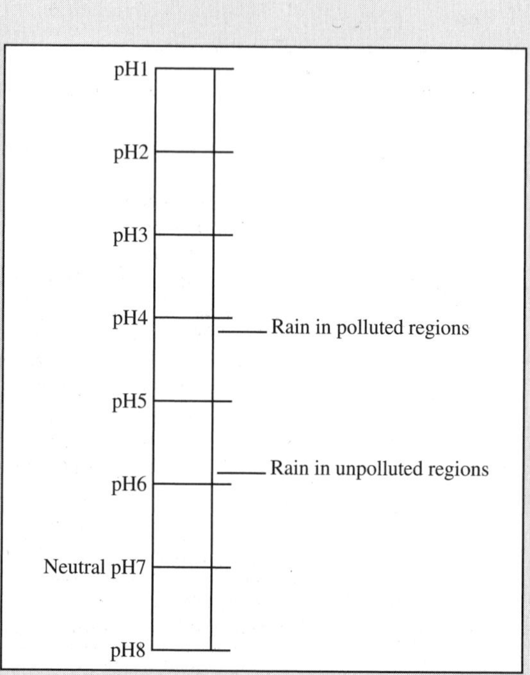

(b) Many local authorities dispose of solid domestic waste by placing it in a tip. Suggest as fully as possible why this refuse should then be covered by a layer of soil. (3 marks)

(SEG 94 Sample papers)

2. The diagram below represents the processes which take place at a sewage works.

Rotating sprinkler bar
Primary settlement tank
Air
Filter bed with stones covered by bacteria
To river
Secondary settlement tank
Methane
To a farm
Sludge

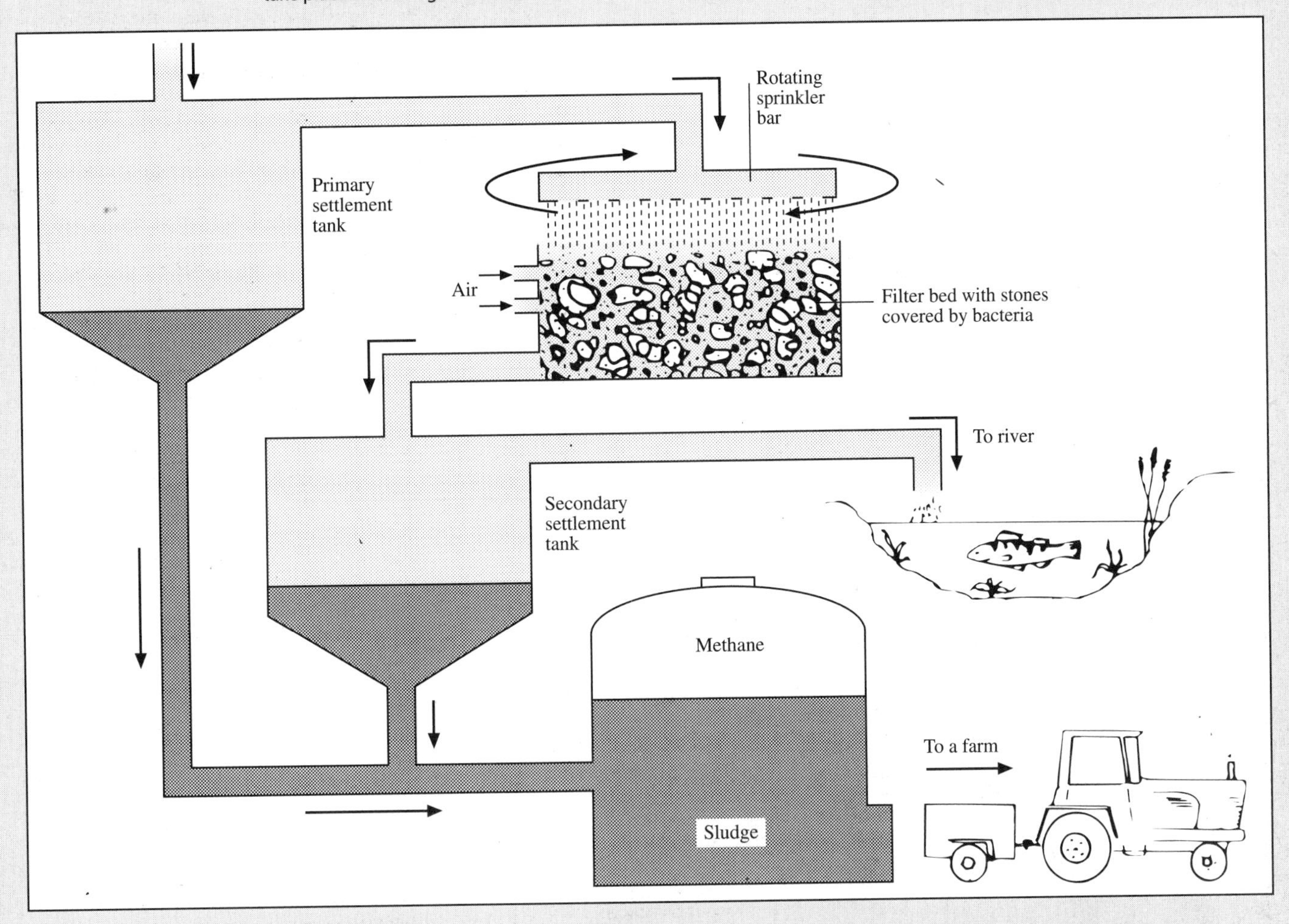

(a) Describe the function of the settlement tanks. (1 mark)

(b) Describe the function of the following in the filter bed:
(i) Bacteria
(ii) Stones
(iii) Air. (6 marks)

(c) Give ONE use of each of the following:
(i) Methane
(ii) Sludge. (2 marks)

(d) The table below shows some of the things which enter and leave the sewage works. After processing the amount of each is changed. Complete the table below by writing MORE or LESS in each box. The first one has been done for you.

	Carbohydrates	*Bacteria*	*Proteins*	*Nitrates*
In raw sewage	More			
Leaving after processing	Less			

(3 marks)

(e) If a large quantity of disinfectant entered the sewage works what effect could this have on the efficiency of the process? Give a reason for your answer. (2 marks)
(ULEAC 93)

3. The figure below shows the stages in the treatment of water to make it safe to drink.

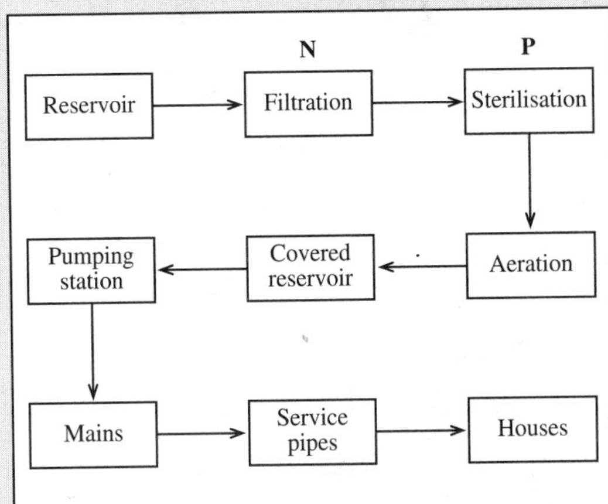

(a) Name TWO things the filter removes from the water at point N. (1 mark)

(b) What substance is normally added to the water at stage P to make it safe? (1 mark)

(c) Why should water be sterilised before drinking? (1 mark)

(d) Give TWO reasons for storing the water in a covered reservoir. (2 marks)
(MEG 93)

Answers to self-check questions

The following guide answers have been devised by the authors. They are entirely the responsibility of the authors and have neither been provided nor approved by the exam boards:

Chapter 1: Qs 1, 2, 3; Chapter 2: Qs 1, 2, 3, 4, 5; Chapter 3: Qs 1, 2, 3, 4; Chapter 4: Qs 1, 2, 3, 4, 6, 7; Chapter 5: Qs 1, 2, 3, 4; Chapter 6: Qs 1, 2, 3, 4, 5, 6, 7, 8; Chapter 7: Qs 1, 2, 3, 4, 5; Chapter 8: Qs 1, 2, 4, 5, 6, 7; Chapter 9: Qs 1, 2, 3; Chapter 10: Qs 1, 2, 3; Chapter 11: Qs 1, 2, 3; Chapter 16: Q 6; Chapter 17: Q 1; Chapter 18: Q 12; Chapter19: Qs 1, 2, 3, 4, 5; Chapter 20: Qs 1, 2, 3, 4, 5, 6, 8, 9; Chapter 21: Qs 1, 2; Chapter 22: Q 1; Chapter 23: Qs 1, 2; Chapter 24: Qs 1, 2, 3; Chapter 26: Q 2.

The Associated Examining Board/University of Cambridge Local Examinations Syndicate/Midland Examining Group/University of London Examinations and Assessment Council/Northern Examinations and Assessment Board bear no responsibility for the example answers to questions taken from their past question papers which are contained in this publication.

The rest of the answers are those that have been provided by the boards in the published mark schemes.

Chapter 1

1. (a) See page 2, Fig. 1.3 (6 marks)
   (b) Nucleus – contains the chromosomes which control the cell's activities; nucleolus – makes ribosomes; chromosomes – control the cell's activities; nuclear envelope – keeps nuclear contents from the rest of the cell/controls what enters and leaves the nucleus; nuclear pore – allows certain substances into and out of the nucleus; mitochondria – produce ATP; ribosomes – protein synthesis; rough endoplasmic reticulum – protein synthesis; smooth endoplasmic reticulum – transports substances within the cytoplasm; cell surface membrane – only allows certain substances into and out of the cell/cell recognition (9 marks)

2. Plant cell has: vacuole; chloroplasts (sometimes); cell wall (3 marks)

3. (a) Tissue – collection of cells of a similar structure and function;
   (b) Organ – collection of different tissues grouped together in one part of the body to perform a particular function;
   (c) Organ system – collection of organs which work together (3 marks)

Chapter 2

1. (a) Anabolism – building up reactions
   (b) Catabolism – breaking down reactions (2 marks)

2. See page 7, Fig. 2.1 (3 marks)

3. (a) Solution C (1 mark)
   (b) Decrease in size due to net water loss (1 mark)
   (c) Osmosis (1 mark)
   Diffusion of water through a partially permeable membrane (2 marks)
   (d) Weaker/hypotonic solution – B; therefore net flow of water in by osmosis; swells and bursts due to weak membrane (3 marks)

4. (a) Any relevant method, e.g. add a known volume of water to the measuring cylinder. Add the raisins. Note the change in volume which is due to the volume of the raisins (2 marks)
   (b) Raisins in an isotonic solution; no net flow of water in or out due to osmosis therefore no volume change (2 marks)
   (c) Water is very weak (hypotonic) therefore net flow of water in by osmosis. This causes swelling of raisins (2 marks)
   (d) Very strong solution is hypertonic therefore net flow of water out by osmosis. This causes the raisins to shrink (2 marks)

5. (a) 35°C (1 mark)
   (b) pH; substrate concentration; enzyme concentration (3 marks)
   (c) 15°C – rate would increase; 35°C is warmer therefore enzyme + substrate molecules moving faster; therefore more chance of colliding; 60°C – rate would be zero; due to denaturation of enzymes, i.e. their active site shape has been lost (5 marks)

Chapter 3

1. (a) Proteins; fats; carbohydrates; vitamins; salts; water; dietary fibre (7 marks)
   (b) Carbon; hydrogen; oxygen; nitrogen (2 marks)
   (c) (i) Add 2 cm^3 of the sample to 2 cm^3 of Benedict's solution; boil; red/brown precipitate (3 marks)
   (ii) Add 1 cm^3 of sodium hydroxide to 2 cm^3 protein solution; add fresh 1% copper sulphate drop by drop; purple/violet colour (3 marks)
   (d) DCPIP (1 mark)

2. (a) (i) Starch / cellulose / glycogen
   (ii) Maltose / sucrose / lactose
   (iii) Glucose / fructose / galactose (3 marks)
   (b) Fatty acids and glycerol (2 marks)

(c) (i) Globular – round in shape; fibrous – straight (1 mark)
(ii) Essential – cannot be made by the body therefore must be taken in with food; non-essential – can be made by the body (1 mark)
(d) (i) Sight – in dim light
(ii) Bone / teeth formation
(iii) Blood clotting (3 marks)
(e) (i) Bones / teeth
(ii) Haemoglobin production (2 marks)

3. (a) Incisors; canines; premolars; molars (4 marks)
(b) Mixture of saliva, bacteria and food on teeth (1 mark)
(c) (i) Cavity in a tooth due to the enamel / dentine being dissolved by acid. (1 mark)
(ii) Bacterial toxins cause inflammation of the gums where the gum and tooth meet (1 mark)
(d) Brushing regularly; diet; use of toothpaste (particularly one with fluoride); regular check ups by the dentist (4 marks)

4. (a) (i) A liver; B stomach; C duodenum / ileum / small intestine (3 marks)
(ii) lipase / amylase / protease (1 mark)
Lipase – converts fats to fatty acids and glycerol / amylase – converts starch to maltose (sugar) / protease – converts peptides / proteins to amino acids (1 mark)
(b) (i) So that variable would not affect the reaction (1 mark)
(ii) Enzyme worked best at pH 7.0 and 8.0; enzyme worked but took longer at pH 6.0 and 9.0; enzyme did not work at pH 5.0 and 10.0 (3 marks)
(iii) Do experiment at pH 7.0 or 8.0; repeat at temperatures above 50°C; compare to the results in the table (3 marks)

Chapter 4

1. (a) Any two of: red blood cell no nucleus – white blood cell has; red blood cell no granular cytoplasm – white blood cell has; red blood cell has haemoglobin – white blood cell hasn't (2 marks)
(b) Red blood cell transports oxygen – white blood cell doesn't; white blood cell protects the body by phagocytosis – red blood cell doesn't (2 marks)

2. Platelets produce thromboplastin; this converts prothrombin to thrombin; thrombin converts fibrinogen to fibrin; this is a mesh / network; traps blood cells especially red blood cells; these dry out and form a scab (6 marks)

3. (a) Plasma minus fibrinogen (1 mark)
(b)

Blood group	Antigen	Antibody
A	A	β
B	B	α
AB	AB	–
O	–	α & β

(4 marks)

c) Group A has A antigens and β antibodies; serum of group B will have α antibodies; when A antigens meet α antibodies agglutination occurs (3 marks)

4. See page29, Fig. 4.4 (2 marks)

5. (a) (i) Artery (1 mark)
(ii) Vein (1 mark)
(b) Capillaries (1 mark)
(c) From intestines to liver (1 mark)
(d) Acts as a pump (1 mark)
(e) (i) Family history (1 mark)
(ii) Blood vessels (coronary) have fatty deposits laid down inside them; causes a blockage; cardiac muscle becomes starved of food and oxygen therefore dies (3 marks)
(iii) Any two e.g.
diet – eat less saturated fat; exercise more; stop smoking (2 marks)

6. (a) (i) F; G; C; A (4 marks)
(ii) 1 is a coronary artery that supplies the cardiac / heart muscle with food; and oxygen; If there is a lack of these the muscle will die (3 marks)
(iii) From pulmonary artery to aorta (1 mark)
(iv) Aorta to pulmonary artery; pressure in the aorta greater than that in the pulmonary artery (2 marks)
(v) Some oxygenated blood in the aorta; will go back to the lungs (2 marks)
(b) Smaller lumen; more muscle; more elastic tissue (3 marks)

7. Through open tricuspid valve; into right ventricle; into pulmonary artery; through open semi-lunar valves; to lungs; into pulmonary vein; back to left atrium; through open bicuspid valve into right ventricle (8 marks)

Chapter 5

1. (a) (i) Increases volume of bell jar; pressure in the bell jar decreases; pressure inside the balloons decreases; air therefore moves in from atmosphere (4 marks)
   (ii) A – trachea; B – bronchi; C – ribs/intercostal muscles/thorax; D – thoracic cavity; E – diaphragm (5 marks)
   (iii) Diaphragm is dome shaped at rest not flat; lungs much larger than balloons; bell jar cannot move; no pleural membranes; thoracic cavity too large (5 marks)
   (b) (i) Breathe deeper; breathe faster; greater carbon dioxide concentration in expired air (2 marks)
   (ii) Decrease in breathing rate (1 mark)

2. (a) (i) Volume breathed in and out in one cycle. (2 marks)
   (ii) Fill a bell jar with water; place on wedges in a trough of water; record the initial volume of water in the bell jar; breathe out normally for 1 breath; using a tube going to the bell jar; record the decrease in volume (Tidal Volume) (6 x 1/2) (3 marks)
   (b) (i) G
   (ii) E
   (iii) D
   (iv) F (4 marks)
   (c) (i) Volume of each breath =0.5 dm^3 (see trace); subject breathes at a rate of 16 breaths per minute; therefore the subject breathes in $16 \times 5\ dm^3 = 8\ dm^3$ per minute.; for five minutes the subject therefore breathes in $8 \times 5\ dm^3 = 40\ dm^3$ (2 marks)
   (ii) Volume of each breath =1.0 dm^3 (see trace); subject breathes at a rate of 21 breaths per minute; therefore the subject breathes in 21 dm^3 per minute; for 2 minutes the subject therefore breathes in $2 \times 21 = 42\ dm^3$ (2 marks)
   (d) Diaphragm contracts; external intercostal muscles contract; ribs move up; ribs move out; volume in lungs/thorax increases; pressure in thorax/lungs decreases; air taken in from atmosphere; abdominal muscles relax; no upward pressure on diaphragm (9 marks)

3. Place a lighted candle in a gas jar of inspired air; time how long it takes to go out; using downward displacement of water obtain a sample of expired air in a gas jar; repeat as above; candle will go out in a shorter time in the expired air (6 marks)

4. (a) (i) Trachea (1 mark)
   (ii) Pulmonary artery (1 mark)
   (b) A: bronchiole; B: blood capillary; C: Alveolus (air sac) (3 marks)
   (c)

Oxygen	Carbon dioxide	Nitrogen	Water vapour
20.7 less	0.04 more	78.0 same	low more

(4 marks)

Chapter 6

1. Excretion – removal of the waste products from metabolism; defecation – removal of undigested waste material (2 marks)

2. Longer loop of Henlé allows more water to be reabsorbed; therefore preventing dehydration (2 marks)

3. Urea – waste nitrogenous compound; urine – mixture of urea, water and salts (2 marks)

4. (a) Decreases water content and therefore volume; yellow brown in colour (2 marks)
   (b) Decreases water content and therefore volume; yellow brown in colour (2 marks)
   (c) Increased urea concentration; from the greater concentration of amino acids (2 marks)

5.

Renal artery	Renal vein
1 high oxygen	low oxygen
2 low carbon dioxide	high carbon dioxide
3 high urea	low urea
4 more glucose	less glucose

(3 marks)

6. (a) (i) Water; salts (2 marks)
   (ii) Proteins are too large to be ultra-filtrated (2 marks)
   (iii) Urea (1 mark)
   (iv) Liver (1 mark)
   (v) Deamination (1 mark)
   (vi) All of the glucose is reabsorbed in the first coiled tubule (2 marks)
   (b) Compare with Fig. 6.1 on page 47 (6 marks)

(c) (i) C
(ii) D
(iii) E
(iv) D (4 marks)
(d) E – loop of Henlé
G – collecting duct (2 marks)

7. (a) Blood separated from dialysis fluid by a partially permeable membrane; dialysis fluid contains same concentration of salts and glucose as a normal persons blood therefore no net flow; no urea in dialysis fluid therefore this moves from the blood into the fluid; protein molecules are too large therefore remain in the blood (4 marks)
(b) If the person was a diabetic (1 mark)

8. (a) Compare with Fig. 6.3 on page 48 (5 marks)
(b) Compare with Fig. 6.3 on page 48 (5 marks)

Chapter 7

1. (a) (i) Dead outer layer (cornified); sebum (2 marks)
(ii) Dead outer layer containing keratin which is waterproof; temperature receptors which will modify behaviour (2 marks)
(iii) Germinal layer; contains melanin (2 marks)
(b) (i) Too high a body temperature leads to denaturation of proteins; dehydration; too low a body temperature would mean metabolism, e.g. respiration would occur too slowly; therefore would produce insufficient energy (3 marks)
(ii) Any three relevant answers, e.g. Less blood in the circulation; constrict (close up) arterioles; make more use of the shunt vessels; raise hairs (try to avoid as useless in humans); wear more clothes/cover exposed area; Move to a warmer area (3 marks)
(iii) Consequences: sweat is evaporated; uses heat from the body therefore has a cooling effect; can lead to dehydration
Value: maintains a constant body temperature; ensures survival (5 marks)
(c) Removes some microbes from hands; less microbes will therefore reach the food; less microbes have a chance to flourish and cause food poisoning (3 marks)

2. (a) (i) B
(ii) Blood vessels dilated (2 marks)
(b) (i) A
(ii) Body needs to keep warm so little blood wanted near the skin surface (2 marks)
(c) Temperature receptor detects how hot the skin surface is (1 mark)

3. (a) As the external temperature decreases the metabolic rate increases (and vice versa) (1 mark)
(b) 7200 kJ per 24 h (2 marks)
(c) Lose more heat to the surroundings; therefore must produce more heat to keep body temperature constant (2 marks)
(d) Sweat less; less blood in circulation; constriction of arterioles; use of shunt vessels; raise hairs; wear more clothes (any 4) (4 marks)
(e) 6525 kJ per 24 h (2 marks)
(f) Any relevant answer, e.g. sweating;excrete sweat onto the skin's surface; uses heat from the body to evaporate this therefore has a cooling effect (3 marks)

4. (a) Pancreas (1 mark)
(b) Liver (1 mark)
(c) Extreme thirst; passing a lot of urine – two symptoms
Low ADH level means less water reabsorbed from the urine. More urine is excreted leading to a sensation of thirst as less water in body (3 marks)
(d) Would be digested (1 mark)
(e) High insulin leads to low blood sugar level; too low a respiratory rate particularly in the brain leading to unconsciousness (2 marks)

5. (a) Sweat from sweat gland; along duct onto skin surface/epidermis; evaporates; uses heat from the body/skin; skin therefore cooled (5 marks)
(b) Blood from the core at approximately 37°C; blood in skin capillaries; is cooled. (3 marks)

Chapter 8

1. (a) (i) Rubbery / tough / flexible. (1 mark)
(ii) Lubrication / nutrition (1 mark)
(iii) Strong; slightly elastic (2 marks)
(b) (i) Spinal cord (1 mark)
(ii) Muscle plus ligament attachment (1 mark)
(iii) Prevent bone rubbing against bone / shock absorber (1 mark)
(c) (i) Left arm: A contracted; B relaxed
Right leg: E contracted; F relaxed;
H contracted; G relaxed
Left leg: C relaxed: D contracted (4 marks)
(ii) C (1 mark)

2. (a) A – increases surface area for muscle / ligament attachment; B – protection of spinal cord; C – support of the neural arch / protection of spinal cord / hold disc in place (3 marks)
(b) Spinal cord (1 mark)

3. (a) (i) A – femur; B – pelvic girdle (2 marks)
(ii) movement / locomotion / support / production of blood cells (1 mark)
(iii) Cartilage; synovial fluid (2 marks)
(iv) Osteoporosis / osteoarthritis (1 mark)

(b) (i) No attack by the immune system; plastic – light; metal – very strong; both can be shaped / moulded (3 marks)
(ii) Elbow – hinge – movement in one plane when flexing / extending; hip – ball and socket – movement in more than one plane as it rotates (2 marks)
(c) (i) Painful therefore wish to reduce this; probably get worse – want to try to avoid (2 marks)
(ii) Age 12 therefore started / about to start puberty where there is a great deal of growth; do not wish to affect this particularly in one place (2 marks)

4. (a) (i) A (1 mark)
(ii) Relax (1 mark)
(b) muscles must work antagonistically; i.e. when one contracts the other relaxes and vice versa. (2 marks)

5. (a) (i) Any two of: corns – hardened skin; bunions – swollen joint at the base of the big toe; hammer toes – big toe pushed inwards / crushes others (2 marks)
(ii) Strain Achilles tendon; strain on back as they lead to bad posture (2 marks)
(iii) Bones in young children contain a lot of flexible cartilage therefore badly fitting shoes can deform the feet. (2 marks)
(b) Failure to follow the instructions could prevent each vertebra supporting the one above it; stretch the discs between the vertebrae too much; (both lead to damage to the vertebral column) may lead to a slipped disc where the spinal nerve is trapped. (3 marks)
(c) Any drawing e.g. elbow joint (see Fig. 8.9 on page 65)
1 for drawing.
6 x 1/2 for the labels: two bones e.g. humerus / ulna; ligament; cartilage; synovial membrane; synovial fluid
1 for each function e.g. ligament – holds bone to bone;
cartilage – prevents bone rubbing on bone;
synovial fluid – lubricates the joint, nourishes cartilage (6 marks)

6. (a) Some fibres (cells) in the muscles are contracted (1 mark)
(b) Muscles maintained in a permanently active state so can contract rapidly when needed; keeps the body upright and the internal organs in position (2 marks)
(c) Any three e.g. minimum energy needed by muscles to keep the body upright; less fatigue in the neck; no chance of a deformed vertebral column; no compression of / blood vessels / breathing system / digestive system; no chance of flat feet (3 marks)
(d) Reduces the leverage exerted by the heavy object (2 marks)
(e) Keep the backbone as straight as possible; always bend from the knees to allow the legs to take the weight; use your legs and hips to help support the weight (3 marks)

7. (a) Compare with Fig. 8.7 on page 63.
1/2 for each bone to max of 5 (5 marks)
(b) (i) Knee; elbow (2 marks)
(ii) Shoulder; hip (2 marks)

Chapter 9

1. (a) (i) G
(ii) H
(iii) B
(iv) J
(v) I (5 marks)
(b) (i) Impulse passes down sensory neurone (A) by a reversal of charge on the inside and outside;
At rest: positive on the outside, negative on inside;
Impulse: negative on the outside, positive on inside;
Travels over synapse (gap) by the release of a chemical / neurotransmitter which stimulates the neurone (F) (4 marks)
(ii) Slowed down the response; alcohol inhibits the chemical at the synapse (2 marks)
(c) (i) A – Balance / Posture;
B – Any relevant answer e.g. thought/ memory/learning.
C – Any relevant answer e.g. control of heart beat – breathing. (3 marks)
(ii) Pituitary gland (1 mark)
(iii) Any three, e.g. Hair; cranium; skull; bones meninges; membranes; cerebrospinal fluid cushions the brain against blows; sense organs, e.g. eyes which allow the person to take defensive / offensive action (3 marks)
(iv) Larger surface area therefore can have more cells therefore more capacity to think, learn etc. (2 marks)

2. (a) Rapid, automatic unvarying response to a specific stimulus (2 marks)
(b) Assists the baby in finding the nipple therefore helping in breast feeding. (2 marks)
(c) Tap just below the knee stretches to stretch receptor in the thigh muscle; impulse sent to the spinal cord via a sensory neurone; enters the spinal cord via the dorsal root; moves over a synapse to a motor neurone; impulse leaves via the ventral root; goes to the thigh muscle / quadriceps and causes contraction. Lower leg moves up (6 marks)
(d) (i) They dilate / increase; then return to normal 1 hour after (2 marks)
(ii) Left (1 mark)
(iii) Right side of the brain governs the left side of the body and vice versa (2 marks)

3. (a) Both involve a stimulus; both involve a change in organs (2 marks)
(b) Message carried by nerves / in blood / no hormones involved in nervous system / hormones involved in endocrine system (1 mark)

Chapter 10

1. (a) (i) Y – Cornea;
Z – Iris (2 marks)
(ii) Ciliary muscle contracts;
suspensory ligaments slacken;
lens becomes short and fat;
converse when the ciliary muscles relax (4 marks)
(b) (i) Lens in the eye becomes opaque / cloudy (1 mark)
(ii) Blurred – only allows some light from an object onto retina;
blindness – lets no light from an object onto retina (2 marks)
(iii) Few eye hospitals;
lack of money for treatment (2 marks)
(iv) Setting up of temporary operating theatres;
surgeons moving round the country (2 marks)
(v) Need glasses to focus light; onto the retina / fovea (2 marks)

2. (a) (i) Ciliary muscles relax;
suspensory ligaments become taut;
lens becomes long and thin;
far object (player scoring a goal) is focused on retina / fovea (4 marks)
(ii) Cones stimulated in retina;
in fovea;
nerve impulse produced;
impulse goes along a sensory / receptor / afferent neurone to the brain (3 marks)
(b) (i) 160 000 per mm^2 (1 mark)
(ii) Fovea / yellow spot (1 mark)
(iii) Blind spot;
where the neurones of the optic nerve leave the eye (2 marks)
(iv) Highest density of rods at Z;
rods work in dim light (2 marks)
(v) Cones give you colour vision;
not working in dim light (2 marks)

3. (a) see Fig. 10.15 on page 84 (7 marks)
(b) Vibrations transmitted in perilymph in vestibular canal;
Reissner's membrane vibrates;
endolymph in middle canal vibrates;
basilar membrane vibrates;
sensory hairs in organ of Corti stimulated;
nerve impulses generated in the auditory nerve (6 marks)
(c) Infection causes fluid which may block the tube and middle ear;
therefore no way of equalising pressures between middle and outer ear;
eardrum / ear ossicles therefore do not vibrate;
vibrations therefore not transmitted to inner ear (4 marks)
(d) When the head moves the cupula also moves;
stretches the sensory cells;
nerve impulses generated and sent to the brain which interprets them in terms of position (3 marks)

Chapter 11

1. (a) Reduce risk of cancer of ovary; reduce risk of cancer of the lining of the womb; reduce benign breast disease; irregular periods generally replaced by regular bleeding; periods generally lighter; premenstrual syndrome commonly eliminated (4 marks)
(b) Pill taken daily for 21 days; then a gap of 7 days during which period occurs (2 marks)
(c) Statistical evidence; shows that if you take the combined oral contraceptive pill; you are more likely; to experience various disorders of the circulatory system; such as strokes, heart attacks and blood clots (4 marks)
(d) Glad the pain likely to be much less; concerned about the possibility she might have sexual intercourse (2 marks)

2. (a) (i) Penis fills with blood; stiffens/becomes erect; able to enter the vagina (3 marks)
(ii) Prostate gland, testis, bladder (2 marks)
(iii) After puberty; presence of pubic hair (2 marks)
(iv) Urethra (1 mark)
(b) (i) Sperm cell has tail; egg cell has large volume of cytoplasm/surrounded by a jelly-like coat/other smaller cells (2 marks)
(ii) Each cell has 23/the haploid number of chromosomes in its nucleus (2 marks)
(c) Fusion/joining; of two gametes/sperm and egg; to give rise to a zygote (3 marks)

3. (a) (i) Hold testes/keep them cool
(ii) Produces secretions/proteins and salts that are added to the sperm
(iii) Carries sperm/semen (3 marks)
(b) (i) Hormone (1 mark)
(ii) Rises; due to its secretion by corpus luteum; following ovulation (3 marks)
(iii) High levels of oestrogen and progesterone; results in thickening of the lining of the uterus; low levels of both these hormones towards end of cycle/a couple of weeks after ovulation; leads to menstruation/loss of the lining of the uterus (4 marks)
(c) Any four points:
folded wall of uterus; provides large surface area/villi; which makes it easier for the embryo to implant; good blood supply; to provide oxygen and nutrients; and remove carbon dioxide and other waste products from the developing embryo/fetus (max. 4 marks)

Chapter 12

1. (a) (i) Umbilical cord/amniotic fluid/placenta/needle of syringe (1 mark)
   (ii) Stage 1:
   syringe penetrates uterus wall/syringe;
   penetrates amniotic membrane;
   syringe sterile/abdomen (skin) made sterile;
   embryo/fetal cells contained
   (max. 2 marks)
   Stage 2:
   fluid transferred to dish;
   lid parted slightly to avoid microbes from air/dish covered;
   nutrient agar or medium used;
   dish turned over if qualified by water avoidance
   (max. 2 marks)
   Stage 3:
   diagram; cells grown;
   temperature within the range (35–40)°C
   (max. 2 marks)
   Stage 4:
   cells placed on slide/use a slide;
   stain/dye;
   microscope focussed
   (max. 2 marks)
   (total 8 marks)
   (b) (i) 46/23 pairs (1 mark)
   (ii) Normal (1 mark)
   (iii) Down's Syndrome/Mongolism (1 mark)
   (iv) Sex of A female and B male; twins; non-identical/not produced from the same ovum
   (max. 2 marks)
   (v) 2 sperms and 2 ova (1 mark)

Chapter 13

1. (a) (i) 139 cm (1 mark)
   (ii) Male (1 mark)
   (iii) Selecting and adding the ten figures correctly (1534 cm); dividing by 10 (1534/10); 153.4 cm; value inserted into table (accept value calculated) (4 marks)
   (b) (i) Use of scale provided (not own scale); plotting figures for males accurately; plotting figures for females (accept candidate's value); joining points accurately; identifying curves
   (5 marks)
   (ii) 13–13.2 years (accept value on graph)
   (1 mark)
   (iii) 12–14 years (1 mark)
   (c) Onset of puberty earlier in females (1 mark)

Chapter 14

1. (a) (i) Vegetable burger (1 mark)
   (ii) 18 g (1 mark)
   (iii) Liver/muscles (1 mark)
   (iv) Glycogen (1 mark)
   (b) Contains more fibre;
   reduces risk of constipation/aids movement of materials through gut/reduces risk of bowel cancer;
   contains less fat;
   lowers risk of atherosclerosis/heart attack/becoming overweight;
   higher protein content;
   (more) material available for growth/repair;
   Any two reasons with appropriate explanations – 2 marks each (4 marks)

2. (a) Mr Smith (1 mark)
   (b) Milk (1 mark)
   (c) 11 400 – 1800 (kJ); 9600 (2 marks)
   (d) Lucy has commenced puberty/girls commence puberty first; this involves a growth spurt; non-identical twins; (therefore) different alleles; Lucy bigger/more sporty/has higher metabolic rate
   (max. 2 marks)
   (e) He will get fatter/become overweight/become obese/store more fat/develop heart disease
   (1 mark)

3. (a) (i) Men (1 mark)
   (ii) In men approximately same numbers light and heavy/slightly less were heavy smokers; in 1982/in recent years a bigger difference developed with more light smokers;
   In women many more were light smokers
   (3 marks)
   (iii) Slow decline at first then a more rapid decline in numbers/bigger decline in numbers; greater knowledge about effects of smoking/more non-smoking areas at work/at recreation places/more public awareness about dangers of smoking (3 marks)
   (b) Any two of: cancer; bronchitis; heart disease
   (2 marks)
   (c) Breathe in other people's smoke/other people's smoke can enter their lungs (1 mark)

4. A
Hazard: girl's hair close to Bunsen flame;
Action: tie hair back (2 marks)
OR
Hazard: test tube held vertical;
Action: hold test tube at an angle
B
Hazard: (elbow almost in) liquid spilt on bench;
Action: mop up spills (2 marks)
C
Hazard: liquid splashes could get into eyes;
Action: wear goggles/eye protection (2 marks)
D
Hazard: test tube rack on edge of bench/overhanging edge of bench;
Action: make sure equipment does not overhang edge of bench (2 marks)
OR
Hazard: Bunsen standing directly on bench;
Action: place Bunsen on heatproof mat
OR
Hazard: beaker could fall off tripod;
Action: support beaker with clamp stand

Chapter 15

1. (a) (i) Accept nos. between range (1600–1799) (1 mark)
(ii) Day 1; day 7 (2 marks)
(b) (i) White cells/phagocytes/lymphocytes (1 mark)
(ii) [Note to score here method must link to b(i)] engulfment/phagocytosis/antibody production/killing or agglutination of bacteria (2 marks)
(c) Peter;
not fighting the disease successfully (2 marks)
(d) (i) Virus/HIV (1 mark)
(ii) Sexually/blood transfusion/clear description of either/sharing (dirty) needles/from mother to fetus (1 mark)

2. (a) (i) Protozoa/protoctista (1 mark)
(ii) Unicellular/reproduces by binary fission/capable of forming spores (1 mark)
(b) Parasitism; (1 mark)
lives in salivary glands of mosquito/lives in RBCs/liver cells of human/feeds off other cells/host (1 mark)
(c) Injected into bloodstream;
when female mosquito feeds;
plasmodium in saliva/salivary glands; ANY TWO (2 marks)
(d) Little/no water;
mosquitoes need water to breed (2 marks)

Chapter 16

1. (a) (i) Dead/weakened disease-causing organisms/bacteria/viruses/toxins (1 mark)
(ii) Clear description of correct sequence of events;
making use of all information in diagram;
vaccine/organisms attached to white blood cell;
white blood cell produces antibody;
antibody released/enters blood/remains in blood/in body of person;
destroys/attaches to bacteria next infecting body (6 marks)
(b) Any three of:
Sneeze/cough into tissue/handkerchief;
good ventilation/air conditioning;
room temperature not too high;
take medication to reduce sneezing/coughing;
people with colds/influenza stay at home (3 marks)

2. (a) Some bacteria still live/spores not killed/spores still alive;
bacteria/spores then develop/reproduce/bacteria increase in numbers (2 marks)
(b) All bacteria and spores killed (1 mark)
(c) In freezer bacteria do not reproduce;
in refrigerator bacteria still able to reproduce/reproduce slowly (5 marks)

3. (a) (i) A disease causing organism; R (reject) – a named example only (1 mark)
(ii) An organism which transmits/carries pathogen/carries disease organism but not affected by it (1 mark)
(iii) Protozoa/protista/protoctista (1 mark)
(iv) Any point with explanation:
eggs laid in stagnant water;
remove water/speed up flow insect cannot breed;
larva/pupa hangs from surface of water;
add oil/poison/insecticide/pesticide to water surface;
R (reject) – fungicide;
larva feeds on bacteria;
add *B. thuringiensis* to water;
adult rests in dark places;
spray insecticide/pesticide there (2 marks)
(b) (i) Number of sufferers increases;
anti-malarial drugs no longer effective (2 marks)
(ii) Presence of resistant gene/genetic mutation (1 mark)
(c) Protein (on cell surface) which stimulates a reaction (1 mark)

(d) Any three points:
antigens produced can be extracted/purified;
could be injected into person before infection/used as a vaccine;
stimulates antibody formation;
gives active/long term immunity;
safe as it does not require injection of parasite (max. 3 marks)

4. (a) Accept any sexually transmitted disease and look for the points indicated. Most will probably choose AIDS/HIV. Any six of:
AIDS/HIV infection/name of disease;
attacks white blood cells/area of body affected;
damages immune system/effect on body;
reduced ability to produce antibodies;
during incubation period/when symptoms subside/carrier may not realise they are infected;
carrier infectious to others;
loss of friends/partners/social stigma financial problems;
likely to need long term medical care support/counselling;
carrier may be afraid to seek help (max. 6 marks)

(b) Any two points:
avoiding promiscuity;
using a condom/Femidom; R (reject) contraceptive if unqualified;
health education programmes/counselling of patients; celibacy; R (reject) references to drugs/needles (max. 2 marks)

5. C; A; D; B (4 marks)

6. (a) After 0.5 hours dye has already changed to pink; after 1.0 hour milk is white meaning that dye is colourless; since oxygen has been used up; by bacteria / microorganisms in milk (4 marks)

(b) More bacteria / microorganisms in 4 day-old pasteurised milk; because they have had longer to reproduce; so dye loses its colour more quickly (3 marks)

(c) Sterilised milk contains no bacteria / living microorganisms; so even when 4 days old; freshly opened sterilised milk fails to change the colour of the dye from blue; but if kept in an open jug for 4 days enough bacteria / their spores enter from the atmosphere; and reproduce to change the dye from blue to pink within 1.5 hours (5 marks)

(d) Shaking would introduce oxygen from the atmosphere; obscuring differences between the treatments (2 marks)

Chapter 17

1. (a) Any two, e.g.
chloroplast; nucleus; cytoplasm; vacuole; cell wall (2 marks)

(b) Possesses many nuclei (1 mark)

(c) Similarity to plant: possesses a chloroplast/ possesses cell wall;
similarity to animal: possesses a flagellum/ possesses contractive vacuoles (2 marks)

(d) Several nuclei (1 mark)

(e) (i) *Saccharomyces*; *Chlamydomonas* (2 marks)

(ii) Any relevant answer, e.g.
number of nuclei/ flagellum/ contractile vacuole (1 mark)

Chapter 18

1. Making cheese: fungi / bacteria;
Making bread: fungi;
Making vinegar: bacteria;
Making yoghurt: bacteria;
Pollination: insects;
Sewage disposal: bacteria; (6 marks)

Chapter 19

1.

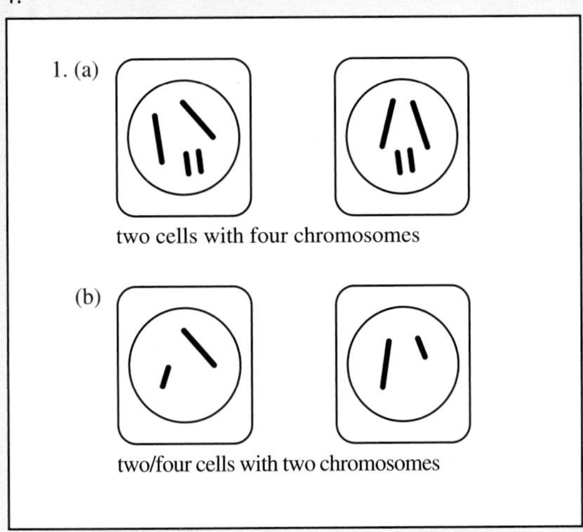

(5 marks)

2. (a) (i) Long, thin, threadlike structures found in the nucleus; that contain genes (2 marks)
   (ii) Two cells (elongated) are about to divide into two (or relevant answer) (1 mark)
   (iii) Cells have the same number of chromosomes; no gamete formation visible (2 marks)
   (iv) Ovary; testis (2 marks)
   (b) (i) Grandmother (1 mark)
   (ii) 30% (1 mark)
   (iii) Carries H – dominant allele for woolly hair along with h – recessive allele for straight hair (1 mark)

3. (a) Eye colour/ blood groups/ types of hair; no graduations between them e.g. brown or blue (2 marks)

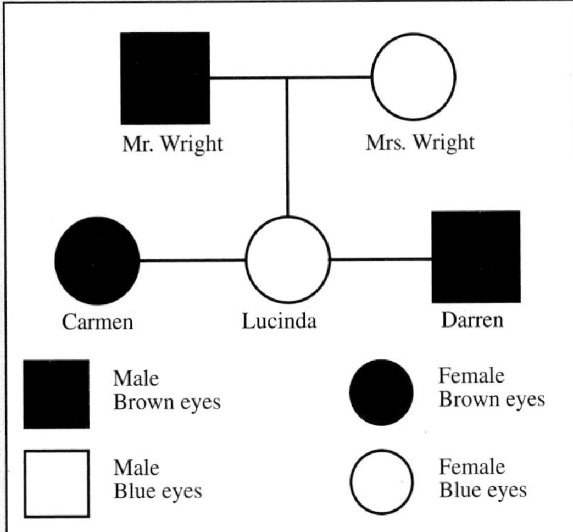

(b)

(4 marks)

(c) (i)

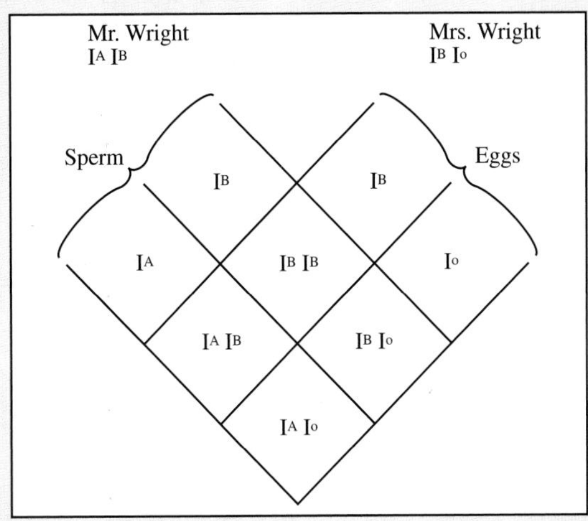

(2 marks)

(ii) Carmen I^AI^o
Darren $I^B I^B$ or $I^B I^o$ (2 marks)

(d) (i)

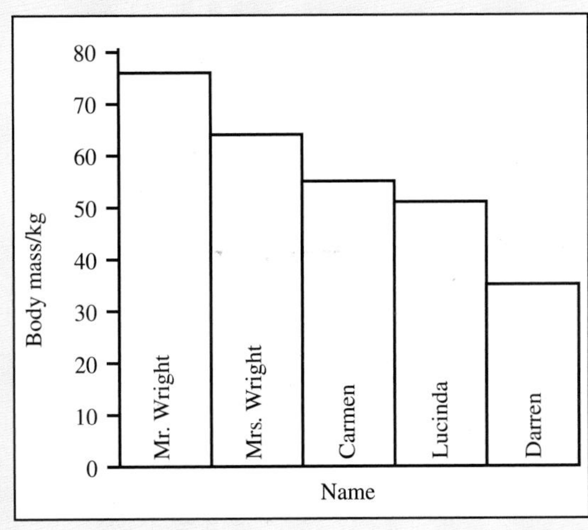

(4 marks)

(ii) Age/ height/ build (1 mark)

4. (a) DNA/ deoxyribonucleic acid; gametes; haploid; meiosis; zygote; male; female (6 marks)
   (b) (i) Mr Smith Bb
   Mrs Smith bb (2 marks)
   (ii) Mr Smith produces two types of gamete, B or b;
   Mrs Smith produces one type of gamete b;
   Offspring will therefore be Bb (brown eyes); or bb (blue eyes) (4 marks)

5. Mother has genotype of X^nX^n;
Father has genotype of X^NY;
To produce a daughter with sex chromosomes XX
One X comes from mother, i.e. X^n;
One X comes from father, i.e. X^N;
All daughters will therefore be X^NX^n i.e. have normal vision (5 marks)

Chapter 20

1. (a) A phosphate;
   B deoxyribose sugar;
   C nitrogen base (3 marks)
   (b) Nucleotide (1 mark)
   (c) Thymine (1 mark)
   (d) Uracil (1 mark)
   (e) The production of mRNA with a complementary nitrogen base sequence to the strand of DNA exposed after it has unzipped (2 marks)
   (f) tRNA – Amino acids line up on the mRNA;
   amino acids join to form a protein (2 marks)

2. Isolate the required gene;
   Insert it into a vector (carrier);
   Place it into a host (3 marks)

3. (a) Restriction enzymes
   (b) DNA ligase (2 marks)

4. Can re-use therefore cheaper (1 mark)

5. Penicillin;
   larger clearer zone around this disc, i.e. less bacterial growth (2 marks)

6. Less space; carried out all the year round; production is very high; genetically identical plants, etc. (3 marks)

7. (a) Inoculation (1 mark)
   (b) Agar is non-living;
   viruses need living cells in order to survive (2 marks)

8. (a) To mix / distribute;
   Penicillium best contact with food / oxygen (2 marks)
   (b) Temperature monitored by probe;
   if too high more cooling water / less steam is added;
   if too low less cooling water / more steam is added;
   correct reference values (max. 3 marks)
   (c) (i) 21.5 g per litre / 17.5 g per litre (1 mark)
   (ii) increases slowly then more rapidly;
   growth rate slows
   then negative growth / no growth / some dies;
   reference to at least three correct times (max. 3 marks)
   (iii) Follows similar pattern but time lag (1 mark)
   (iv) 80 hours (1 mark)

9. (a) One correct reference to mechanism, e.g.
   unwinding strands / mRNA;
   use of base code;
   enzymes / protein fermentation (3 marks)
   (b) (i) 1,5,7,13 (1 mark)
   (ii) Meiosis; chromosome number halves therefore some bands lost (2 marks)
   (iii) Yes;
   some of the child's bands (2, 6, 8, 14) are not from mother, all of these come from the husband (2 marks)

Chapter 21

1. (a) ✓ —;
   — ✓;
   ✓ —;
   ✓ —;
   — ✓; (5 marks)
   (b) Identical twins (1 mark)

2. Inherited variation in the bacterial population;
   some are resistant to penicillin some are not due to gene mutation;
   struggle for existence – avoiding being killed by the antibiotics;
   survival of the fittest – those resistant to the antibiotic survived treatment;
   natural selection – nature, in this case, the introduction of the antibiotics, has selected those most able to survive and reproduce whilst rejecting those least fit. (5 marks)

Chapter 22

1. (a) More of them (1 mark)
   (b) More of them (1 mark)
   (c) Light; darker in tree crop; (there might also be differences in water content, temperature, nutrient levels and pH) (2 marks)
   (d) Succession; to trees (2 marks)
   (e) More attractive; to drivers / walkers (2 marks)
   (f) Cost of maintenance (1 mark)

Chapter 23

1. (a) Carbon dioxide concentration with units (%) on horizontal axis; rate of photosynthesis on vertical axis; sensible scales (to use up most of the available graph paper); smooth, thin line drawn accurately through points/thin, straight lines drawn accurately to join neighbouring points (4 marks)
   (b) Up to a carbon dioxide concentration of 0.6% rate of photosynthesis is directly proportional to carbon dioxide concentration; above a carbon dioxide concentration of 0.6% rate of photosynthesis begins to flatten off/rate of photosynthesis no longer increases with increasing carbon dioxide concentration once the carbon dioxide concentration reaches 1.0% (2 marks)
   (c) Light intensity; temperature; wavelength of light; water supply; nutrient availability; internal factors (e.g. number of chloroplasts) (2 marks)
   (d) Warmer/less likely to suffer from frost damage; less competition from other plants; less likely to suffer from drought (2 marks)

2. (a)

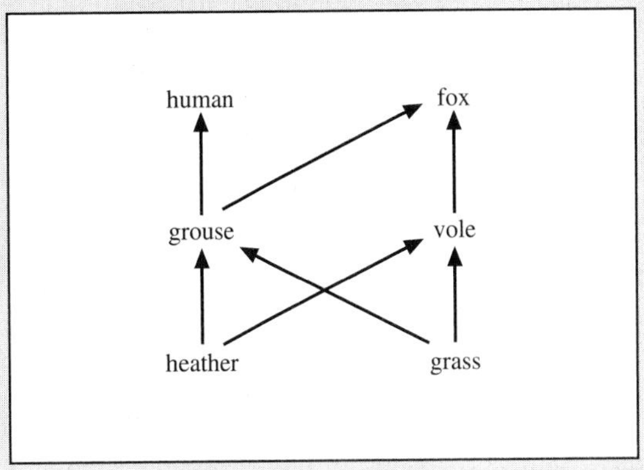

(5 marks)

   (b) Shelter/hiding place/nesting site/nesting material (1 mark)
   (c) (i) Decrease (1 mark)
   (ii) Heather and grass might increase (1 mark)

Chapter 24

1. (a) (i) It is used in photosynthesis; some of the glucose/starch/carbohydrate made remains in the producers/grass and is used for growth; the rest is respired; some of the grass is eaten by bullocks; the rest is eaten by other organisms/is decomposed (4 marks)
   (ii) 6.25% (1 mark)
   (b) One less step in the food chain; energy losses from producers to farm animals avoided (2 marks)
   (c) (i) 15.2 million hectares (1 mark)
   (ii) On average each person in the world has available 0.38 hectares of agricultural land; on average a person on a mixed diet needs 0.62 hectares of agricultural land to support themselves; on average a person on a strict vegetarian diet needs 0.08 hectares of agricultural land (3 marks)
   (iii) It decreases in height (1 mark)
   (iv) Less meat eaten would decrease the area of land used for feeding animals; and increase the land available for growing plant food for humans; more people can be supported by the same area of land if they eat less meat (3 marks)

2. (a) Arrow heads point upwards (i.e. bean → aphid, etc.) (1 mark)
   (b) Bean (1 mark)
   (c) Respiration/heat energy/not all the products of one level of a food chain eaten by the level above (1 mark)

3. (a) 49 (1 mark)
   (b) Lines correctly extended; 1999-2000 (2 marks)
   (c) Solar; wave/tidal; wind; hydroelectric; geothermal; wood (2 marks)
   (d) Gas is cheaper; gas produces less pollution; gas does not need to be imported; Electricity Generating Companies keen to diversify/not rely on only one fuel (2 marks)

Chapter 25

1. (a) Increasing in amount/eq (1 mark)
   (b) (i) Plants/green plants/producers/photosynthetic organisms (1 mark)
   (ii) Photosynthesis (1 mark)
   (c) Low carbon dioxide: plants photosynthesising (a lot); in summer/spring due to higher temperature/more light;
   less combustion (of fossil fuels);
   high carbon dioxide: low photosynthesis/high respiration; in winter/autumn
   (only if qualifying photosynthesis) due to low temperature/low light;
   more combustion (of fossil fuels) (4 marks)
   Note: no more than 3 marks for high or for low.

2. (a) 4 (1 mark)
   (b) Protein/ammonia/nitrates (1 mark)
   (c) Plant eaten by animal/digestion (1 mark)
   (d) No plant matter to decompose/to form ammonia/to form nitrates back into soil; must be added for growth of next crop (4 marks)

3. (a) (i) Evaporation at A; urination/defecation at B (accept non-jargon equivalent) (2 marks)
   (ii) Rain; snow; hail and run off; spring; stream: any two (2 marks)
   (b) (i) X: photosynthesis/making food
   Y: respiration/using food (2 marks)

(ii) Rabbit eats grass; fox eats rabbit (2 marks)
(iii) Less CO_2 removed by process X or similar (2 marks)
(iv) Nitrogen (accept any element except noble gas) (1 mark)

Chapter 26

1. (a) 20 000 (1 mark)
   (b) 18 000 (2 marks)
   (c) Rise; because large proportion of people of reproductive age; small proportion of old people (3 marks)

2. (a) Recycle aluminium cans; fit catalytic converters to cars (2 marks)
   (b) 10.0 g carbon monoxide per kilometre × 20 000 kilometres = 200 kg (2 marks)
   (c) Burning of low grade coal (1 mark)
   (d) (i) 'Acid rain kills' = sulphur dioxide; 'greenhouse effect' = carbon dioxide (2 marks)
   (ii) Most people see stamps/advertising effective/makes people think/Royal Mail trusted (1 mark)
   (iii) Fewer animals in the lake; oxygen level of lake drops; lake less attractive; toxins released by decaying plants (2 marks)

3. (a) (i) coal tip waste/slag/waste from mine/sewage – if qualified in (ii) (1 mark)
   (ii) run-off, e.g. inefficient works/storm overflow/ through tributaries/smaller steams/ slumping/sliding/dust blown in (1 mark)
   (b) pollution increased downstream;
   from confluence of streams to West;
   because more coal tip waste;
   numbers – reduced;
   and types of animals reduced/less variety plants/animals;
   bacteria increase; named e.g. of animal reduced in number (5 marks)
   (c) (i) Pumping station should be located anywhere upstream of upper left hand tributary/anywhere unpolluted if qualified in (ii) near city (1 mark)
   (ii) Water here unpolluted/clean;
   score = 9/no sewage works/coal mine/tips (2 marks)
   (d) Run off from roads;
   factory effluent;
   litter, household rubbish (2 marks)
   any named source

Chapter 27

1. (a) (i) Carbon monoxide;
   more cars/more factories/more household fires (2 marks)
   (ii) 55% (1 mark)
   (iii) 15% (1 mark)
   (iv) More sulphur dioxide in air in polluted regions;
   dissolves in rain;
   producing (sulphurous/sulphuric) acid (3 marks)
   (b) Three of: prevents pests/flies/rats/mice etc. reaching it;
   prevents material blowing away;
   prevents children/people reaching it;
   helps compaction for decomposition (3 marks)

2. (a) Allow solids to settle/allow less dense material to be run off/separate solid from liquid (1 mark)
   (b) (i) Bacteria: break down/decompose/digest; organic matter/sewage/effluent using enzymes (max. 2 marks)
   (ii) Stones: increase surface area; to hold bacteria/ for bacteria to work/for enzymes to work; slow down fluid/ensures contact with bacteria/ensures contact with enzymes; allows air entry (max. 2 marks)
   (iii) Air: allows aerobic; respiration; encourages bacterial growth; speeds up breakdown (max. 2 marks)
   (max. 6 marks)
   (c) (i) Methane: fuel
   (ii) Sludge: fertiliser/soil conditioner/compost/ enhanced growth (2 marks)
   (d) (Bacteria) less, more
   (Proteins) more, less
   (Nitrates) less, more (3 marks)
   (e) (Some) bacteria or microbes killed by disinfectant; process disrupted/slowed down/less efficient (2 marks)

3. (a) Two of: algae; insect larvae; other small animals; some bacteria; fine particles; clay particles; R (reject) anything large (2 marks)
   (b) Chlorine (1 mark)
   (c) Destroy pathogens/make it safe (1 mark)
   (d) Two of: Prevent (re)contamination by pathogens; prevent dust getting in; avoid contamination with (bird droppings) but, must be QUALIFIED; give chlorine time to work (2 marks)

Answers to in-text questions

Chapter 1

1 (a) Both contain nucleus; both have a cell surface membrane; both contain cytoplasm;
(b) Only plant cell has a cell wall; only plant cell has chloroplasts; only plant cell has a large vacuole containing sap.

2 Nucleus; mitochondrion; smooth endoplasmic reticulum; rough endoplasmic reticulum.

3 It is not all used in each cell/each cell uses only part of the genetic material.

4 Epithelial tissue; muscle tissue; nervous tissue; connective tissue.

Chapter 2

1 Those in a gas – they move fastest in this state.

2 The reaction involving glucose is catabolic – a large molecule is broken down; the reaction involving ATP is anabolic – ATP is built up from two smaller molecules.

3 The cell does not use its own energy to make the ions or molecules move.

4 (a) Net flow from left to right by diffusion;
(b) Net flow from right to left by diffusion;
(c) Each side will have the same concentration of water. Each side will have the same concentration of glucose.

5 Prevent them moving from one side to the other.

6 Our blood becoming more dilute than our red blood cells – we cannot repair burst red cells but crenated red cells will still carry oxygen.

7 Lipase.

8 The reaction $A + B \rightarrow AB$ (look at the shape of the active site and of the molecules A to D).

9 The acid slows the action of the bacterial enzymes because it is not their optimum pH.

Chapter 3

1 Plant cell walls.

2 32.

3 Epiglottis – closes larynx; soft palate – closes off the nasal cavity.

4 Kills harmful bacteria.

5 (a) Increased;
(b) Increase.

Chapter 4

1 Diffusion.

2 (a) In solution in the plasma;
(b) As oxyhaemoglobin in the red blood cells.

3 (a) Can safely donate blood to anyone;
(b) Can safely accept blood from anyone.

4 (a) Decrease;
(b) Increase.

5 Prevent backflow of blood from the ventricles to the atria.

6 Prevent backflow of blood from the pulmonary artery and aorta to the ventricles.

7 Prevent the bicuspid and tricuspid valves turning inside out.

8 Has to pump the blood all round the body; the right ventricle only pumps it to the lungs.

9 Short distance to move the blood; also aided by gravity.

10 A left atrium; B bicuspid (mitral) valve; C cardiac muscle of left ventricle.

11 (a) Rises when ventricles contract and falls when they relax;
(b) Through the arterioles.

12 Smaller lumen in artery; more muscle in artery; more elastic fibres in artery.

13 e.g. water; inorganic ions; glucose; amino acids; vitamins; urea.

Chapter 5

1 It would die because it could not do any work.

2

	Aerobic	Anaerobic
1	Yes	No
2	A lot	little
3	Carbon dioxide and water	Animals: lactate; plants: ethanol + carbon dioxide
4	Mitochondria	Cytoplasm

3 Any three, e.g. cirrhosis of the liver; overweight/obesity; violence; financial strains, etc.

4 1: Diffuses through capillary wall; 2: Diffuses through alveolar wall; 3: Diffuses through mucus/moisture; 4: Diffuses into alveolar space.

5 Large surface area; good blood supply; thin walls.

6 (a) decreases;
(b) increases.

Chapter 6

1 Most of our faeces is material that has never been digested and absorbed so it is not a waste product from metabolism. But, remember it contains small amounts of bile pigments that are waste products of metabolism.
2 Collecting ducts, pelvis, ureters, bladder, urethra.
3 The cortex has many more capillary networks around the nephrons than does the medulla. The blood in these capillary networks makes the cortex darker.
4 They are too big to get through the glomerulus.
5 Urea is more concentrated in the ultrafiltrate; all the glucose is reabsorbed; not possible by passive diffusion therefore another mechanism must be involved.
6 Other substances (including water) have been reabsorbed but urea has not.
7 The only time that this child could remove the surplus salt or water from her/his blood is when on the dialysis machine.
8 If untreated, the sufferer would lose too much water from their blood.

Chapter 7

1 (a) Net flow of water out leading to crenation;
(b) Net flow of water in leading to lysis (bursting).
2 Respiration.
3 (a)

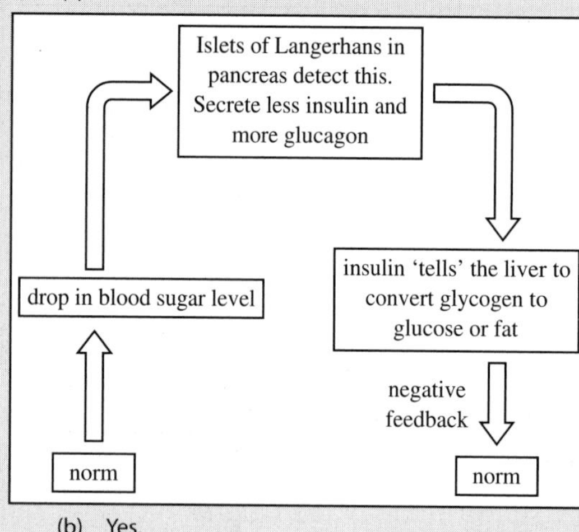

(b) Yes.
4 Place 2 cm^3 of urine in a test tube and add an equal volume of Benedict's solution.
Boil. A positive test would be an orange/red/brown precipitate.
5 It would be digested as it is a protein.
6 Liver no longer responds to insulin.
7 Temperature regulation; excretion; prevents infection; prevents dehydration; prevents damage; detects stimuli e.g. pain.
8 Need less insulation.
9 (a) Less/no sweat produced;
(b) Hairs become erect;
(c) Arterioles and shunt vessels constrict therefore less blood gets to the surface. Less heat is lost;
(d) Less blood in the circulation;
(e) Metabolic rate increases;
(f) More adipose tissue therefore more insulation;
(g) Shivering will occur.
10 (a) Any three of: drink cold drinks; swimming; remove certain clothes; wear different clothes; seek shade;
(b) Any three of: drink hot drinks; wear warmer clothes wear more clothes; use heating.

Chapter 8

1 Rigid skull could damage the baby's brain/the mother's uterus and vagina during birth.
2 A = neural spine; B = transverse process; C = centrum; D = neural canal; E = neural arch.
3 (a) Pelvic girdle/sacrum;
(b) Between the two halves of the pelvic girdle;
(c) Elbow/shoulder.
4 1 = femur/bone; support/movement/locomotion/ supply of calcium
2 = cartilage; prevents bone rubbing on bone
3 = (striated) muscle; causes movement/locomotion
5 Alimentary canal/iris of eye/blood vessels (arteries and veins but not capillaries)/ureters/urethra/sperm ducts/ oviducts/uterus/vagina.
6 (a) Straightens/extends;
(b) Bends/flexes;
(c) Extensor;
(d) Flexor.
7 (a) Anaerobic respiration;
(b) Lactate;
(c) Lactate is acidic (sometimes referred to as lactic acid) and causes a burning sensation.
8 A simple closed fracture.

Chapter 9

1 Stimulus – ring of telephone → receptor – ear → sensory nerve → central nervous system → motor nerve → effector – muscles that allow you to pick up the telephone.
2 Any three, e.g. reflex is usually faster; reflex involves a smaller number of neurones; reflex does not involve memory; reflex does not require thought; the stimulus in the reflex always produces the same response; not necessarily the case in voluntary.
3

Reflex	Stimulus	Recepter	Response	Purpose
1 Withdrawal of hand	Pin prick	Pain recepters in skin	Arm muscles contract	Protection against further damage
2 Production of saliva	Sight, smell of food	Retina in eye or olfactory cells in nose	Salivary glands produce more saliva	More efficient digestion
3 Blinking	Object approaching eye	Retina	Eyelid muscles contract	Protects the eye
4 Narrowing (constriction) of pupils	Bright light	Retina	Circular muscles in iris contract	Protects the retina
5 Knee jerk	Pressure below the knee	Stretch receptors in the thigh muscle	Thigh muscle contracts, straightening the leg	Helps to keep balance; walking

4 Slow down.
5 Protection; Nutrition.
6 Anything relevant, e.g. control of breathing/digestion.
7 Any two e.g. nervous – by means of depolarisation/hormonal – by means of chemicals; nervous – along nerve fibres/hormonal – in the blood stream; nervous – action over quickly/hormonal – action longer lasting.

Chapter 10

1 Touch – dermis; pain – epidermis; pressure – dermis; temperature – dermis.
2 Finger tips/lips/tongue/genitals.
3 (a) You are aware of smell and taste; awareness is a function of the cerebrum of the brain;
(b) Sensory/receptor/afferent neurones.
4 Iris – controls amount of light entering the eye; retina – is light sensitive; choroid – supplies the cells with nutrients and oxygen/prevents internal reflection; optic nerve – transmits impulses from the eye to the brain; cornea – bends the light during focusing/allows light through; lens – bends the light during focusing; ciliary muscle – changes shape of lens during focusing; conjunctiva – protects the cornea; scleroid – tough, protective layer/prevents light entering.
5

Unaccommodated	Accommodated
Relaxed	Contracted
Taut	Slack
Long and thin	Short and fat
Long	Short
Far	Near

6 Sensory/receptor/afferent.
7 Hammer; anvil; stirrup/malleus; incus; stapes
8 Sensory hairs in the organ of Corti may be damaged as basilar membrane vibrates too much; ear ossicles may vibrate too much and become damaged; ear drum may burst.

Chapter 11

1 To control the movement of things into (penis, sperm); and out of (blood, baby) the body.
2 Epididymis is where sperm mature; sperm duct carries sperm to the penis; urethra carries either semen or urine to the end of the penis.
3 One.
4 The levels of oestrogen and progesterone are rising.
5 The levels of oestrogen and progesterone are both low.
6 Mature.
7 Testis; epididymis; sperm duct; urethra/penis; vagina; uterus (or womb); oviduct (or Fallopian tube).
8 Intra-uterine device; progestogen-only pill (sometimes).
9 Contraception involves the prevention of pregnancy; abortion occurs weeks or months after a woman becomes pregnant.

Chapter 12

1 Mitosis.
2 Approximately $\times$ 20.
3 Approximately $\times$ 15.
4 Diffusion.
5 Diffusion.
6 Half the fetus' genes come from its father.
7 Slow down growth of the fetus; because it would receive less oxygen from the mother.
8 Belly button/navel.
9 No; monozygotic twins are genetically identical, but males and females are not.
10 50%/0.5.

Chapter 13

1 Puberty.
2 Approximately 50 cm; approximately 70 cm per year; greater than at any other age.
3 Three years.
4 Better nutrition/less disease.
5 (a) 23–27%;
(b) 12–16%.
6 40 years with one egg every 4 weeks (13 a year); equals 520 eggs.
7 Approximately 9 + 4 = 13 periods missed each pregnancy plus lactation; so number of eggs produced equals 520 minus 3 $\times$ 13; equals 480.

Chapter 14

1 Swimming (hard).
2 (a) Five times;
(b) 22%.
3 Exercise makes the heart bigger/stronger/increases the volume of heart muscle; so it pumps more blood each time it contracts; so at rest fewer contractions per minute provide all the blood needed by the body.
4 Slightly under one and a half.
5 If in a group, the person in danger can be helped/ambulance called.

Chapter 15

1 1.2%.
2 Immunity to existing strains builds up; so few people develop influenza; until a new strain arises; when many people are susceptible.
3 Gonorrhoea; tuberculosis; cholera; food poisoning.

Chapter 16

1 Keep away all pathogens/disease-causing organisms; as person unable to produce antibodies.
2 Passive immunity; appropriate antibodies present immediately.
3 Active immunity; lymphocytes have learnt how to make the appropriate antibody.
4 Prevents HIV passing from patient to dentist; and from dentist to patient; through cuts.
5 Slows decay of food; as most microorganisms are aerobic/require oxygen.
6 Oxygen makes haemoglobin red; people like steak to look red.

Chapter 17

1 Non-living – living organisms lose these features when they die.
2 Any three of: cell surface membrane; cell wall; ribosomes; food granules.
3 Kingdom; phylum; class; order; family; genus; species.
4 Animalia; Vertebrate; Chordate; Mammal; Primate; Hominidae; *Homo sapiens*.

Chapter 18

1 Heat; released by respiration of decomposers.
2 Decrease.
3 They would soon break down/organisms would die; no nutrients; being recycled/released by decomposers.
4 No; fungi do not photosynthesise.
5 Release of sewage increases chance of *Entamoeba* entering drinking water supply/food; and so spreading to other people; rather than being confined to sewage system.
6 Oxygen is produced by plants; in photosynthesis.
7 Light to be carried by the wind; huge amounts because most of it never reaches the female part of a flower of the same species.
8 Colour to attract insects; nectar to make the visit worth it for the insect.

Chapter 19

1 (a) Become more muscular/larger;
(b) Environment.
2 2n = 6; n = 3.
3 Any relevant answer, e.g. germinal layer of skin/cells of bone marrow.
4 It must have been copied/ replicated / duplicated.
5 Four.
6 Egg cells and sperm cells.
7 Ovaries and testes.
8 (a) Restriction enzyme;
(b) DNA ligase.
9 (a) a;
(b) AA;
(c) aa;
(d) Aa;
(e) (i) free ear lobes;
(ii) fixed ear lobes;
(f) if a person had an A allele he/she would have free ear lobes;
(g) organisms are diploid, i.e. must have two copies of each gene;
(h) the point on the chromosome where a particular gene is always found;
(i) AA and Aa.
10 Because it is homozygous.
11 1 in 4 chance/ 25% chance/ 0.25 (all ways of saying the same thing).
12 (a) RR or Rr;
(b) rr.
13 Children could be produced with blood groups that are different from either parent.

Chapter 20

1 TTA GGC AAC.
2 (a) Three;
(b) UAG CAG CCU;
(c) AUC GUC GGA.
3 TAG CAA AGG.
4 Gas exchange/diffusion.
5 Insecticide.
6 Decrease it/make it cheaper.
7 No nucleus (therefore no DNA).
8 Restriction enzymes.

Chapter 21

1 No. As long as they had fewer offspring (e.g. because they had so little food that they failed to ovulate), natural selection would still occur.
2 The seeds will have to contain five 'large' alleles and five 'small' alleles, e.g. AA BB Cc dd ee; AA Bb CC dd ee; Aa BB CC dd ee; aa BB CC Dd ee; Aa Bb Cc Dd Ee, etc.
3 Haemophilia, eye colour and cystic fibrosis.
4 Mutation. The other sources of variation occur during sexual reproduction.
5 A mutagen increases the rate of mutation. It may be radiation (e.g. radioactivity, X rays, ultraviolet radiation) or a chemical (e.g. mustard gas).
6 It would disappear from the population through natural selection.
7 Places where malaria is endemic, e.g. southern India and parts of Africa.
8 (a) 47;
(b) With 47 chromosomes, cells cannot divide by meiosis to produce gametes.
9 Variation in a single feature.
10 They were less conspicuous on the trunks of trees and so were less likely to be eaten by birds.
11 Gene mutation.
12 Pollution from the industrial revolution had caused the lichens on tree trunks to be killed and soot had blackened these bare trunks. The melanic moth was now inconspicuous. The speckled form was more conspicuous and so more likely to be eaten by birds.
13 Clean Air Acts have resulted in less pollution, so lichens grow once more on the tree trunks.

Chapter 22

1 A lake.
2 (a) Sedges; rush; water crowfoot; arrowhead; water lily; duckweed;
(b) Tadpole; water snail;
(c) Caddis fly larva;
(d) Dragonfly; dragonfly nymph; leech; great diving beetle larva; water boatman; frog; stickleback.
3 Temperature (colder in northern Scotland); wind (windier in northern Scotland); water content (higher in northern Scotland).
4 During the day plants take up carbon dioxide from the water; in photosynthesis; as a result carbon dioxide levels in water drop; since carbon dioxide dissolves in water to form a weak acid; this means that the water becomes less acidic; and so the pH rises; at night no photosynthesis occurs; but carbon dioxide is released into water; as a result of respiration; so pH falls.
5 Other woodmice (competition, to mate with, offspring); insects (food); herbs (food); weasel (predator); dormice (competition); fleas (parasites).
6 More slowly; takes time for soil to build up; soil in secondary succession may already contain seeds.
7 Grass would grow longer; seeds; of shrubs and trees would invade; succession would occur; eventually resulting in a wood.

Chapter 23

1 Six.
2 One.
3 Photosynthesis requires an input of energy.
4 When there is no carbon dioxide there is no photosynthesis; at low carbon dioxide concentrations the rate of photosynthesis is directly proportional to the carbon dioxide concentration; at a carbon dioxide concentration of about 0.1% the rate of photosynthesis levels off; above this increasing carbon dioxide concentration has no effect on the rate of photosynthesis.
5 Rate of photosynthesis fastest at a concentration of about 0.1%; rather than natural level in atmosphere of 0.035%; burning paraffin releases carbon dioxide; raises concentration of carbon dioxide in the greenhouse; increases rate of photosynthesis; plant grows faster/yields bigger crop.
6 Below about 35°C, the higher the temperature, the greater the rate of photosynthesis; rate of photosynthesis approximately doubles for every 10°C increase in temperature; at about 35°C the rate of photosynthesis reaches a peak; above 35°C the rate of photosynthesis decreases steeply; reaches zero at approximately 45–50°C.
7 Enzymes involved in photosynthesis work faster; activation energy less.
8 Enzymes denatured; plant killed.
9 When there is no light, there is no photosynthesis; initially the rate of photosynthesis is directly proportional to the light intensity; at high light intensities the rate of photosynthesis levels off.
10 (a) Blue;
(b) Green.
11 (a) To reduce water loss when the stomata are open;
(b) Desert plants have a maximum rate of photosynthesis that is lower than other plants; because with few stomata, they cannot get much carbon dioxide into their leaves.
12 Yes.
13 Mutualism.
14 (a) Herbs might increase; because bank voles eat herbs;
(b) Owls might decrease; because owls eat bank voles;
(c) Woodmice might increase; because bank voles and wood mice compete for food/herbs;
(d) Moles are unlikely to be affected; because there are no links in the food web that connect bank voles and moles.

Chapter 24

1 Lost as heat; in respiration.
2 (a) C;
(b) A;
(c) B.
3 Not all the rabbits caught by foxes; a fox does not eat every part of a rabbit; foxes cannot convert rabbit meat into fox meat with 100% efficiency.
4 Number per unit area.
5 Pyramids of energy measured in flow of energy per unit area per unit time; e.g. kilojoules (kJ) per square metre (m^{-2}) per year ($year^{-1}$).
6 Carnivores obtain all their energy from eating herbivores; some of the herbivore production goes in respiration/heat loss and to decomposers; therefore energy reaching carnivores less than that leaving the herbivores.
7 Energy used to power cars/other forms of transport; power factories; power lights/generate electricity; manufacture goods; heat homes/elsewhere.
8 Coal; oil; gas.
9 (a) Solar power; wind power; hydroelectric power; wave power; wood;
(b) When trees are not replaced or are used faster than they can grow.

Chapter 25

1 (a) Increase;
(b) Decrease;
(c) Decrease.
2 Plant more trees/stop cutting down and burning trees; reduce use of fossil fuels.
3 Waterlogged soils contain less oxygen than non-waterlogged soils.
4 Waterlogging reduces the levels of nitrate in the soil; most plants obtain their nitrogen from the soil as nitrate; nitrate availability usually limits plant growth.
5 Transpiration; evaporation.
6 Trees act as a sponge/slowly release water to the ground; vegetation protects soil from running water; plant roots and humus bind soil particles together.
7 Legumes have root nodules; contain nitrogen-fixing bacteria; increase nitrogen/nitrate levels in the soil; when ploughed back into the soil and allowed to decompose.
8 Rise in oxygen levels; prevent aerobic organisms (e.g. fish) from dying; increase rate of decomposition.

Chapter 26

1 (a) 20 million;
(b) 40 million;
(c) 80 million.
2 Shortage of food/starvation/famine; shortage of space; shortage of water/drought; disease; fighting/wars.
3 250 000 people per day × 365 days; = approximately 90 million people a year.
4 Exponential.
5 Around 1600 years BP/400 AD/Dark Ages; approximately 650 years BP/1375 AD/Black Death; approximately 350 years BP/1650 AD.
6 20th.

7 (a) Births; immigration;
(b) Deaths; emigration.

8 (a) Population size would remain constant;
(b) Population size would increase;
(c) Population size would decrease.

9 (a) Hungary;
(b) Germany;
(c) Kenya.

10 (a) 20–29;
(b) Women;
(c) 30–34.

11 90–95 million.

12 Acid rain in Scandinavia caused by air pollution in the UK.

13 Biodegradable.

14 Non-biodegradable.

Chapter 27

1 Adding limestone helps to neutralise the acid; raises the pH.

2 (a) Cheap/out of sight/not near people;
(b) Containers may break open/radioactivity may leak out/may contaminate fish/other marine organisms.

3 Carbon dioxide.

4 Most of the nitrates, phosphates; and organic matter have been removed; by the bacteria and protozoa.

5 Fluorine helps prevent tooth decay.

6 Smell of refuse; noise of dust carts; risk of infection; danger to children; nuisance of blown rubbish; lower house prices/opposition from residents.

7 Trees.

Index

Page numbers in **bold** type show where terms that appear frequently are defined or fully explained.

Acknowledgements

Illustrations and other printed matter

The authors and publishers are grateful to the following for permission to reproduce copyright material. If any acknowlegement has been omitted, this will be rectified at the earliest possible opportunity.

4.3, page 29: Macmillan Press Ltd
4.9, page 32: Reprinted by permission of Oxford University Press
4.13, page 34: Macmillan Press Ltd
13.1, 13.2, 13.3, page 103; 13.9, page 109: B. Bogin, *Patterns of Human Growth*, 1988, Cambridge University Press
14.10, 14.11, page 121: Dorling Kndersley
18.1, page 144: Daniels Publishing
22.2, page 185: J.L.Chapman and M.J.Reiss, Ecology, Principles and Applications, 1992, Cambridge University Press
26.3, page 215: Optimum Population Trust
26.4, page 216: Steve Kinzett, POPTRAN Project, Sir Davd Owen Population Centre, University of Wales, Cardiff
Page 237 (photograph in Q3): Mr A. Brinded
Page 253: Crown copyright, reproduced by permission of the Forestry Commission
Past examination questions are reproduced by kind permission of the following Examination Boards:
Midland Examining Group (MEG)
Assocated Examining Board (AEB/SEG)
University of London Examinations & Assessment Council (ULEAC)
Northern Examinations and Assessments Board (NEAB)

Photographs

1.2, page 1: J. C. Levy/Science Photo Library
1.3, page 2: Don Fawcett/Science Photo Library
1.5a, page 4: Science Photo Library
1.5b, page 4: Bruce Iverson/Science Photo Library
1.5c, page 5: Manfred Kage/Science Photo Library
1.5d, page 5: John Burbidge/Science Photo Library
1.5e, page 5: Eric Grave/Science Photo Library
3.7, page 21: James Stevenson/Science Photo Library
3.13, page 25: Martin/Custom Medical Stock Photo/Science Photo Library
4.6, page 30: Biophoto Associates
4.10, page 32: Biophoto Associates
5.4, page 40: Biophoto Associates
6.5, page 48: Astrid and Hans-Frieder Michler/Science Photo Library
6.10, page 52: Simon Fraser, Royal Victoria Infirmary, Newcastle upon Tyne/Science Photo Library
6.12, page 53: Chris Priest/Science Photo Library
8.10, page 65: Science Photo Library
8.16, page 69: SIU/Science Photo Library
8.17, page 70: James Stevenson/ Science Photo Library
9.1, page 71: Sporting Pictures
10.5, page 80: Astrid and Hans-Frieder Michler/Science Photo Library
10.11, page 82: Science Photo Library
11.4, page 88: John Burbidge/Science Photo Library
11.7, page 89: Science Photo Library
11.10, page 90: Network/Paul Love
11.13, page 92: John Urling Clark
11.15, page 93: Nature magazine
12.1, page 95: Professor P. M. Motta/Science Photo Library
12.5, page 96: BSIP Bajande/Science Photo Library
12.9, page 98: CNRI/Science Photo Library
12.12, page 99: Taeke Henstra/Petit Format/Science Photo Library
12.14 top and bottom, page 101: Rex Features
12.15a, page 102: Eye Ubiquitous/Roger Chester
12.15b, page 102: Rex Features
13.4, page 106: J. Allan Cash
13.11, page 110: Michael Reiss
14.1, page 113: Telegraph Colour Library
14.2, page 113: Eye Ubiquitous
14.3, page 113: Telegraph Colour Library
14.7, page 118: Rex Features/Rick Colls
15.1, page 125: Hattie Young/Science Photo Library
15.2, page 127: Jonathan Watts/Science Photo Library
15.5, page 128: Custom Medical Stock Photo/Science Photo Library
15.6, page 129: Rex Features
16.2, page 131: Phillippe Plailly/Science Photo Library
16.4, page 134: Adam Hart-Davis/Science Photo Library
16.5, page 134: Gideon Mendel/Network
18.6, page 146: Holt Studios/Nigel Cattlin
18.9, page 147: Martin Dohrn/Science Photo Library
18.11, page 148: Holt Studios/Nigel Cattlin
18.12, page 149: Holt Studios/Nigel Cattlin
18.13, page 149: Holt Studios/Nigel Cattlin
18.14, page 150: Marcelo Brodsky/Science Photo Library
19.5, page 153: M. Hirons/Geoscience Features
20.6, page 165: T. Tracy/Telegraph Colour Library
20.13, page 169: David Parker/Science Photo Library
21.1, page 178: Bruce Coleman/Mark N. Boulton
21.5, page 180: Alfred Pasieka/Science Photo Library
21.7a and b, page 181: Bruce Coleman/Kim Taylor
22.1, page 184: Holt Studios/Nigel Cattlin
22.4, page 186: Holt Studios/Nigel Cattlin
22.7, page 189: Holt Studios/Nigel Cattlin
22.9, page 190: Holt Studios/Nigel Cattlin
23.1, page 191: Tony Craddock/Science Photo Library
23.13, page 197: Dr Jeremy Burgess/Science Photo Library
23.14, page 197: Dr Jeremy Burgess/Science Photo Library
23.15, page 197: Geoff Tomkinson/Science Photo Library
24.7, page 201: J. Allan Cash
24.8, page 202: Jerry Mason/Science Photo Library
24.9, page 203: Martin Bond/Science Photo Library
24.11, page 204: Holt Studios/Nigel Cattlin
25.4, page 208: Heather Angel
25.6, page 210: Holt Studios/Nigel Cattlin
25.7, page 210: Holt Studios/Nigel Cattlin
26.2, page 214: J. Allan Cash
26.6, page 217: Environmental Picture Library/Robin Culley
26.8, page 220: David Campione/Science Photo Library
26.10, page 220: W. Eugene Smith/Magnum
26.11, page 221: Environmental Picture Library/Chris Westwood
27.1, page 222: Mark Edwards/Still Pictures
27.2, page 223: US Department of Energy/Science Photo Library
27.6, page 226: J. Allan Cash